Pain management
From basics to clinical practice

To Lisa for her patience and support.

Commissioning Editor: Timothy Horne
Development Editors: Linda Bennett/Lulu Stader
Project Manager: Elouise Ball
Designer: Sarah Russell
Illustrator: Samantha Elmhurst
Illustration Manager: Merlyn Harvey

Pain management
From basics to clinical practice

Edited by

John Hughes

Consultant in Anaesthetics and Pain Management
The James Cook University Hospital
Middlesbrough, UK

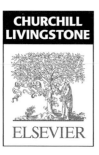

EDINBURGH LONDON NEW YORK OXFORD PHILADELPHIA ST LOUIS SYDNEY TORONTO 2008

CHURCHILL
LIVINGSTONE
ELSEVIER

An imprint of Elsevier Limited

© 2008, Elsevier Limited.

The right of John Hughes to be identified as the editor of this work has been asserted by him in accordance with the Copyright, Designs and Patents Act 1988.

No part of this publication may be reproduced, stored in a retrieval system, or transmitted in any form or by any means, electronic, mechanical, photocopying, recording or otherwise, without the prior permission of the Publishers. Permissions may be sought directly from Elsevier's Health Sciences Rights Department, 1600 John F. Kennedy Boulevard, Suite 1800, Philadelphia, PA 19103-2899, USA: phone: (+1) 215 239 3804; fax: (+1) 215 239 3805; or, e-mail: *healthpermissions@elsevier.com*. You may also complete your request on-line via the Elsevier homepage (http://www.elsevier.com), by selecting 'Support and contact' and then 'Copyright and Permission'.

First edition 2008

ISBN 9780443103360

British Library Cataloguing in Publication Data
A catalogue record for this book is available from the British Library

Library of Congress Cataloging in Publication Data
A catalog record for this book is available from the Library of Congress

Notice
Knowledge and best practice in this field are constantly changing. As new research and experience broaden our knowledge, changes in practice, treatment and drug therapy may become necessary or appropriate. Readers are advised to check the most current information provided (i) on procedures featured or (ii) by the manufacturer of each product to be administered, to verify the recommended dose or formula, the method and duration of administration, and contraindications. It is the responsibility of the practitioner, relying on their own experience and knowledge of the patient, to make diagnoses, to determine dosages and the best treatment for each individual patient, and to take all appropriate safety precautions. To the fullest extent of the law, neither the Publisher nor the Authors assume any liability for any injury and/or damage to persons or property arising out or related to any use of the material contained in this book.

 your source for books, journals and multimedia in the health sciences

www.elsevierhealth.com

Working together to grow libraries in developing countries

www.elsevier.com | www.bookaid.org | www.sabre.org

ELSEVIER   BOOK AID International   Sabre Foundation

The publisher's policy is to use paper manufactured from sustainable forests

Printed in China

Foreword

Pain is a ubiquitous human experience and one of the commonest reasons for a patient to consult. Knowledge about the pathophysiology of the pain experience is growing. It is important that undergraduate medical students, postgraduate doctors and other health care professionals can easily access this new information, so that they can better understand, assess and manage pain.

Acute pain results from disease or trauma and often resolves either with healing or with treatment of the underlying condition. Better management of acute pain is vital from a humanitarian viewpoint. Chronic pain is a complex condition involving a myriad of nociceptive mechanisms in the peripheral and central nervous system. Psychosocial and environmental factors also play a role in the pain experience and these influences need to be better understood and validated by clinicians.

Mechanisms and treatment of acute and chronic pain need to be taught at undergraduate and postgraduate level to all health care professionals who may be involved in patient care. This includes doctors, nurses, physiotherapists, pharmacists, occupational therapists and clinical psychologists. All these people will come into contact with people in pain and have an important role to play in its better management.

Communication with patients with pain is vital, but can be difficult. Society tends to understand the Cartesian model of pain and has not moved on. Introducing new concepts to patients is essential but challenging as they, too, need to understand more about their pain.

This text is an exciting development into undergraduate and general health care professional education. It has a clear and accessible style and the key learning points summarise the important topics of each chapter and reinforce the prime messages that will be of practical benefit to all clinicians.

Beverly Collett
Assistant Medical Director
Consultant in Pain Management & Anaesthesia
Leicester Royal Infirmary NHS Trust
Leicester, UK

Preface

Pain is one of the most common symptoms experienced by patients. It is incumbent on all healthcare professionals to recognise this and to have an understanding of the basic mechanisms, both physiological and psychological, that underpin our understanding of pain. It is important to build on this basis and to develop the techniques of assessment and management planning that are essential in attempting to alleviate the pain or suffering that goes with it.

Education about pain, especially for budding doctors, should commence in medical school and for nursing and other allied professionals at a similar point in their education. Historically, inadequate attention has been paid to this area of teaching, both at undergraduate and graduate level, and this text is aimed at filling that void.

The aims of this book are to introduce the concepts of pain from a basic science perspective and to develop it into the biopsychosocial model that is modern pain management. There is little assumed knowledge and it is hoped it will help those who look after patients who are suffering. Nursing and allied professionals, who are developing a deeper understanding of pain management, may also find this text useful before moving onto the larger more comprehensive books on the subject.

John Hughes

Acknowledgements

I would like to acknowledge the support and help from Mary Law who took the seed and helped develop it into the project it is. Following that Linda Bennett who has guided me through the process from commissioning authors to completion. Without her this text would not have made it this far.

A special word of thanks to Jenny Hyland (a then 4th year medical student), who has critically commented on the rough and finished chapters as they came in. That input has been invaluable in shaping the final version of the text.

Contents

Contributors   xi

Abbreviations   xiii

Definitions   xv

1. Introduction   1
   John Hughes

2. Neurophysiology   6
   Sanjay Varma

3. Neuroanatomy   20
   John Hughes

4. Neuropharmacology   28
   Paul L. Chazot

5. Peripheral mechanisms   48
   Paul Farquhar-Smith

6. Central mechanisms   65
   Christopher Coe

7. Non-pharmacological interventions   80
   Alistair Dodds

8. Non-steroidal anti-inflammatory drugs and paracetamol   91
   Andrew Lloyd

9. Local anaesthetics: other membrane stabilisers   118
   Amit Kumar

10. Opioids   130
    Gemma Udhaykumar

11. Adjuvant and miscellaneous drugs used
    in pain management   143
    Dilip Kapur

12. Peripheral interventions   159
    Donald Graham

13. Pain as a clinical entity   187
    Gwenda Cavill

14. Epidemiology of pain   201
    Paul Wilkinson and Nilofer Sabrine

15. Pain assessment   213
    Ashish Gulve

16. Psychological impact of chronic pain   230
    Claire Davies

17. Interventions in pain management   242
    Sam Eldabe and Sivakumar Raghavan

18. Management strategies   263
    Keith Milligan

19. Pain, ethics and research   277
    Andrew Skinner

    Index   285

Contributors

Gwenda Cavill
Consultant in Anaesthesia and Pain Management
Wansbeck General Hospital
Ashington, UK

Pain as a clinical entity

Paul Chazot
Acting Head
Centre for Integrative Neuroscience
School of Biological and Biomedical Sciences
Durham University
Durham, UK

Neuropharmacology

Christopher Coe
Consultant in Anaesthesia and Pain Management
Wansbeck General Hospital
Ashington, UK

Central mechanisms

Claire Davies
Clinical Psychologist
Welsh Regional Spinal Cord Injury Centre
Rookwood Hospital
Cardiff, UK

Psychological impact of chronic pain

Allistair Dodds
Consultant in Anaesthesia and Pain Management
Sunderland Royal Hospital NHS Trust
Sunderland, UK

Non-pharmacological interventions

Sam Eldabe
Consultant in Anaesthesia and Pain Management
The James Cook University Hospital
Middlesbrough, UK

Interventions in pain management

Paul Farquhar-Smith
Consultant in Anaesthetics, Pain and Intensive Care
The Royal Marsden NHS Foundation Trust
London, UK

Peripheral mechanisms

Donald Graham
Consultant in Anaesthesia and Pain Management
Doncaster Royal Infirmary
Doncaster, UK

Peripheral interventions

Ashish Gulve
Consultant in Pain Management and Anaesthesia
The James Cook University Hospital
Middlesbrough, UK

Pain assessment

John Hughes
Consultant in Anaesthetics and Pain Management
The James Cook University Hospital
Middlesbrough, UK

Introduction

Neuroanatomy

Dilip Kapur
Senior Consultant in Pain Management
Flinders Medical Centre
Adelaide
Australia

Adjuvant and miscellaneous drugs used in pain management

Amit Kumar
Consultant in Anaesthetics and Pain Management
Sunderland Royal Hospital NHS Trust
Sunderland, UK

Local anaesthetics: other membrane stabilisers

Andrew Lloyd
Specialty Registrar in Anaesthesia
The James Cook University Hospital
Middlesbrough, UK

Non-steroidal anti-inflammatory drugs and paracetamol

Keith Milligan
Clinical Director of Pain Management
The James Cook University Hospital
Middlesbrough, UK

Management strategies

Sivakumar Raghavan
Specialist Registrar in Anaesthesia
The James Cook University Hospital
Middlesbrough, UK

Interventions in pain management

Nilofer Sabrine
Research Associate/Paediatrician
Comparative Biology Centre
University of Newcastle
Newcastle Upon Tyne, UK

Epidemiology of pain

Andrew Skinner
Consultant Anaesthetist
The James Cook University Hospital
Middlesbrough, UK

Pain, ethics and research

Gemma Udhaykumar
Final Year Medical Student
The James Cook University Hospital
Middlesbrough, UK

Opioids

Sanjay Varma
Consultant in Pain Management and Anaesthesia
Sunderland Royal Hospitals NHS Trust
Sunderland, UK

Neurophysiology

Paul Wilkinson
Consultant in Pain Management
Royal Victoria Infirmary
Newcastle Upon Tyne, UK

Epidemiology of pain

Abbreviations

AA	Arachidonic acid
ACC	Anterior cingulate cortex
ACE	Angiotensin converting enzyme
AMPA	Alpha-amino-3-hydroxy-5-methyl-4-isoxazole propionic acid
Asics	Acid-sensing ion channels
ATP	Adenosine triphosphate
BBB	Blood–brain barrier
bd	Twice daily (medication instructions)
BDNF	Brain-derived neurotrophic factor
BK	Bradykinin
BNF	British National Formulary
BPI	Brief Pain Inventory
cAMP	Cyclic adenosine monophosphate
CB	Cannabinoid receptors 1 and 2
CBT	Cognitive behavioural therapy
CCF	Congestive cardiac failure
CGRP	Calcitonin gene-related peptide
CHD	Coronary heart disease
COX	Cyclooxygenase generic
COX1	Cyclooxygenase 1 specific
COX2	Cyclooxygenase 2 specific
CRPS	Complex regional pain syndromes
CSF	Cerebrospinal fluid
CVA	Cerebrovascular accident
DRG	Dorsal root ganglia
ED50	Effective dose for 50% of the population
EPSP	Excitatory post synaptic potential
GABA	Gamma-aminobutyric acid
GDP	Guanosine diphosphate
GI	Gastrointestinal tract
GPCRs	G-protein-coupled receptors
G-proteins	Guanine nucleotide binding proteins
GTP	Guanosine triphosphate
HAD	Hospital Anxiety and Depression Scale
HRQL	Health-related quality of life measures
IASP	International Association for the Study of Pain
IDDS	Implantable intrathecal drug delivery systems
IL-1beta	Interleukin-1beta
IPSP	Inhibitory post synaptic potential
im	Intramuscular injection
IV or iv	Intravenous injection
IVRA	Intravenous regional anaesthesia
LD_{50}	Lethal dose for 50% of the population
LGICs	Ligand-gated ion channels
LTB4	Leukotriene B4
LTP	Long-term potentiation
mAChR	Muscarinic acetylcholine receptor
MAO	Monoamine oxidase
MAOI	Monoamine oxidase inhibitors
mGlu	G protein-coupled metabotropic glutamate receptor
MI	Myocardial infarction
M6G	Morphine-6-glucuronide
NAPQ1	N-acetyl-p-amino-benzoquinoneimine
NGF	Nerve growth factor
NK1	Neurokinin 1 receptors
NMDA	N-methyl-D-aspartate
NNH	Numbers needed to harm
NNT	Numbers needed to treat
NO	Nitric oxide
NRS	Numerical rating scale
NSAIDs	Nonsteroidal anti-inflammatory drugs
NTS	Nucleus tractus solitarius
OA	Osteoarthritis
PAD	Primary afferent depolarisation

PAG	Periaqueductal grey matter	**SP**	Substance P
PCA	Patient-controlled analgesia	**TCAs**	Tricyclic antidepressants
PCEA	Patient-controlled epidural analgesia	**tds**	Three times daily (medication instructions)
PDGF	Platelet-derived growth factor receptors	**TENS**	Transcutaneous electrical nerve stimulation
PET	Positron emission tomography	**TNFalpha**	Tumour necrosis factor alpha
PG	Prostaglandin in a generic sense	**TRPV1**	Transient receptor potential channel 1
PGE$_2$	Prostaglandin E$_2$ specific, others also exist	**TTX**	Tetrodotoxin
PKA	Protein kinase A	**VAS**	Visual Analogue Scale
PKC	Protein kinase C	**Vd**	Volume of distribution
PoM	Prescription only medicine	**VGSCs**	Voltage gated Na$^+$ currents
PPIS	Present Pain Intensity Scale	**VGSC**	Voltage gated Na$^+$ channels
qds	Four times daily (medication instructions)	**VMAT**	Vesicular monoamine transporter
REC	Research Ethics Committee	**VNS**	Verbal numerical scale
RFTC	Percutaneous radiofrequency thermocoagulation	**VR1**	Vanilloid receptor 1
RhA	Rheumatoid arthritis	**VRS**	Verbal Rating Scale
RTKs	Receptor tyrosine kinases	**WDR**	Wide dynamic range neurones
RVM	Rostroventral medulla	**WHO**	The World Health Organization
SCS	Spinal cord stimulation	**5HT**	5-hydroxytryptamine. A family of receptors for the neurotransmitter serotonin
SMP	Sympathetically maintained pain		
SNRIs	Serotonin/noradrenaline (norepinephrine) reuptake inhibitors		

Definitions

Below is a list of common definitions used within this text. Many are those described by The International Association for the Study of Pain (IASP) who published a Classification of Chronic Pain [1] that provides a useful taxonomy and set of current definitions.

Addiction Is a syndrome and pattern of substance misuse. There are specific psychiatric definitions that involve a compulsive psychological and physiological need for a substance. The sufferer us unable to control their behaviour.

Affective Related to feelings, moods and emotions.

Afferent Nerves that carry impulses from the periphery to the central nervous system.

Affinity A drug's tendency or ability to combine with a receptor. This is different to efficacy, as it does not imply any response by the receptor.

Agonist An agent that binds to a receptor producing a maximal effect.

Algogens Pain-producing substances.

Allodynia Pain due to a stimulus that is not normally painful.

Anaesthesia Absence of all sensory modalities (including touch, temperature, movement and pain).

Anaesthesia dolorosa Pain in an anaesthetic area. When pain is felt in an area that is otherwise numb or desensitised.

Analgesia Absence of pain in response to a stimulus that would normally be painful.

Analgesic An agent that produces analgesia.

Antagonist An agent that binds to a receptor producing no response.

Antidromic The conduction of nerve impulses in the opposite direction to normal.

Arthralgia Pain in a joint.

Bioavailability The amount of administered drug that reaches the systemic circulation.

Causalgia Pain described as 'burning' usually following a nerve injury.

Central pain Pain initiated or caused by a primary lesion or dysfunction in the central nervous system.

Clearance rate The volume of plasma cleared of drug per unit time.

Cognitive In psychology is often referred to as mental functions or processing. Is often used loosely with regard to human processing of information.

Deafferentation pain Pain due to loss of sensation of an afferent fibre or fibres.

Decussate To cross to the other side as seen with nerves entering the spinal cord on one side and ascending on the other side.

Dependence Is where a drug is required to be taken in order to prevent a physiological withdrawal response. This may be physical or physiological.

Dorsal root ganglia The dorsal root ganglia are where the cell bodies of primary afferent neurons reside.

Downregulation	Where a cell reduces the number of receptors to reduce its sensitivity to a hormone or neurotransmitter.
Dysaesthesia	An unpleasant abnormal sensation, whether spontaneous or evoked.
Efferent	Nerves carrying impulses from the central nervous system to the periphery.
Efficacy	An agent's ability to produce an effect. Different drugs may act on the same receptor but produce differing degrees of effect.
Endogenous	Produced from within the body.
Eutectic	When two compounds are mixed producing a substance that behaves with a single set of physical characteristics.
Hydrophilic	Compounds that have an affinity for water.
Hyperaesthesia	Increased sensitivity to stimulation, excluding the special senses.
Hyperalgesia	An increased response to a stimulus that is normally painful.
Hyperpathia	A painful syndrome in which there is an abnormally explosive painful reaction to a stimulus.
Hypoaesthesia	Diminished sensitivity to a stimulus, excluding the special senses.
Hypoalgesia	Diminished response to a normally painful stimulus.
Iatrogenic	Resulting unintentionally from medical treatment.
Intrathecal	Injection through the dural layers into the cerebrospinal fluid.
Ion channels or ionophores	Proteins that form pores through the membrane of cells. They are involved with establishing the voltage gradient across membranes.
Ionotropic receptors	Also known as ligand gated ion channels. These are transmembrane ion channels that open in response to a chemical transmitter.
Kinesophobia	An intense fear of movement
Ligand	A chemical that binds to a receptor. This may have an excitatory effect, inhibitory effect or no effect.
Ligand gated ion channels	These are transmembrane ion channels that open in response to a chemical transmitter.
Lipophilic	Has an affinity for fat. Dissolves in lipids.
Metabotropic receptors	Indirectly act on ion channels by signal transduction mechanisms on the plasma membrane.
Microwave diathermy	Produced by a Magnetron which produces a high-frequency alternating current.
Narcotic	A drug that reduces awareness to sensory impulses, especially pain.
Neuralgia	Pain in the distribution of a peripheral nerve.
Neuritis	Inflammation of a nerve or nerves.
Neuroma	Is a tumour (benign or malignant) of cells in the nervous system. Commonly occurring at the end of damaged nerves (e.g. surgical) with poorly regulated nerve regeneration. They are frequently painful.
Neuropathic or neurogenic pain	Pain initiated or caused by a primary lesion or dysfunction in the nervous system.
Peripheral	Where the lesion or dysfunction is in the peripheral nervous system.
Central	Where the lesion or dysfunction is in the central nervous system.
Neuropathy	Impaired function of a nerve.

Neuropeptides	Peptides (linked amino acids) found in neuronal tissue.
Neurotrophic substance	Chemicals produced by nervous tissue that are involved with nerve cell function and survival.
Nociception	Is the response of the nervous system to a noxious stimulus.
Nociceptive pain	A noxious or unpleasant stimulus activating nociceptors.
Somatic	Where the pain is related to superficial structures (e.g. skin, bone, tendons, muscle, connective tissue).
Visceral	Where the pain is related to one of the viscera (e.g. heart, bowels, bladder).
Nociceptor	A receptor preferentially sensitive to a noxious stimulus or to a stimulus, which would become noxious if prolonged.
Noxious stimulus	A stimulus that is capable of potential or actual damage to a body tissue.
Opiate	Naturally occurring opioids. The alkaloids found in opium.
Opioid	An agent that binds to opioid receptors.
Pain	An unpleasant sensory and emotional experience associated with actual or potential tissue damage, or described in terms of such damage.
Pain threshold	The least intensity of a stimulus at which a subject experiences pain.
Pain tolerance level	The greatest level of pain a subject is prepared to tolerate.
Paraesthesia	An abnormal sensation, whether spontaneous or evoked.
Partial agonist	An agent that binds to a receptor but does not produce full activation.
Phantom pain	Pain in a part of the body that has been surgically removed or is congenitally absent.
Pharmacodynamics	How drugs evoke their pharmacological responses or how the drug affects the body. This includes therapeutic and toxic effects.
Pharmacokinetics	How the body acts upon drugs. This includes the absorption, distribution and elimination (metabolism and excretion) of drugs.
Pharmacophore	The set of structural features in a molecule that is recognised as a receptor site and is responsible for that molecule's biological activity.
Pro-drug	Is a drug that is inactive on its own and has to be metabolised for the active agent to be produced.
Proprioception	The special awareness of movement and the spatial orientation of the body.
Psychogenic	Thought of as being in the mind. Of psychological origin rather than physiological.
Psychotropic	Usually a drug that acts on the brain causing alterations in mood, behaviour, consciousness and perception.
Radicular pain or radiculalgia	Pain in the distribution of a sensory nerve root or roots.
Radiculitis	Inflammation of one or more nerve roots.
Radiculopathy	Disturbance of function in the distribution of one or more nerve root areas.
Referred pain	Pain localised not to the site of its cause but to an area that may be adjacent to or at a distance from that site (e.g. shoulder tip pain caused by diaphragmatic irritation).
Rubefacient	Rub into skin to alter or mask pain.
Somatic	Relates to the areas of the body under voluntary control as opposed to the viscera or mind. Pertaining to the skin and muscle.

Tachyphylaxis	A decreasing response to a given dose of drug following its initial administration.
Tolerance	Increases in drug dose are required to have the same effect.
Trigger point	A hypersensitive area (site) within a muscle or connective tissue.
Upregulation	Is where a cell increases the number of receptors to increase its sensitivity to a hormone or neurotransmitter.
Voltage-gated ion channels	Are ion channels that are activated by changes in the potential difference across the membrane within the region of the ion channel.
Withdrawal	Is a syndrome that manifests when a drug is stopped or the dose reduced in patients who have been habitual users of the drug.

Reference   1. Merskey H, Bogduk N (eds) *Classification of Chronic Pain.* 2nd edn. Seattle: IASP Press; 1994.

John Hughes

Introduction

Pain is an experience that is common to us all whilst also being unique to the individual. Here we will explore the structures, mechanisms and science that are involved in the perception of unpleasant stimuli, as well as the interpretation of these at a psychological level that results in the experience of pain. This provides the basis for understanding how individuals perceive pain and where interventions may be of benefit. In the second part of the text patient assessment is considered, before dealing with the development of management plans aimed at alleviating the pain and the associated distress.

A working definition is important in understanding that pain has both biological and psychological components. The International Association for the Study of Pain (IASP)[1] defines pain as:

"An unpleasant sensory and emotional experience associated with actual or potential tissue damage, or described in terms of such damage."

- This definition emphasises that pain is unpleasant, with both sensory and emotional components.
- This allows for the same noxious stimulus resulting in different severities of pain under differing emotional situations (e.g. the knocks and bumps seen on the playing fields of rugby, hockey, football, etc., that do not appear to be noticed compared to the response that would occur if the same stimuli were received when walking down the high street).
- There does not have to be tissue damage to experience pain (e.g. heat from a fire or cooking hob felt on the hand is experienced as painful without any damage being done to the skin).
- Finally, pain is described using terms that signify tissue damage (e.g. sharp, stabbing, burning).

Other definitions have their advantages, but all should encompass the biological, psychological and social components. Table 1.1 includes several

TABLE 1.1 Pain definitions (this table includes a variety of definitions to contrast with that from the IASP)

Source	Definition
IASP	An unpleasant sensory and emotional experience associated with actual or potential tissue damage, or described in terms of such damage
www.doctorsforpain.com/patient/terminology.html	Sensation of discomfort, distress, or agony, resulting from the stimulation of specialised nerve endings. It serves as a protective mechanism (induces the sufferer to remove or withdraw)
New Oxford American Dictionary 2004 (© Apple 2005)	Physical suffering or discomfort caused by illness or injury A feeling of marked discomfort in a particular part of the body Mental suffering or distress
encyclopedia.worldvillage.com/s/b/Pain	Is both a sensory and emotional experience, generally associated with tissue damage or inflammation. Pain is ultimately a perception, and not an objective bodily state

definitions that can be compared to that of the IASP. As a result the management of pain has to allow for interventions that involve all these dimensions.

Pain is common and a feature of the majority of consultations in primary care and the sole feature in many. Often the pain is part of an underlying condition and resolves with it. Under these circumstances it could be considered specific to that condition and thus classified from a disease-specific angle.

There are other circumstances where the pain persists well beyond the recovery of the initiating event (e.g. postherpetic neuralgia following shingles) when the pain becomes the problem in its own right.

When looking at the underlying neurophysiology and neuroanatomy there are common pathways and mechanisms involved in the sensing, transmission, processing and interpretation of nociceptive activity. The same interventions may be used with benefit for pains relating to different disease states (e.g. postherpetic neuralgia and painful diabetic neuropathy). This leads to a mechanistic approach to pain processing. It also allows for the psychological and social influences that impact on all pain states.

From this mechanistic approach there are three broad types of pain to be considered, all having different influences on pain pathways:

1. Somatic pain, which relates to a noxious stimulus activating nociceptors. The pain is related to the area involved by the stimulus (e.g. pain after surgery, broken bone).
2. Visceral pain, where the nociceptive stimulus is affecting one of the viscera (e.g. renal colic, angina).
3. Neuropathic pain, where there is a lesion or dysfunction in the nervous system (e.g. painful diabetic neuropathy).[1] The site may be felt in a somatic or visceral distribution.

The first two types of pain fit into a concept that pain is as a result of injury and thus equates to harm, often followed by an intervention (e.g. rest) that allows healing to occur.

Neuropathic pain continues after any healing is complete. Under these conditions rest or avoidance of the painful area will not allow resolution of the pain. This is where the pain does not equate to harm and is more difficult to conceptualise.

Some degree of pain or discomfort is expected following injury or surgery and it is assumed to reduce and go as the injury recovers. This is easily described as acute pain.

Chronic pain is taken to mean pain that does not settle as the acute insult recovers or as pain persisting for more than 3 or 6 months. The incidence of moderate to severe chronic pain is as high as 1 in 5 of the population. The pain limits the independence of 30% of sufferers and 50–60% have interference with their ability to exercise, sleep, socialise, undertake household chores, walk or have sexual relationships.[2] Table 1.2 gives an idea of the frequency of neuropathic pain in the population.[3] This represents a huge problem for society as it has direct social and economic implications running into billions of pounds. The cost to health services is only part of the effect, time lost from work, reduced productivity, role of carers, etc., should also be considered. Pain management, therefore, has an important role in reducing the suffering of patients and reducing the social and financial cost to society.

The assessment of patients has to encompass the medical components of where the pain is, when it started, how it has changed with time and what it is like now. A description of what it 'feels like' (for the patient) is essential to understand the impact on the sufferer and to help assess the type of pain being experienced. There are scoring systems to measure pain and suffering (e.g. visual analogue scale, hospital anxiety and depression scale). The impact on sleep, mood, coping, relationships and activities of daily living are important elements of assessment for both initial evaluation and to assess the effect of interventions. Along with this, an understanding of the patient's expectations of therapy helps develop a constructive doctor–patient relationship. This allows for realistic therapeutic goals to be set. The general medical health of the patient influences decision-making, as does a full current and past drug history. A thorough history, therefore, provides an understanding of the physical, psychological and social components of the patients' illness. An examination may then be considered to help confirm the clinical impression from the history.

The role of investigations may be important in the acute setting when the cause of the pain is directly linked to its management (e.g. fractures). In the chronic setting investigations may already have been done, then a thorough review of the notes would be more appropriate in the first instance. Investigations that are then considered appropriate should have a direct influence on management and if not should be avoided.

TABLE 1.2 Estimated incidence of neuropathic pain in the USA based on a population of 270 million		
Condition	Numbers of patients	Frequency in population (1in x)
Painful diabetic neuropathy	600 000	450
Postherpetic neuralgia	500 000	540
Cancer associated	200 000	1350
Phantom pain	50 000	5400
MS	51 000	5294
Post CVA (central)	15 000	18 000
Low back pain (10% of 21 million cases)	2 100 000	128
Total neuropathic pains	3 781 000	71

Data from: Bennett GJ. Neuropathic pain. In: Borsook (ed.) Molecular neurobiology of pain. Seattle: IASP Press; 1997.

When considering management options it is important to maintain a broad perspective. Acute pain can be approached in an expectant manner with interventions aimed at reducing the pain significantly with the expectation that with time the pain will ease. In the chronic setting this is an unrealistic goal, as the pain often persists indefinitely. Here the approach is to minimise the impact of the pain or for the patient to achieve the best quality of life they can despite the limitations set upon them. The emphasis thus moves away from the purely medical model (of drugs and injections) to encompass the psychological, social and environmental issues surrounding the pain.

The assessment is, therefore, multidimensional and interventions or strategies to minimise the impact of the pain have to follow a similar structure. Simple manoeuvres such as heat, cold, support, massage and movement, often done by patients at home, can be very effective. The psychological impact of pain may be better managed by understanding what the patient feels about their pain and how it impacts on their life and how they cope. Pain has an emotional component that does not respond well to pharmacological intervention, for example, patients with cancer pain may have a fear of dying and this fear will influence their pain. Drugs will not address the fear that has to be assessed alongside the nociceptive and neuropathic elements of the pain.

Mobility, posture and ability to exercise will impact on quality of life and the pain. Movement may provoke pain, but inactivity can do the same. Here the role of physiotherapy is vital in helping the patient to optimise their mobility and regain the confidence to exercise within their limitations, often after prolonged periods of relative inactivity. This may be linked with goal setting, allowing the patient to perform tasks of daily living. Simple aids may significantly affect the ability to live independently and this is where occupational therapy has a role. Other commonly used non-drug interventions include transcutaneous electrical nerve stimulation (TENS) and acupuncture.

Within the medical model there are drugs that may be used independently or in combination. These are broadly divided into simple analgesics, co-analgesics and other agents (Table 1.3). Injections form part of the armoury and may involve local anaesthetic agents or, occasionally, neurolytic drugs (e.g. phenol). There are surgical interventions that may be beneficial (e.g. surgery for spinal disk entrapment syndromes). Other interventions may include implanting devices that stimulate the spinal cord (spinal cord stimulators) or

TABLE 1.3 Broad classification of the common drug classes used in pain management	
Simple analgesics	Paracetamol
	Non-steroidal anti-inflammatory drugs (ibuprofen)
	Weak opioids (codeine)
	Strong opioids (morphine)
Co-analgesics	Tricyclic antidepressants
	Anticonvulsants
	Membrane stabilisers (e.g. mexiletine)
	Novel agents (e.g. ketamine)
Others	Muscle relaxants (e.g. baclofen)
	Anxiolytics (e.g. diazepam)

pumps that are implanted and deliver drugs directly into the cerebrospinal fluid surrounding the spinal cord.

The use of complementary therapies has grown significantly over recent years with some individuals claiming tremendous benefit. This has not in the main been backed up with any good scientific research and thus makes it difficult to assess the true value or otherwise of these interventions.

Pain and its management are, therefore, multidimensional and have to be approached in this fashion. The text aims to expand on the mechanisms, whilst encompassing the emotional components and demonstrating where interventions may be of benefit. Understanding the mechanisms along with the assessment process allows a structured approach to develop individualised management strategies. Knowledge of the epidemiology and size of the problem will reinforce the importance of good pain management at an individual, social and global level.

KEY POINTS

- Pain is common in 1 in 5 of the population
- There are sensory and emotional components to pain
- Assessment has to include psychological and physical elements
- Understanding the mechanisms will help plan management options
- Pain is not the same as harm
- Not all pain can be eradicated

References

1. Merskey H, Bogduk N (eds). *Classification of Chronic Pain,* 2nd edn. Seattle: IASP Press; 1994.
2. IASP. *Unrelieved pain is a major global healthcare problem.* Press Release, 2004 (cited 2004 October). Available from: *http://www.iasp-pain.org/Global%20Day2004.html.*
3. Bennett GJ. Neuropathic pain: an overview. In: Borsook D (ed.) *Molecular Neurobiology of Pain.* Seattle: IASP Press; 1997: 109–113.

Sanjay Varma

Neurophysiology

Neurone – basic functional unit of the nervous system

A nerve cell consists of five to seven processes called *dendrites* that extend outwards from the cell body. A typical neurone has a long fibrous *axon* that originates from the *cell body*. The axon divides into terminal branches, each ending in a number of knobs called *terminal buttons* or *axon telodendria*. Axons of some neurones are *myelinated*. The myelin sheath envelopes the axon except at its ending and at the *node of Ranvier* (Fig. 2.1).

The nerve cell has a low threshold for excitation from stimuli that may be mechanical, chemical or electrical. A propagated stimulus is called an *action potential* (or a nerve impulse). These are the only electrical responses of the neurone and are the main language of the nervous system. They are due to changes in the conduction of ions across the cell membrane and are produced by alterations in the ion channels.

Membrane potentials

Resting membrane potential

When two electrodes are placed, one into the interior of the axon and the other placed on the surface of the same axon, a constant potential difference is observed across the membrane. The inside is negative relative to the outside when the cell is at rest. This is called the resting membrane potential (RMP). The internal potential is about -70 mV compared to the outside of the membrane. In reality, the RMP does fluctuate slightly with time.

Action potential

Nerve signals are transmitted by action potentials (APs), which are rapid changes in the membrane potential that spread along the nerve fibre membrane. Each AP

Fig. 2.1   Motor neurone

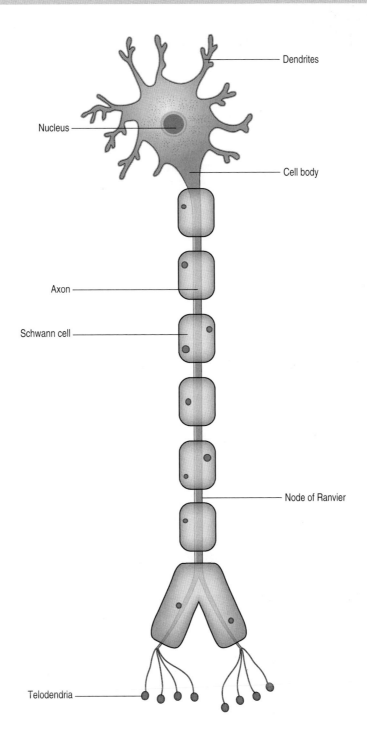

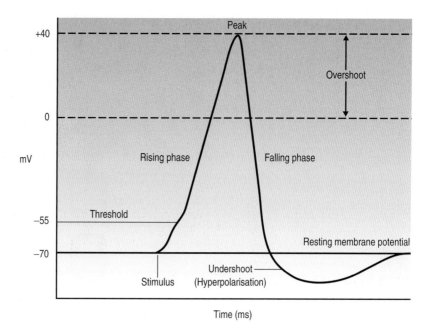

Fig. 2.2 Schematic action potential

begins with a sudden change from the normal negative RMP to a positive potential and ends with an almost equally rapid change back to the negative potential. To conduct a nerve signal, the AP moves along the nerve fibre until it comes to the fibre's end (Fig. 2.2).

Ionic basis of resting membrane potential

Sodium ions (Na^+) are actively transported out of the neurone and potassium ions (K^+) are actively transported into the cells. Potassium ion moves out of the cell and sodium ion moves in, but because of potassium channels, potassium ion permeability at rest is greater than sodium ion permeability. Therefore, potassium ion generally maintains the resting membrane potential.

Inside the axons are many negative charged ions that cannot go through the membrane channels. These are the anions of protein molecules and organic phosphate compounds. Because these ions cannot leave the interior of the axon, any deficit of positive ions inside the membrane leaves an excess of these impermeable negative ions, which are responsible for the negative charge inside the fibre when there is a deficit of positively charged potassium and other positive ions.

Ionic fluxes during an action potential

Depolarisation

During this stage of the AP the membrane becomes very permeable to sodium ions, allowing them to enter into the interior of the axon. The normal polarised state of -70 mV is immediately neutralised by inflowing sodium ions, with the result that the membrane potential rises rapidly in the positive direction. This is called depolarisation and takes place with the help of activated voltage-gated sodium channels.

Repolarisation

This stage starts within a fraction of a millisecond after the membrane becomes highly permeable to sodium ions; the sodium channels begin to close and the potassium channels open more than in the resting phase. There is, therefore, rapid diffusion of potassium ions out of the neurone to re-establish the normal negative RMP. This is called the repolarisation of the membrane.

The effect of this is for the membrane potential to become even more negative than the original RMP for a few milliseconds following the action potential; this is called 'after hyperpolarisation' or undershoot. This is due to the potassium ion channels remaining open for several milliseconds after the repolarisation of the membrane is complete.

Role of calcium ions. A deficit of calcium ions in the extracellular fluid activates the sodium ion channels resulting in increased excitability of nerve and muscle cell. Conversely an increase in the extracellular calcium concentration stabilises the membrane by decreasing excitability.

Propagation of action potential

In the preceding paragraph we discussed the AP as it occurs at one spot on the membrane; however, an AP elicited at any one point on an excitable membrane usually excites the adjacent portion of the membrane, resulting in the propagation of the AP over the membrane and hence along the axon.

All or none law

For an action potential to occur the stimulus (which may take several forms) has to elevate the resting membrane potential to threshold. If threshold is reached an action potential is propagated with a constant amplitude and form regardless of the strength of the stimulus. An action potential fails to occur if the stimulus is subthreshold in magnitude. The AP is, therefore, all or none in character and is said to obey the 'all or none law'.

Nerve fibre types and function

Gasser and Erlanger divided mammalian nerve into A, B and C groups.[1] Group A is further subdivided into α, β, γ and δ fibres. In general, the greater the diameter of a given nerve fibre, the greater its speed of conduction. The large axons are concerned primarily with proprioceptive sensation, somatic motor function, conscious touch and pressure, while the smaller axons transmit pain, temperature and autonomic impulses. In Table 2.1 the various types of nerve fibres are listed with their diameters, conduction velocity and functions.

C-fibres that enter the dorsal root of the spinal cord conduct some impulses generated by touch and other cutaneous receptors in addition to impulses generated by pain and temperature receptors. Apart from variation in speed of conduction and fibre diameter, the various classes of fibres in peripheral nerves differ in their sensitivity to anaesthetics and hypoxia. This has a clinical and physiological significance. Local anaesthetic drugs depress transmission (of action potentials) in C-fibres before they affect the touch fibres in group A. Conversely, pressure on a nerve (or nerve root as it leaves the spinal canal) can cause a loss of conduction in large-diameter motor, touch and pressure fibres while pain sensation remains relatively intact. This can be seen in

TABLE 2.1 Nerve fibre types in mammalian nerve

Fibre type	Function	Conduction velocity (m/s)	Fibre diameter (mm)
A (myelinated)			
α	Proprioception; somatic motor	70–120	12–20
β	Touch, pressure, motor	30–70	5–12
γ	Motor-to-muscle spindles	15–30	3–6
δ	Pain, cold, touch	12–30	2–5
B (myelinated)	Preganglionic autonomic	3–15	<3
C (unmyelinated)			
Dorsal root	Pain, temperature, some mechanoreception, reflex responses	0.5–2	0.4–1.2
Sympathetic	Postganglionic sympathetics	0.7–2.3	0.3–1.3

individuals who sleep with their arms under their heads or over the back of a chair for long periods, causing traction or compression of the nerves in the arms (often associated with deep sleep and alcohol intoxication, the syndrome is commonest at weekends and has acquired the interesting name of Saturday night or Sunday morning palsy).

Synaptic and junctional transmission

Synapses are junctions where the axon or some other portion of one cell (presynaptic cell) terminates on the dendrites, soma or axon of another neurone or muscle cells (the post synaptic cell). There is a clear synaptic cleft between the presynaptic and postsynaptic membrane, typically with a width of 20 nm (Figs 2.3 & 2.4).

Fig. 2.3 Neuromuscular junction

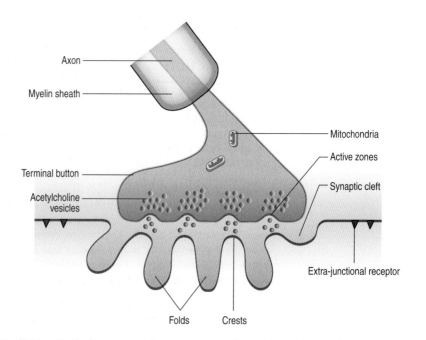

Fig. 2.4   Neuronal synapse

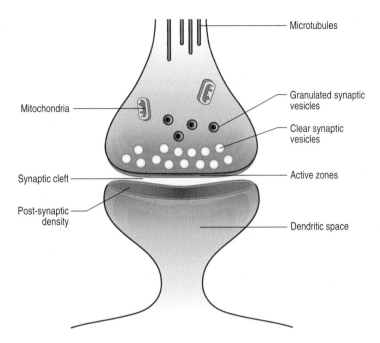

The transmission at most synaptic junctions is chemical; the impulse in the presynaptic axon causes secretion of a neurotransmitter such as acetylcholine. This chemical mediator binds to receptors on the surface of the postsynaptic cell, and triggers events that open or close channels in the membrane of the postsynaptic cell.

The transmitter is rapidly removed from the synaptic cleft by diffusion, metabolism or reuptake into the presynaptic neurone.

Transmission from nerve to muscle resembles the chemical synaptic transmission from one neurone to another. The specialised area where a motor nerve terminates on a skeletal muscle is called the neuromuscular junction.

The presynaptic terminal has numerous mitochondria; there are also membrane-enclosed vesicles, which contain the neurotransmitter. These vesicles with neurotransmitters are synthesised in the Golgi apparatus in the neuronal cell body and migrate down the axon to the endings by axoplasmic transport.

The postsynaptic terminal has numerous smaller folds to increase the surface area with many receptors to which neurotransmitter binds.

The events occurring at the synapse are as follows: the action potential reaches the presynaptic terminal opening voltage-gated calcium channels. This results in calcium influx that triggers the release of vesicles into the synaptic cleft; the released neurotransmitter then binds to the receptors in the surface of the postsynaptic terminal.

Synapses permit conduction of impulses in one direction only from presynaptic to postsynaptic neurones. There are two kinds of chemical synapses, excitatory and inhibitory, which are differentiated by the effects of the neurotransmitter on the postsynaptic cell.

Excitatory chemical synapses

At an excitatory synapse, the postsynaptic response to the neurotransmitter is depolarisation, bringing the membrane potential closer to the threshold.

This is brought about by the opening of postsynaptic membrane ion channels thus increasing the concentration of sodium, potassium and other small positively charged ions. These ions are then free to move according to the electrical and chemical gradients across the membrane.

There is both an electrical and a concentration gradient driving sodium into the cell, while for potassium the electrical gradient opposes the concentration gradient. Opening channels that are non-specific to all small positively charged ions, therefore, results in the simultaneous movement of a relatively small number of potassium ions out of the cell and a larger number of sodium ions into the cell. Thus the net movement of positive ions is into the postsynaptic cell causing a slight depolarisation. This potential change is called an excitatory postsynaptic potential (EPSP). Its only function is to bring the membrane potential of the postsynaptic neurone closer to threshold. A single action potential in the presynaptic nerve will not produce sufficient excitation in the postsynaptic nerve to reach the threshold.

Inhibitory chemical synapses

At inhibitory synapses, the potential change in the postsynaptic neurone is a hyperpolarising graded potential called an inhibitory postsynaptic potential (IPSP). Activation of an inhibitory synapse lessens the likelihood that the postsynaptic cell will depolarise to threshold and generate an action potential. When an impulse arrives at an inhibitory synapse, the released transmitter activates receptors on the postsynaptic membrane that open chloride (Cl^-) or potassium channels, sodium ion channels are not affected. The chloride channels allow chloride ions to enter the cell producing hyperpolarisation and thus an IPSP. The potassium channels that are opened allow potassium ions to leave the cell thereby causing hyperpolarisation and an IPSP.

Of the thousands of synapses on any one neurone, probably hundreds are active simultaneously. The membrane potential of the postsynaptic neurone at any moment is, therefore, the result of all the synaptic activity affecting it at that moment. A depolarisation of the membrane towards threshold occurs when excitatory synaptic input predominates and a hyperpolarisation occurs when inhibitory input predominates. An action potential will occur if the balance of activity causes the membrane potential to reach threshold.

The nervous system needs both excitatory and inhibitory connections. In particular, the way in which our muscles are generally arranged in pairs that oppose one another implies that excitation of one muscle is usually associated with inhibition of the other by a process of reciprocal innervation. For example the tendon reflex, here the reflex contraction of the muscle (protagonist) that is stretched is accompanied by a relaxation of its antagonist. In this case, the inhibition of the corresponding motor neurone is brought about by branches of the afferent fibres from the stretch receptors which, after entering the dorsal cord, send excitatory branches to interneurones, they in turn form inhibitory synapses with the motor neurones in the ventral horn resulting in inhibition of the antagonist muscle (Fig. 2.5). A great amount of information has accumulated concerning the synthesis, metabolism and mechanism of action of these neurotransmitters and is well beyond the scope of this chapter.

Fig. 2.5 Tendon reflex

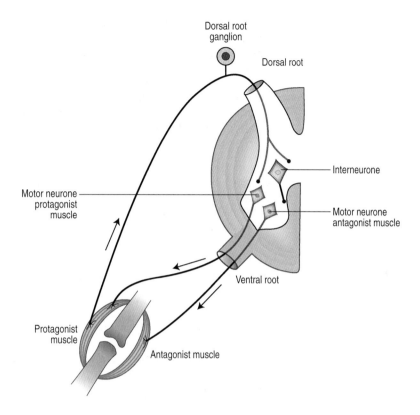

Neurotransmitters

Acetylcholine

Acetylcholine is a major neurotransmitter at the neuromuscular junction and in the brain. Neurones that release acetylcholine are called cholinergic neurones.

Acetylcholine is synthesised from choline and acetyl coenzyme-A in the cytoplasm of synaptic terminals and stored in synaptic vesicles. After it is released from the presynaptic membrane it activates receptors on the postsynaptic membrane; the concentration of acetylcholine at the postsynaptic membrane decreases due to action of the enzyme acetylcholinesterase and by simple diffusion away from the synapse, this results in the halting of receptor activation.

Acetylcholinesterase is located on the pre- and postsynaptic membranes and rapidly destroys acetylcholine, releasing choline and acetate. The choline is then transported back into the presynaptic axon terminals where it is reused to synthesise new acetylcholine.

There are two types of acetylcholine receptors (both respond to acetylcholine) and they are distinguished by their responsiveness to two different drugs:

1. Nicotinic receptors respond to the drug nicotine. These receptors are present at neuromuscular junctions. Nicotinic receptors are also found in the brain where they are important in cognitive function and behaviour.

2. Muscarinic receptors are stimulated by the mushroom poison muscarine. These receptors are coupled with a G-protein, which then alters the activity of a number of different enzymes and ion channels. These are prevalent at cholinergic synapses in the brain and at the junction of neurones that innervate many glands and organs, notably the heart. Atropine is an antagonist of muscarinic receptors, having many clinical uses.

Biogenic amines

The biogenic amines are synthesised from amino acids and contain an amino group (R-NH2). Common examples are: dopamine, noradrenaline (norepinephrine), serotonin and histamine. Adrenaline (epinephrine), another biogenic amine is not a common neurotransmitter, but is a major hormone secreted by the adrenal medulla.

Catecholamines

Dopamine, noradrenaline (norepinephrine) and adrenaline (epinephrine) all contain a catechol ring and an amino group, and are thus called catecholamines, they are formed by hydroxylation and decarboxylation of the amino acid tyrosine. Synthesis of the catecholamines begins with reuptake of tyrosine by axon terminals and its conversion to L-dopa by the enzyme tyrosine hydroxylase. Depending on the enzymes present in the terminal, any one of the three catecholamines may ultimately be released. Presynaptic autoreceptors strongly modulate synthesis and release of the catecholamines.[2]

After activation of the postsynaptic receptors, the catecholamine concentration in the synaptic cleft declines mainly due to reuptake into the presynaptic neurone by active transport. The neurotransmitter is also broken down in both the extracellular fluid and the axon terminal by an enzyme called monoamine oxidase (MAO). Monoamine oxidase inhibitors (MAOIs) have a clinical role as they increase the amount of norepinephrine and dopamine in a synapse by slowing their metabolism and are used in the treatment of mood disorders (e.g. depression).

There are two major classes of receptors for noradrenaline (norepinephrine) and adrenaline (epinephrine):

- α-adrenoceptors
  - these are further classified into α1 and α2
  - α1 act postsynaptically to either stimulate or inhibit activity at different types of potassium channels
  - α2 act presynaptically to inhibit norepinephrine release
- β-adrenoreceptors
  - β-receptor channels have three subclasses, β1, β2 and β3.

Serotonin

Serotonin is synthesised from tryptophan, an essential amino acid. Serotonin-releasing neurones innervate virtually every structure in the brain and spinal cord, and operate via at least 16 different receptors. In general, serotonin has an excitatory effect on pathways that are involved in the control of muscles, and an inhibitory effect on pathways that moderate sensations. The activity of serotonergic neurones is highest during states of alert wakefulness and lowest during sleep.

Serotonergic pathways contribute in emotional states such as mood and anxiety. They also contribute to motor activity, sleep and regulation of reproductive behaviour.

Serotonin uptake blockers, such as paroxetine, are thought to act in the treatment of depression by inactivating the 5-hydroxytryptamine (5-HT) transporter system resulting in the increase in synaptic concentrations of serotonin.

Amino acid neurotransmitters

In addition to neurotransmitters that are synthesised from amino acids, several amino acids themselves function as neurotransmitters. The amino acid neurotransmitters are by far the most prevalent neurotransmitters in the central nervous system.

Glutamate

This is the most common neurotransmitter at *excitatory synapses* in the brain and spinal cord (responsible for 75% of excitatory transmitter in the brain).

Metabotropic glutamate receptors modify the activity of presynaptic terminals. Two important subtypes of glutamate receptors are ionotropic receptors (i.e. ligand gated ion channels) found in postsynaptic membranes. They are designated as AMPA receptors (identified by their binding to α-amino-3hydroxyl-5methyl-4isoxazole propionic acid) and NMDA receptors (which bind to *N*-methyl-D-aspartate). Cooperative activity of AMPA and NMDA receptors has been implicated in a phenomenon called long-term potentiation (LTP). This mechanism couples frequent activity across a synapse with lasting changes in the strength of signalling across that synapse. This is then thought to be a cellular process underlying learning and memory formation. The proposed mechanism is that an action potential in the presynaptic neurone results in the release of glutamate from presynaptic terminals that bind to both AMPA and NMDA receptors in the postsynaptic membrane (Fig. 2.6). When glutamate binds with the AMPA receptor, the channel becomes permeable to both sodium and potassium ions, owing to a higher influx of sodium ions, a depolarisation EPSP results in the postsynaptic cell. By contrast, the NMDA receptor channel is blocked by a magnesium ion and when open mediates calcium ion influx. The NMDA receptor channel requires more than glutamate binding to remove the magnesium ion and become activated. NMDA receptors require a significant depolarisation by the current passing through AMPA channels to move the blocking magnesium ion and start the influx of calcium ions. At low-frequency stimulation there is insufficient summation of AMPA receptor EPSPs to provide activation of NMDA receptor.

With activation of NMDA receptors there is an increased calcium ion flux and a second messenger cascade in the postsynaptic cell is activated resulting in activation of protein kinases, which increases the sensitivity of the postsynaptic neurone to glutamate. The second messenger system also activates long-term enhancement of presynaptic glutamate release, this results in each action potential causing a greater depolarisation of the postsynaptic membrane.

Ketamine and phencyclidine block NMDA receptors, producing amnesia and a feeling of dissociation from the environment.

NMDA receptors have been implicated in mediating a phenomenon called excitotoxicity. This is due to the injury or death of some brain cells resulting in release of glutamate thereby causing excessive stimulation of AMPA and

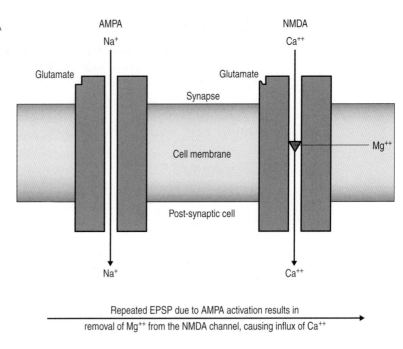

Fig. 2.6 AMPA and NMDA receptor channel

NMDA receptors on adjacent neurones. The excessive stimulation of these receptors results in accumulation of toxic intercellular levels of calcium ions, which results in further destruction of neurones causing progressive damage.

Gamma-aminobutyric acid

Gamma-aminobutyric acid (GABA) is the major *inhibitory* neurotransmitter in the brain. With few exceptions, GABA neurones in the brain are small interneurones that dampen activity within a neural circuit. At the postsynaptic membrane GABA may bind to ionotropic or metabotropic receptors. The ionotropic receptors increase chloride ion fluxes into the cell, resulting in hyperpolarisation of the post-synaptic membrane. The receptor also binds compounds such as barbiturates, ethanol and benzodiazepines. Benzodiazepines decrease anxiety, reduce seizures and induce sleep by increasing chloride flux through the GABA receptors.

Glycine

Glycine is the major neurotransmitter released from *inhibitory* interneurones in the spinal cord and brain stem. It binds to ionotropic receptors on postsynaptic cells that increase influx of chloride ions, hyperpolarising or stabilising the resting membrane potential.

Glycinergic neurones are essential for maintaining a balance between excitatory and inhibitory activity in the spinal cord integrating centres that regulate skeletal muscle contraction. Strychnine is an antagonist of glycine and poisoning with this drug results in widespread hyperexcitability throughout the nervous system as evidenced by convulsions, spastic contraction of skeletal muscles and, ultimately, death due to impairment of the muscles of respiration.

Substance P

Substance P is a polypeptide belonging to a group called tackykinins. It is found in high concentration in the endings of primary afferent neurones in the spinal cord, and acts as a mediator at the first synapse in the pathway for slow pain (see below). Upon injection into the skin it causes redness and swelling, and it is the mediator released by nerve fibres that is responsible for the axon reflex. It is also found in the nigrostriatal system where it may play a role in neuroendocrine regulation.

Opioid peptides

The brain and gastrointestinal tract contain receptors that bind morphine. The search for endogenous ligands for these receptors led to the discovery of closely related pentapeptides called enkephalins, which bind to these receptors. These and other peptides that bind to opioid receptors are called opioid peptides. This group also includes β-endorphins and dynorphins. Examples of commonly used opioids include: morphine, methadone, fentanyl and oxycontin.

Somatic sensations – pain

Pain is a protective mechanism for the body, it occurs whenever any tissue is being damaged, and it causes the individual to react and move away from the pain stimulus. Note the definition for chronic pain, which is more inclusive. The discussion here is to look at the effect of a painful stimulus.

Pain receptors and their stimulation

Pain receptors are free nerve endings (that is, they do not have specialised endings that respond to pain, unlike mechanoreceptor Pacinian corpuscles) and are widespread in the superficial layers of the skin as well as in certain internal tissues such as: the periosteum, atrial walls, joint surfaces and the falx and tentorium of the cranial vault. Most other deep structures are not extensively supplied.

The stimuli that excite pain receptors can be *mechanical, thermal or chemical*. Substances such as bradykinin, serotonin, histamine and potassium ions may excite chemical pain. In addition prostaglandin and substance P enhance the sensitivity of pain endings but do not directly excite them.

In contrast to most other sensory receptors in the body the pain receptors adapt very little and sometimes not at all. Furthermore, the intensity of pain is also closely correlated to the rate of tissue damage.

Tissue ischaemia and muscle spasm as causes of pain

Pain results as a consequence of blocked blood flow. The onset of pain is proportional to the rate of metabolism of the tissue. For instance, if a blood pressure cuff is placed around the forearm and inflated until the arterial blood flow ceases, exercising the muscles in the forearm can cause severe muscle pain within 15 to 20 s, without exercising the muscle the pain may not start for 3 to 4 min. The suggested cause for pain during ischaemia is thought to be due to accumulation of large amounts of lactic acid in the tissues, formed as a consequence of anaerobic metabolism and accumulation of chemical agents such as bradykinin and proteolytic enzymes released due to cell damage.

Muscle spasm is also a common cause of pain. The pain results partially from direct effect of muscle spasm in stimulating mechanosensitive pain receptors. Another mechanism is a direct compression of blood vessels leading to ischaemia. Muscle spasm increases the rate of metabolism in muscle tissues, thus making the ischaemia even greater and resulting in release of pain-inducing chemical substances.

Pain transmission into the central nervous system

Pain receptors are free nerve endings that use two separate pathways for transmitting pain signals into the central nervous system. They are the *fast* and *slow* pain pathways.

Fast pain pathways

Fast pain is elicited by mechanical or thermal stimuli and is carried by Aδ fibres at a velocity of between 6 and 30 m/s. They provide a rapid perception of damaging influences, which makes an individual react immediately to remove them to safety. Aδ fibres terminate mainly in lamina I of the dorsal horns, which excite second order neurones of the neospinothalamic tract. These give rise to longer fibres that cross immediately to the opposite side of the spinal cord through the anterior commissure and then pass upwards to the brain stem in the anterolateral column. Few fibres terminate in the thalamus and some continue to the somatosensory cortex. Glutamate is the excitatory neurotransmitter involved.

Slow pain pathway

Slow pain is elicited by chemical, mechanical or thermal stimuli and is carried by C-fibers travelling at a slower rate of 0.5–2 m/s. The slow pain tends to become greater over time and makes the person continue to respond to the cause of the pain. Impulses travel in peripheral slow C-fibres, which terminate in the dorsal horn in laminas II and III (substantia gelatinosa).

Most of the signals then pass through one or more additional short fibre neurones (interneurones) within the dorsal horn before entering lamina V of the dorsal horn. Here the last neurone in the series gives rise to long axons that mostly join the fibres from the fast pain pathway, passing first through the anterior commissure to the opposite side of the cord, then upwards to the brain in the anterolateral pathway and terminating either in the thalamus (very few) or (mostly) at the reticular nucleus of the medulla and pons, tectal area of mesencephalon and periaqueductal grey region.

Alteration to the nervous system in response to injury

When an axon is cut, the proximal end forms a swelling called a neuroma. Neuromata may also form as a result of partial damage to a neurone. Neuromas exhibit spontaneous electrical activity due to alterations in the quantity and distribution of ion channels. The rate of ectopic (spontaneous) firing is dependent on the metabolic, chemical and physical environment of the nerve.

These peripheral changes are accompanied by central changes. It has been shown in the dorsal horn of the cord that repetitive C-fibre activation leads to an augmented response to subsequent C-fibre input: so-called 'wind-up'. Another response seen in the spinal cord is central sensitization; this is characterised by enhanced transmission of nociceptive information, sensitivity to non-nociceptive input and spontaneous impulse generation. The central changes involve alterations in the neurochemistry of NMDA, neurokinin and nitric oxide.

Structural reorganisation may also occur in the dorsal horn with the generation of new C-fibre afferent terminals in lamina II of the substantia gelatinosa and sprouting of Aβ mechanoreceptor afferents into lamina II (they normally terminate in lamina III and IV). This may be the mechanism of touch-evoked pain.

There is also evidence for the reorganisation in the thalamus, subcortical and cortical structures of the brain.

KEY POINTS

- Nerves have a negative internal resting potential
- Action potentials are all or none events
- Synaptic transmission is usually chemical
- Neurotransmitters can be excitatory or inhibitory
- A threshold membrane potential has to be reached for an action potential to propagate
- Neurones have multiple synapses and the response depends on the balance of ESPS and ISPS

References

1. Gasser HS, Erlanger J. The role played by the sizes of the constituent fibers of a nerve trunk in determining the form of its action potential wave. *Am J Physiol* 1927; **80**(3): 522–547.
2. Raiteri M. Presynaptic autoreceptors. *J Neurochem* 2001; **78**(4): 673–675.

John Hughes

Neuroanatomy

Introduction

Pain is an experience that has emotional components as well as the anatomical localisation of the stimulus and a physiological grading of intensity. Pain is what is perceived when the noxious stimulus has been integrated and processed by the brain.

The anatomy of nociceptive pathways is not exact, as there are many connections between individual nerves. The spinal cord is arranged so that there is convergence of information before it is integrated prior to passing via ascending pathways to the brain. The brain processes the nociceptive information further before the individual can perceive pain. Therefore, there are no pain pathways. There are pathways that transmit nociceptive information that ascends to multiple sites in the brain before being forwarded on to the higher centres, where it is believed the perception of pain occurs.

The understanding of which areas in the brain are involved with the perception of pain is increasing, but a full understanding of the localising and emotional components has yet to be elucidated.

Nerves are not simply wires that transmit information from the periphery to the centre. They have a principal axon, but also multiple dendrites that communicate with other local cells. There is, thus, a concept of a balance between excitatory and inhibitory influences on a neurone, which determine if that neurone will fire off an action potential or not. Physiologically neurones are capable of changing their response to stimulation.

The pathways described are those that transmit noxious stimuli, but they may also carry other information. There are ascending pathways from the periphery to the centre, but also descending pathways from the brain to the spinal cord.

Peripheral neuroanatomy

The peripheral nociceptors are simple bare-ending nerve fibres. They do not have specialised endings unlike muscle spindles or mechanoreceptors, such as Pacinian corpuscles. Nociceptors are classified as: Aδ fibres, which are small diameter, lightly myelinated and C-fibres, which are not myelinated (see Chapter 2). Nociceptors are found in most body tissues (skin, muscles, joints, viscera), but not the brain itself.

The nociceptor neurones pass in the peripheral nerves and enter the spinal cord at the dermatomal level ascribed by their insertion. The cell bodies of these neurones are in the dorsal root ganglion with the primary synapse in the dorsal horn of the spinal cord (Fig. 3.1).

The dorsal root ganglion has all the cell bodies of the peripheral nerves in it. This is, therefore, a site where there can be physiological interactions between nerves. This is an area of increasing interest and is involved with the peripheral processing of neural information.

Spinal cord

There is more understood about spinal cord processing of nociceptive inputs than there is of the higher centres. This encompasses the connections between nerves and the biochemical interactions between them. It is clear that there are descending pathways from the brain that modulate spinal cord processing. Here the aim is to look at these processes in a simplified manner to gain an understanding of the concepts of the organisation of the nociceptive pathways.

Rexed lamina of the spinal cord

In 1952 Rexed[1] described an organisation of the grey matter of the spinal cord in the cat. Physiological studies have shown this to be a useful functional organisation as well (Fig. 3.2). Axons enter the dorsal horn of the spinal cord at a level

Fig. 3.1 Peripheral input to the spinal cord

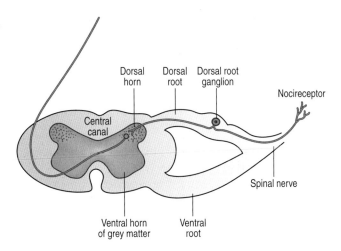

Fig. 3.2 Anatomy of the spinal cord

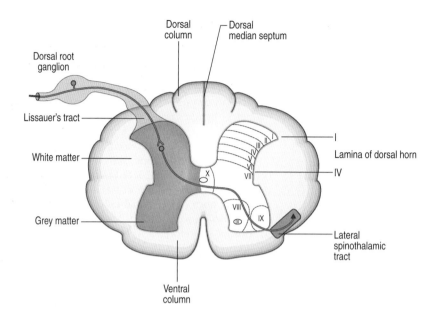

that correlated to the embryological origin of the area or tissue innervated. Dermatomal maps of the body show the cutaneous areas and their associated spinal level.

Lamina I and II

Nociceptor afferents (except visceral) enter the dorsal horn and terminate in lamina I with some in lamina II. The majority of cells terminating here respond to noxious stimuli and all of them are small-diameter neurones. There are many small interneurones (nerve cells that communicate between afferent neurones and ascending neurones to the higher centres) in lamina II that respond to the primary afferent nociceptors. These cells appear to modulate the primary afferent input in lamina I, but also in lamina V. They, therefore, have their axons and dendrites that travel between these lamina.

Lamina V

Lamina V has primary visceral nociceptor afferents entering it. The neurones in this lamina respond to noxious and non-noxious inputs and to neurones of all sizes. The cells in this lamina are thus termed wide dynamic range neurones.

There is a convergence of input in lamina V (e.g. nociceptive and touch input from the skin as well as visceral input). This arrangement is further complicated as the wide dynamic range neurones also respond to stimulation from adjacent spinal levels (Fig. 3.3).

This anatomical arrangement of the spinal cord gives the possibility for referred pain to be explained. Visceral afferents enter the cord at the same spinal level as somatic afferents. With wide dynamic range neurones having input from both modalities it is possible for pain from the viscera to be preserved in an appropriate dermatomal distribution (e.g. pain of angina being

Fig. 3.3 Dorsal horn organisation of primary afferents

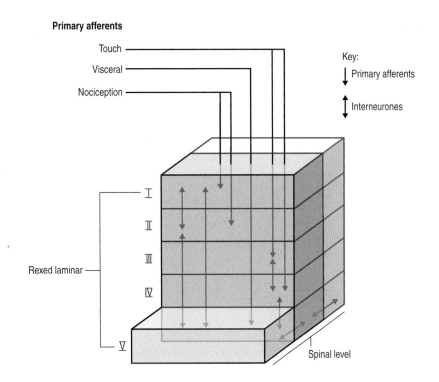

Primary afferents

Touch

Visceral

Nociception

Key:

↓ Primary afferents

↕ Interneurones

I

II

III

IV

V

Rexed laminar

Spinal level

preserved in the arm). There are several theories as to the exact mechanism. This also leads to the possibility of one afferent modality influencing another modality.

Gate control theory

Melzack and Wall postulated this in 1965[2] and, although understanding has improved and there have been modifications, it remains valid. These interactions, especially at a chemical (neurotransmitter) level remain to be fully elucidated.

In essence (Fig. 3.4), nociceptor afferents stimulate second-order neurones that project nociceptive information to higher centres. Mechanoreceptor

Fig. 3.4 Gate control theory modified

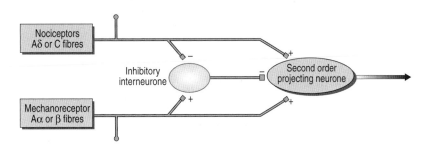

Nociceptors Aδ or C fibres

Inhibitory interneurone

Second order projecting neurone

Mechanoreceptor Aα or β fibres

primary afferents (large myelinated fibres) have dendrites that stimulate inter-neurones, which themselves inhibit second-order nociceptor projection neu-rones. This is the theory behind the mechanism for transcutaneous electrical nerve stimulation (TENS) and why rubbing an area that has been knocked reduces the pain perceived.

Ascending pathways

Following spinal cord integration of afferent inputs there are neurones (often called second-order neurones) that cross the midline and transmit this informa-tion to the higher centres via ascending pathways. Some of these second-order neurones respond solely to nociceptive inputs, but many are also responsive to other modalities (mechanical and temperature). The classical ascending path-way ascribed to pain is the spinothalamic pathway (see Fig. 3.2). Other ascend-ing pathways that are also involved in pain modulation include the spinomesencephalic, spinoreticular and dorsal column pathways.

Spinothalamic pathway

This pathway has cells that originate in lamina I, IV and V, cross the midline in the anterior commissure and ascend in the anterolateral spinothalamic path-way. The majority of neurones terminate in the ventral nucleus of the thala-mus. From there projections are sent to the somatosensory cortex (location, intensity and duration of stimulus).

Some neurones terminate in the medial thalamus where projections are sent to cortical, limbic and motor areas. It is postulated that these projections influence the emotional and motor responses to painful stimuli (of affective elements of pain). The medial thalamus is itself influenced by emotional states, which may explain why the response and perception of pain are altered by emotion.

Some of these fibres also project to the periaqueductal grey (PAG) and hypothalamus.

Spinomesencephalic pathway

This pathway ascends to terminate in the superior colliculus and PAG. These systems are considered important in the modulation of afferent nociceptive input rather than being essential for the perception of pain.

The superior colliculus is thought to be involved with the behavioural ele-ments of pain perception.

The PAG is involved with descending pathways for pain modulation and influences the autonomic nervous system. This is probably part of the defen-sive function of nociception.

Spinoreticular pathway

This pathway terminates on cells in the medulla and pons with onward projec-tions to the medial thalamus. It is thought that this pathway influences the descending modulation pathways from the medial thalamus along with the spinothalamic pathway.

Dorsal column

The majority of ascending neurones in this pathway are sensory and not nociceptive. They ascend to the cunate and gracile nuclei. This pathway may, however, be important in transmitting visceral nociceptive information.

There are other ascending tracts involved with the transmission of nociceptive information including one that projects to the pons and amygdala, which is considered important in the perception, fear and memory of pain.

Brain

Pain is a complex sensation and is not always proportional to the strength of the stimulus. The nervous system is not hard-wired, but plastic and is modified by previous damage or nociceptive input. For example, the amount of pain perceived following a punch or knock to a normal area of skin is different to the same stimulus if that area has already been bruised or damaged. This modulation is in part peripherally mediated, but there are also central mechanisms that influence the experience of pain. In broad terms, pain has elements that are sensory and localising with other elements that are involved with memory, cognition and affect.

Descending pathways

The PAG projects descending neurones to the medulla, which in turn projects neurones to the dorsal horn of the spinal cord. The PAG is one area of the brain that is rich in opioid receptors and thus involved with the endogenous opioid system. The analgesic effect of morphine is in part due to its action at this level. The descending pathways are, therefore, inhibitory at the dorsal horn reducing ascending nociceptive inputs. There is also a high density of opioid receptors in the dorsal horn at the termination of these descending pathways.

The input to the PAG comes from: the prefrontal cortex, and thus the emotional components of pain, the hypothalamus and the ascending spinomesencephalic pathway. The integration of this information in the PAG influences the autonomic, motor and emotional response to a given threat.

More recently, descending excitatory pathways have been found, and this is an area of current research. They increase the amount of ascending nociceptive information. Their role and location have yet to be fully elucidated.

Cerebral cortex

Pain is a subjective experience, sometimes relating to the stimulus directly, but it may be perceived with no nociceptive stimulus (e.g. neuropathic or psychogenic pain). Newer functional imaging techniques have allowed an insight into the cerebral events that take place with pain perception. Some of the connections postulated are outlined in Figure 3.5. Broadly, the systems can be divided into the sensory elements relating to the site, duration and strength of a stimulus and those relating to the emotional, memory and affective elements of pain. This work is ongoing and in its relative infancy, but has demonstrated that a given noxious stimulus causes specific areas of the cortex to become active. If the context of the stimulus is altered (e.g. diversion of attention or

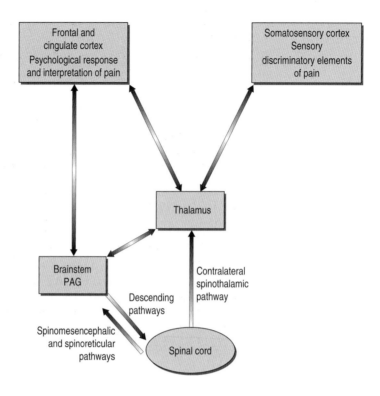

Fig. 3.5 A schematic representation of pain pathways

increasing anticipation) then there are alterations to the areas of the cortex that are active.

This may in time allow a deeper understanding of pain and how the psychological components relate to the physiological responses.

KEY POINTS

- Primary nociceptive afferents are simple bare-ending small neurones (Aδ and C-fibres)
- The dorsal horn of the spinal cord is divided into Rexed lamina with the primary nociceptive afferents terminating in lamina I and II and visceral nociceptors in lamina V
- Lamina V integrates nociceptive and other modalities via wide dynamic range neurones. There is convergence of modality and receptive area
- Spinal level integration explains in part the gate control theory of pain
- Ascending tracts terminate in the midbrain and thalamus for further integration and projection to cortical structures
- Descending pathways especially from the PAG are inhibitory at the dorsal horn of the spinal cord
- Cortical functioning has both localising, emotional and memory components. This is giving an insight to the effect of psychological influences on nociceptive processing and pain perception

References

1. Rexed B. The cytoarchitectonic organization of the spinal cord in the cat. *J Comp Neurol* 1952; **96**(3): 414–495.
2. Melzack R, Wall PD. Pain mechanisms: a new theory. *Science* 1965; **150**(699): 971–979.

Further reading

Basbaum AM, Bushnell C, Devor M. Basic science update: mechanisms of acute and chronic pain. In: Justins DM (ed.) *Pain 2005 an updated review*. Seattle: IASP Press; 2005.

Beaulieu P, Rice ASC. Applied physiology of nociception. In: Rowbotham DJ, Macintyre P (eds). Rice ASC, Warfield CA, Justins D, Eccleston C (series eds). *Clinical pain management*, acute pain. London: Arnold; 2003.

Dostrovsky JO, Heinricher MM, Jones AKP. Central processing of pain. In: Justins DM (ed.) *Pain 2005 an updated review*. Seattle: IASP Press; 2005.

Liebman M. *Neuroanatomy made easy and understandable*. Baltimore: University Park Press; 1997.

McMahon SB. Mechanisms of cutaneous, deep and visceral pain. In: Wall PD, Melzack R (eds) *Textbook of pain*. Edinburgh: Churchill Livingstone; 1994: 129–151.

Matthews EA, Dickenson AH. Pain pathophysiology. In: Dolin SJ, Padfield NL (ed.) *Pain medicine manual*, 2nd edn. London: Butterworth Heinemann; 2004.

Paul L. Chazot

Neuropharmacology

Pharmacology

The term pharmacology derives from two Greek words, *pharmacon* (φάρμακον) meaning 'drug', and *logos* (λόγος) meaning 'study', which combine to define pharmacology as the study of drugs and their effects on living animals. Thus, we can see that a pharmacologist is someone who may be involved in the discovery of new drugs that are to be sold on the clinical market, establishing their mechanism(s) of action and assessing both the efficacy and potential toxicity.

The basic principles of pharmacology can be divided into two discrete aspects:

1. Pharmacodynamics: how drugs evoke their pharmacological responses or how the drug affects the body.
2. Pharmacokinetics: how the body acts upon drugs. This includes the absorption, distribution and elimination.

This chapter will deal with these two key basic elements of pharmacology.

Pharmacodynamics – how drugs evoke their pharmacological responses

In order to induce a pharmacological effect a drug must bind to its target receptor (it is a *ligand* for that receptor). After binding to a receptor, a drug may either activate the receptor, the ligand in this case is termed an *agonist*, or it may block (or antagonise) the receptor, in this latter case it is termed an *antagonist*. Examples of agonist ligands include hormones or neurotransmitters including: β-endorphin, adrenaline (epinephrine), noradrenaline (norepinephrine), acetylcholine, and 5-hydroxytryptamine, which are endogenously expressed in the body.

Morphine, nicotine and salbutamol are exogenous examples of agonist ligands. Examples of antagonist ligands include: naloxone, propranolol, ranitidine and chlorpromazine, all of which are exogenous ligands.

Receptors act as the primary recognition sites for chemical messengers. When an agonist binds to the receptor, the receptor becomes activated and *transduces* the chemical signal into a biological response. Receptors recognise a very limited range of molecules as agonists. For a compound to be useful as a pharmacological tool or a therapeutic drug, ideally, it must bind to only one type of receptor. The complementary physical and chemical properties of the receptor and drug molecule required for binding and activation of the response mean that drugs can act with a great deal of selectivity.

Agonist ligands

Agonist binding can be depicted by a simple equation:

$$\text{Agonist} + \text{Receptor} = \text{Response}$$

and the magnitude of the response is related to the drug dose by applying the simple law of mass-action:

$$E = [A]/[A] + EC_{50}$$

where E = effect, [A] = agonist concentration and EC_{50} = concentration for 50% receptor effect.

This is based on a number of assumptions:

- One agonist molecule interacts with one receptor molecule
- The response is directly proportional to receptor occupancy (50% of receptors occupied = 50% of max. response).

In reality, however, more than one agonist molecule may bind to each receptor (cooperatively) and different agonists may have a similar binding affinity, but different *efficacies*.

The interaction of an agonist with a receptor is a multistage process:

1. Approach of agonist molecule to receptor
2. 'Docking' of agonist molecule with binding site
3. Change in 3D conformation of receptor
4. Coupling of receptor with second messenger
5. Activation of second messenger
6. Physiological response
7. Dissociation of agonist from receptor
8. Conformational change and return to 'resting' state.

The 'docking' process relies on the agonist pharmacophore complementing the structure within the receptor. Using the 'lock-and-key' analogy, for a door to be opened (receptor to be activated), the structure of the key (agonist) must fit the complementary structure of the lock (receptor) (Fig. 4.1).

Agonist dose–response curve

Agonists interact with specific macromolecules (receptors) located usually, but not always, on cell membrane surfaces in order to elicit their biological effects. These receptors are largely responsible for determining the quantitative relationship between dose or concentration of agonist and the respective

Fig. 4.1 Lock and key principle

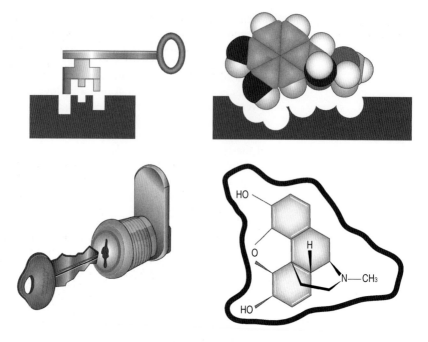

Fig. 4.2 Dose–response curve of concentration against effect

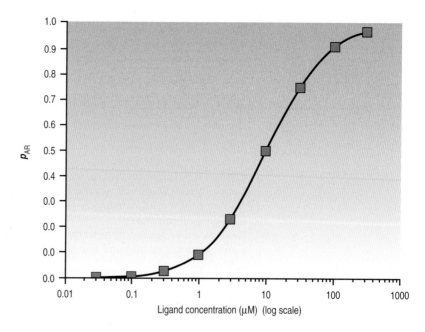

response or effect. This relationship is termed the 'concentration–effect relationship' and is often expressed graphically as the 'concentration–effect curve' (or 'dose–response curve'). Figure 4.2 represents a dose–response curve based on a classic pharmacological experiment described below and in Figure 4.3 that depicts activated and inactivated binding sites.

Fig. 4.3 Activated and inactivated binding sites

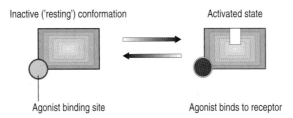

Inactive ('resting') conformation   Activated state

Agonist binding site   Agonist binds to receptor

Practical pharmacology is a fundamental part of the search to find new drugs. The pharmaceutical industry relies heavily on scientists carrying out practical research in the development of new therapeutic agents. For a drug to have an effect it must interact with the body and it is the role of the pharmacologist to investigate where and how these interactions occur.

The organ-bath was first developed in the early 20th century and has been used up to the present day to determine the pharmacological effects of old and new drugs. The guinea-pig ileum is a classic strip of tissue, which possesses a plethora of receptors (drug targets) including muscarinic acetylcholine (mAChR), histamine and even opioid receptors. Stable and reproducible responses are obtained by adopting a consistent experimental procedure. It is important to establish a *dose cycle* at the beginning of the experiment and to maintain it throughout the experiment. The dose cycle depends on the following factors:

- The contact time of the drug
  This is the length of time the drug remains in contact with the tissue preparation. It is usually determined empirically as the time taken for a given concentration of drug to evoke a response that reaches a peak and levels off or even begins to decline. For most agonists on smooth muscle preparations this is about 10–30 s.
- The recovery period
  This is the time it takes for the tissue to recover from the effects of the previous dose of drug, after it has been washed off. This is usually between 1 and 4 min.

The principles of the concentration-dependent response stipulate that the response 'saturates' at high ligand doses, and the action of the agonist is readily reversible. It should be noted that binding affinity and efficacy are independent parameters. Figure 4.4 demonstrates this by looking at the response of an agonist alone and when acting in the presence of an antagonist. Ligands can have a high affinity, but low-efficacy (efficacy less than 1) high-affinity partial agonists, and similarly ligands can have low affinity and be full agonists (efficacy = 1).

Antagonists

Pharmacological antagonism

Many drugs act as agonists and elicit a measurable response. Some, however, produce their therapeutic response by binding to specific receptors, but without eliciting a measurable response, which are termed antagonists (pharmacological efficacy = 0). This should not be confused with 'therapeutic efficacy', as antagonists are effective in a clinical setting (e.g. naloxone in combating opioid agonist overdose). Binding of antagonists to receptors

Fig. 4.4 Effects of agonist alone and when in conjunction with an antagonist

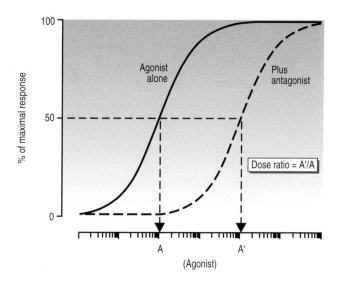

reduces the responses elicited by agonists. Due to the mutual competition between the antagonist and agonist for the same receptor(s), this form of antagonism is termed competitive antagonism. The response elicited by a given concentration of an agonist will be reduced in the presence of an effective concentration of competitive antagonist. Provided both agonist and antagonist bind reversibly to the receptor, the agonist response can be restored (in spite of the continued presence of the antagonist), by increasing the concentration of the agonist. This is the hallmark of competitive, surmountable antagonism (Fig. 4.4). As can be seen, a competitive antagonist reduces the apparent potency of agonist and there is a parallel shift in the dose–response curve to the right. This only applies if the antagonist binds *reversibly*. By definition, an irreversible antagonist does not dissociate from the receptor binding site, consequently an increased concentration of agonist does not displace the antagonist, resulting in a non-parallel shift in the dose–response curve and a suppressed maximal response; here antagonism is said to be 'insurmountable'.

A non-competitive antagonist is one that does not bind to the agonist recognition site, but binds to other sites on a large receptor protein macromolecule or interferes with the intracellular signalling messengers. A non-competitive antagonist thus depresses the maximal response and increasing agonist concentrations do not overcome antagonism. Thus, the net result on a do–response curve is very similar to an 'insurmountable' irreversible competitive antagonist.

Schild analysis is a classic method, first published in 1959 to calculate the potency of competitive antagonists.[1] This is a null method, i.e. it makes no assumptions about the nature of the coupling between receptor binding and the response, it simply assumes that the level of response is associated with the degree of occupation and activation of the receptors by the agonist. There are a number of other assumptions and criteria, including:

- The agonist acts only at a single receptor type
- Binding of both agonist and antagonist is competitive and reversible

- Responses are measured when both agonist and antagonist are at equilibrium with the receptors
- The antagonist causes parallel rightward shifts of the log agonist concentration–response curve with no reduction of the maximum response.

The Schild analysis is based on the Schild equation and the graphical representation of this equation is known as the *Schild plot*.

The Schild equation:

$$(\text{Concentration ratio} - 1) = (\text{Antagonist concentration})/K_B$$

where concentration ratio = concentration ratio for the agonist and K_B = dissociation equilibrium constant for the antagonist. The *Gaddum equation* is the logarithmic transformation of this equation. The Schild plot is a graphical representation of log (concentration ratio − 1) versus log (antagonist concentration) (Fig. 4.5). The intercept on the log concentration axis is equal to the pA_2 value (negative logarithm of the antagonist dissociation constant), while the gradient gives information about the nature of the antagonism. The slope of a Schild plot should equal 1 if all of the assumptions underlying the method of analysis are fulfilled. A slope that is significantly greater than 1 may indicate *positive* cooperatively in the binding of the antagonist, lack of antagonist equilibrium, depletion of a potent antagonist from the medium by receptor binding or non-specific binding (e.g. to glassware, filters or lipid partitioning). A slope which is significantly less than 1 may indicate *negative* cooperatively of the binding, or removal of agonist by a saturable uptake process, or because the agonist is acting at multiple receptor types (this can also result in curvilinear Schild plots). If the slope of a Schild plot is greater than 1, the calculated pA_2 value will be an underestimate of the pK_B (negative logarithm of the antagonist equilibrium dissociation constant) value (i.e. the antagonist is less potent than expected). Conversely, if the slope is less than 1, the calculated pA_2 value will overestimate the pK_B value.

Fig. 4.5   Schild plot

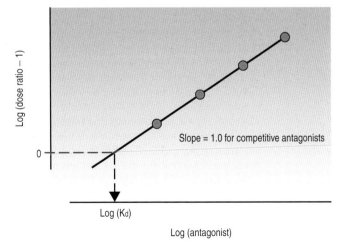

Slope = 1.0 for competitive antagonists

Log (dose ratio − 1)

0

Log (Kd)

Log (antagonist)

Agonist or antagonist?

It should be noted that in some situations, a partial agonist might act as an apparent antagonist. When a partial agonist is applied alone, an agonist action would be noted as described previously, but with a reduction in the evoked maximal response. When a full agonist is applied, a maximum response is evoked, but this can be depressed to give an apparent antagonist effect if a partial agonist is delivered simultaneously.

Thus far, pharmacological antagonism has been described; however, two further types of antagonism can be elicited in the clinic.

Physiological antagonism

This occurs when two different receptors mediate opposed physiological effects (e.g. insulin and glucagon in maintaining sugar balance).

Pharmacokinetic antagonism

This is a third form of antagonism in which one drug alters the systemic blood concentration of the second drug (e.g. phenobarbital and warfarin).

Inverse agonist

The concept of an inverse agonist was first proposed for the benzodiazepine site on the $GABA_A$ receptor, with the discovery of the β-carboline compound class.[2] This type of ligand relies on the concept of constitutive activity (receptors being active in the absence of agonist) and has been observed in both ligand-gated ion and G-protein coupled receptors.[3] Several receptors have a tonic level of activity that can be increased by an agonist. Some antagonists will reduce this tonic receptor activity; they are, therefore, agonists with negative intrinsic activity and are thus called inverse agonists. An antagonist blocks the activity of both types of ligand.

CNS drug targets

Each drug targets a particular type of receptor in the body. Drug receptors are usually proteins that play important roles in normal physiology. Examples of such targets include:

- Enzymes, e.g. monoamine oxidase$_A$ inhibitors (MAOI) for treating depression; cholinesterase inhibitors for treating Alzheimer's disease and dementia with Lewy bodies; cathechol-o-methyl transferase inhibitors for treating movement disorders; cyclo-oxygenase (Cox) inhibitors, NSAIDs (non-steroidal anti-inflammatory drugs) for inflammatory pain
- Re-uptake sites, e.g. 5-HT transporter inhibitors for depression and pain, VMAT-2 (vesicular monoamine transporter) for dystonias and tics
- Voltage-gated ion channels, e.g. voltage-dependent sodium channels (lamotrigine, carbamazepine for epilepsy and pain); voltage-dependent calcium channels for cardiac arrhythmias; chloride channels for cystic fibrosis and sodium channels for local anaesthetics
- Transmitter receptors (for neurotransmitters and hormones). Transmitter receptors represent the largest group of drug targets, and these can be further divided into G-protein-coupled receptors (GPCRs), ligand-gated ion channels (LGICs), kinase-linked receptors (RTKs) and steroid hormone receptors.

G-protein coupled receptors

The GPCRs are the largest group of transmitter receptors with over 1000 members, largely because they include the vast array of olfactory receptors. Some key examples of GPCRs relevant to pain and analgesia include the opioid receptors (e.g. enkephalins), the tachykinin receptors (e.g. substance P), 5-HT and β-adrenergic receptors (e.g. noradrenaline), adenosine receptors and receptors for the endocannabinoids.

Classic features of GPCRs include a 7-transmembrane topology, large intracellular loop domains, which interact with the transducer, the GTP-binding modulatory protein (G-protein), signal transduction through an analogous series of molecular events and mediation of slow neurotransmission and/or an effect on metabolic processes.

GPCRs are classified according to functional criteria and sequence identity. They are further subdivided into three distinct groups based on amino acid identity: rhodopsin/beta-adrenergic receptor-like receptors (Group I); secretin receptor-like receptors (Group II); glutamate/GABA$_B$ metabotropic receptors and related receptors (Group III). GPCRs display both molecular and functional heterogeneity, through ligand selectivity, oligomeric structure, activation and deactivation times, desensitisation kinetics and cellular location. GPCR signal transduction occurs via the heterotrimeric G-proteins, which comprise three subunit types: α, β and γ with several different subunit isoforms adding to the complexity of the system.

Activation by the agonist leads to an exchange of GDP for GTP, the dissociation of α from the β/γ subunits, which then activate various effector enzymes or channels. The intrinsic GTPase activity returns the G-protein to the inactive GDP-bound state, ready for another agonist molecule to bind. The type of G-protein determines which intracellular signal pathways are activated. Examples of effector systems utilised include adenylyl cyclase, to produce cAMP involved in activating protein kinase A; phospholipase C, to produce inositol trisphosphate (IP3) involved in mobilizing calcium stores and diacylglycerol (DAG), involved in activating protein C; thence various Ca^{2+}, Na^+ and K^+ ion channels (Fig. 4.6).[4]

Receptor tyrosine kinases

RTKs are single, transmembrane-spanning, receptor proteins that contain an extracellular ligand binding, dimerisation domains and intrinsic tyrosine kinase activity in the cytosolic domain. RTK members include receptors for several growth factors and insulin. They are classified into at least 14 different subgroups based on their structural organisation. Two major types include: single, transmembrane-spanning proteins that dimerise when ligand binds (e.g. platelet-derived growth factor (PDGF) receptors and epidermal growth factor (EGF) receptors) and two covalently linked dimers (insulin receptor, IGF-1 receptor). These share common structural and functional features, including ligand binding and receptor dimerisation required for autophosphorylation of tyrosine residues (pY) in the cytosolic domain of the receptor. Receptor pY participate in the recruitment of cytoplasmic molecules into receptor-based signalling complexes. The protein modules are coupled directly or indirectly (through adapter proteins) to downstream signalling proteins, including enzymes that control phospholipid metabolism, protein kinases and protein kinase signalling cascades (e.g. MAP kinase pathway), polypeptides that regulate cytoskeletal architecture and cell adhesion and transcription factors, which ultimately lead to changes in activity of particular genes. Interaction of different signalling

Fig. 4.6 G-protein coupled receptors (GPCRs) are seven transmembrane dimeric structures which transduce their signal through a trimeric G-protein

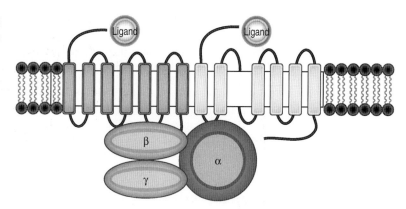

pathways permits the fine-tuning of cellular activities required to carry out complex developmental and physiological processes.

It is important to remember that many signalling pathways are probably working at a modest (basal) level in normal cells, and the balance between them results in a homeostatic state. When this balance is upset, it can lead to more drastic consequences for the cell; for example, cell differentiation or proliferation, growth inhibition or apoptosis.

Ligand-gated ion channels

The LGICs are another important drug target, particularly in the CNS. The two primary neurotransmitters, glutamate and GABA control rapid excitation and inhibition, respectively. These two transmitters activate two distinct families of LGICs, glutamate and GABA$_A$ receptors.[5]

LGICs are multisubunit receptors with three to five subunit types arranged around a central channel pore. Upon activation, Na$^+$/Ca^{2+} cations or Cl$^-$ anions flow into the cell to depolarise or hyperpolarise the neurone, respectively. LGIC glutamate receptors comprise three major types, distinguished by their sensitivity to agonists, AMPA, kainate and N-methyl-D-aspartate (NMDA). These are important potential future CNS targets for treating neuropathic pain, dementias, psychoses and movement disorders. Each type of glutamate receptor has distinct tetrameric or pentameric hetero-oligomeric subtypes, containing subunit combinations, e.g. GluR1/GluR2, GluR5/KA2 and NR1/NR2B for an AMPA, kainate or NMDA receptor. The GABA$_A$ receptor is an important CNS drug target for treating sleep disorders, anxiety and epilepsy. Drugs that target the GABA$_A$ receptor include benzodiazepines, barbiturates, neurosteroids and volatile anaesthetics, each with their own distinct receptor site that is different from the agonist binding site. Drugs generally increase the activity of GABA$_A$ receptors through an allosteric mechanism, to produce an increased inhibitory response in the brain (Fig. 4.7).

Intracellular receptors ('nuclear' receptors)

The nuclear receptors (transcription factors) are unusual in that they are located inside the cell, and so agonists must pass through the cell plasma membrane in order to access the target receptor (e.g. steroid, thyroid hormone receptors). Receptor–agonist complexes are then transported to the nucleus where they bind to specific DNA sequences and thus alter specific gene expression. The net result is either an increase or decrease in protein expression,

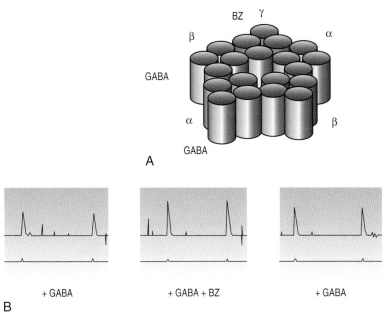

Fig. 4.7 The GABA$_A$ receptor. (A) The GABA$_A$ receptor is the major inhibitory receptor in the human brain. It is a multisubunit protein with an integral chloride ion channel. Most GABA$_A$ receptors are composed of different α, β and γ subunits, which form the distinct binding sites for GABA and benzodiazepines. (B) GABA$_A$ receptor-medicated inhibitory currents in primary cortical neurones in culture, in the absence or presence of a benzodiazepine, e.g. diazepam. Benzodiazepines allosterically increase the affinity for GABA, causing an increase inhibitory current. When the benzodiazepine is removed the current is reduced demonstrating that it is a reversible process. This is how benzodiazepines can act as sedative drugs

which, although slower than other transduction systems, is long lasting (hours, days). A further type of intracellular receptor is the cytoplasmic guanylyl cyclase, which is activated by the membrane-permeable mediator, nitric oxide. It should be noted that some lipid-soluble drugs can affect other intracellular targets, including DNA, RNA and cytoskeletal elements.

Receptor subtypes

Many neurotransmitters bind to different types of receptor. For example, GABA binds both GABA$_A$ (LGIC) and GABA$_B$ (GPCR) in the same brain region, because they are located in different compartments of the neurone (synaptic and extrasynaptic respectively), display a distinct sensitivity to GABA and transduce their signal in very different ways and over a markedly different timescale, thus subserving distinct roles in GABA-ergic transmission. GABA$_A$ receptors are primary and GABA$_B$ are modulatory receptor types.

Drug selectivity

No drug is completely specific for one type of receptor. Selectivity depends on drug dose, where higher doses induce more side effects. This leads to an important pharmacological concept, known as the therapeutic ratio. Highly selective drugs target one receptor, and tend to induce minimal side effects, e.g. benzodiazepines. Poorly selective drugs induce side effects at therapeutic doses, e.g. tricyclic antidepressants (TCAs).

Therapeutic ratio = dose required to induce side effect/therapeutic dose

Receptor plasticity

Repeated drug administration, particularly through long-term chronic use, can lead to receptor adaptation, including receptor down-regulation (reduction in receptors) or up-regulation (increase in receptors). This can lead to drug tolerance resulting in a withdrawal syndrome if the drug is abruptly withdrawn (e.g. opioids, benzodiazepines).

Pharmacokinetics – how the body acts on drugs

There are four aspects of pharmacokinetics, which are termed with the acronym ADME:

Absorption: modes of drug entry into the body
Distribution: movement of drug around the body
Metabolism: chemical changes to drug molecules
Excretion: excretion of drug and/or metabolites.

Absorption – modes of drug entry into the body

There are a number of routes of drug delivery these are divided into:

- *Enteral* routes, via the gastrointestinal (GI) tract
  There are two major enteral routes, termed oral (p.o. – per os) and rectal (p.r.)
- *Parenteral* routes, which are independent of the gastrointestinal tract

  There are a wide selection of parenteral routes, including subcutaneous (s.c.) – under the skin; topical – through skin or other surface (e.g. eye); intradermal (i.d.) – into the skin; intramuscular (i.m.) – into skeletal muscle; intraperitoneal (i.p.) – into peritoneal cavity; intravenous (i.v.) – into blood via a vein; intra-arterial (i.a.) – into blood via an artery; intrathecal (i.t.) – into the cerebrospinal fluid; nasal (inhalation) – by aerosol through bronchioles and sublingual (buccal).

Why so many routes?

The route chosen will be guided by the site of the target organ and receptor, the speed of desired effect and what barriers (membranes) the drug has to cross in order to reach its target. This is defined by the drug characteristics (pharmacodynamics), the pharmacokinetics and the characteristics of the pharmaceutical preparation being used. The aim is to have enough active drug at the receptor site to have the desired effect.

Bioavailability (F) is the proportion of the drug dose, which appears in the systemic circulation (bloodstream) following administration, i.e.:

$$F = (0-1 \text{ or } 0-100\%)$$

Enteral routes

Oral administration. Oral administration is the most common mode of drug delivery. Advantages of the oral route are many-fold: convenience (storage, portability, availability of pre-measured dose), economics, non-invasive, often safer and the lack of need for specialist training. There are, however, a number of disadvantages of the oral delivery route:

- Often erratic and incomplete
- Highly dependent upon patient compliance
- Increased sources of drug–drug and drug–nutrient interactions
- Many drugs are degraded in the gastrointestinal environment.

Following oral administration, bioavailability is mainly determined by: the stability in the gut (gastric acid, intestinal flora) and the extent of *first-pass metabolism*.

What is First-Pass Metabolism? Once an oral drug enters the gut it then passes via the hepatic portal vein to the liver. Extensive drug metabolism can occur in the liver, and if the drug is particularly susceptible to this first-pass metabolism, a low proportion of the oral dose reaches the systemic circulation, i.e. the drug has low oral bioavailability. Drug adsorption from the intestine is affected by a number of factors including:

1. Physicochemical properties of drug
2. Drug formulation
3. Carrier-mediated transport
4. Gastrointestinal motility
5. Splanchnic blood flow.

Rectal administration. The rectal route (using a suppository) is a simple alternative when the oral route is not possible because of vomiting, oral obstruction or variable consciousness of the patient. Its principal advantage is that it can be successfully utilised independent of gastrointestinal tract motility and rate of gastric emptying. This is of considerable importance with the opioid analgesics whose propensity for slowing gastric emptying and ability to induce nausea and vomiting are common problems. Drugs absorbed by this method will be partly via the inferior and middle rectal veins, thus bypassing the portal system and emptying directly into the vena cava. This avoids first-pass metabolism for a proportion of the drug, some of the drug will, however, be absorbed via the superior rectal veins and then transported to the liver via the portal vein. Bioavailability is, therefore, highly variable by this route. It should be noted that many patients have an aversion to rectal administration, so compliance is an issue. Consent to allow rectal administration is also an issue, especially with children.

Parenteral routes
Sublingual/buccal route. Sublingual, meaning literally 'under the tongue' refers to a method of administering substances via the mouth in such a way that they are rapidly absorbed into the blood vessels under the tongue rather than via the digestive tract (Fig. 4.8A). The buccal mucosa is highly vascularised and consequently allows drugs a more direct access to the blood circulation, thus providing direct systemic administration.

Advantages of this route include rapid onset, avoids the first-pass effect and the ability to swallow is not required. Disadvantages include the lack of drugs

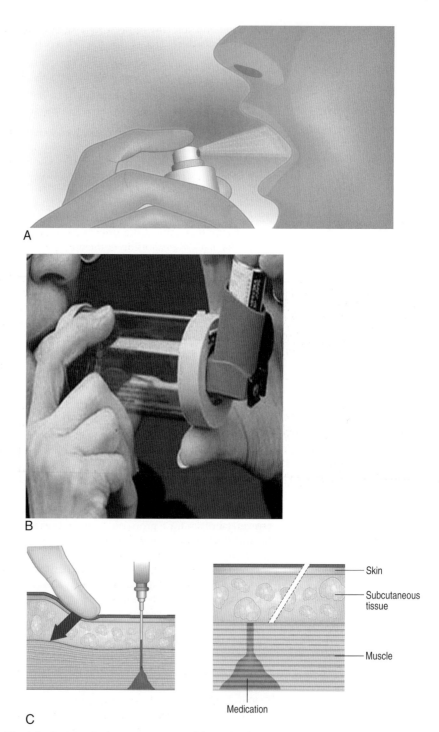

Fig. 4.8 Routes of administration. (A) Sublingual or buccal, (B) inhaled, (C) subcutaneous and intramuscular

that are adequately absorbed by this method, the need for patients to avoid swallowing and compliance can be difficult.

Pulmonary. The pulmonary route is popular for the administration of aerosol drugs in the treatment of respiratory disease; it is also growing in popularity for the treatment for some non-respiratory diseases (Fig. 4.8B). Advantages include the ease of titration, rapid onset of action, particularly for local effects, with maximal benefit and minimal side effects. Disadvantages include the need for a significant degree of patient coordination and variability in delivered dose, most notably patients with significant lung disease may not be able to inhale adequately. This may be partly overcome by nebulised drug delivery, which requires more complex equipment.

Topical. Topical administration comprises a number of different methods, including transcutaneous, intra-nasal and transocular.

The **transcutaneous** route has gained popularity with increasing numbers of drugs being delivered in this manner. Preparations may be in the form of creams for local application or patches (sticking plasters with drug impregnated into a matrix), which are used for the systemic delivery of a drug. The advantages of topical creams are that there are minimal side effects and the drug is applied close to the site of action. The disadvantages are the frequency of application, the inconvenience of creams and their often limited efficacy. The patch preparations often provide systemic levels of agent and thus have similar side effects to orally active preparations. These can be used when the oral route is not available and for some drugs that have high first-pass effect. The advantages include sustained-release formulations (requiring a change of patch every few days) and some gastric side effects may be reduced. The disadvantages include systemic side effects and there can be an allergic reaction to the adhesive in the patch.

The **intranasal** route, although historically utilised only for local effects, is growing in popularity for systemic effects, particularly for drugs that are sensitive to the gastrointestinal environment and/or have high first-pass metabolism. It is now an alternative to intravenous administration, with better safety and patient compliance record. Factors, which influence absorption from the nasal mucosa, include pH, concentration, molecular weight, formulation and condition of nasal mucosa.

The **transocular route** or via the eye is growing in popularity, especially in the delivery of neurotrophic factors, anti-inflammatory drugs and has potential in future gene therapy. It is mainly used for local delivery, but as with the intranasal route can be used for systemic effects.

Subcutaneous. When patients with moderate to severe pain are unable to take opioids by mouth, delivery by subcutaneous continuous infusion is effective.[6,7] This avoids the need for repeated injections that may be painful. Indications for using this parenteral route are an inability to swallow, nausea and/or vomiting, gastrointestinal obstruction or any pathology limiting gastrointestinal absorption. When used for local effects, the subcutaneous route can minimise the systemic side effects and may be as effective as intravenous infusion (Fig. 4.8C). Further advantages include prompt absorption from aqueous solutions, little need for training and it can be used for suspensions. Disadvantages include potential pain and tissue damage, suitable only for small volumes, unappealing appearance and erratic absorption.

Intravenous. The intavenous route of administration offers a number of clear advantages, including rapid achievement of systemic concentration, a precise delivery of dosage and ease of titration. The volume required with delivery is less of a problem compared to other routes. Disadvantages include invasive technique with risk of infection, high initial local concentration, which may result in toxicity and a certain level of skill is required for delivery.

Intramuscular. On the other hand, intramuscular delivery requires relatively less skill for administration and can be used to administer oily vehicles. Disadvantages for this method include variability in bioavailability (variable muscle blood flow), variable speed of onset, the drug may precipitate at the site of administration, the method cannot be used in the presence of abnormal clotting and it can be painful for the patient.

Drug distribution

Movement through membrane barriers (e.g. blood–brain barrier)

There are four main body fluid compartments that a drug can enter:

1. Extracellular fluid, composed of blood plasma and interstitial fluid and lymph
2. Intracellular fluid
3. Transcellular fluid
4. The blood–brain barrier (BBB).

The BBB is formed by tight junctions between the endothelial cells of brain capillaries; lipophilic molecules pass through the BBB, while hydrophilic molecules are poorly accessible due to their lack of ability to pass through the BBB. This barrier can be bypassed by intrathecal administration for hydrophilic drugs. There are active uptake systems within the BBB that transport nutrients and metabolites. Notably the BBB is disrupted by illness, which allows entry of bioactive immune cells and hydrophilic drugs.

Physico-chemical properties of drug

Absorption can occur through four major processes:

1. **Passive diffusion** has a number of features: it does not utilise a carrier, is not saturable, it is driven by the concentration gradient and has a modest structural specificity. Some low-molecular-weight drugs can pass through central pores in the membrane, known as aqueous diffusion, and some highly lipophilic drugs pass directly through the lipid-bilayer, dependent on the respective lipid-aqueous partition coefficient, log p-value (e.g. volatile anaesthetic agents have a high log p and are highly membrane permeable).
2. **Active transport** requires a carrier system, displays structural selectivity and is saturable. This process is both rapid and energy dependent, as the movement occurs against the concentration gradient. Examples of sites of active transport include the choroid plexus in the ventricles of the brain, renal tubular cells and hepatocytes.
3. **Facilitated diffusion** utilises a carrier system, but without the requirement for energy, with movement being along a concentration gradient.

4. **Pinocytosis** is used for very large molecules with molecular weights in excess of 1000 and involves cell engulfment of extracellular material within membrane vesicles.

Factors which affect absorption

- **Solubility:** drugs formulated in aqueous solutions mix more readily with the aqueous phase at absorptive sites. Thus, such formulations are absorbed more readily than those formulated in oily solutions. Drug suspensions require more time to dissolve in the aqueous phase at absorptive sites.
- **pH and pKa:** the pH determines the relative amount of ionised and non-ionised forms of the drug, which therefore governs solubility. The ratio of ionised versus non-ionised forms is related to the pKa (measure of drug acidity) and the surrounding pH using the Henderson-Hasselbalch equation:

$$\text{Log [protonated form/unprotonated form]} = pKa - pH$$

when the pH = pKa, a drug is 50% ionised and 50% non-ionised. Under normal circumstances, only the non-ionised form can cross cell membranes. Therefore, the absorption of a drug depends on its innate pKa and the pH of the environment.

- **Concentration:** highly concentrated drug solutions are absorbed more readily than more dilute drugs.
- **Surface:** organs with a larger surface area (including intestine and lungs) absorb drugs more rapidly than organs with low surface area (e.g. stomach).
- **Contact time:** the longer the contact time, the higher the absorption.
- **Blood flow:** the greater the blood flow, the higher the absorption rates (e.g. high splanchnic blood flow increases intestinal absorption).

Plasma protein binding

Following absorption through the various routes described, a drug then enters the systemic circulation. The bloodstream has the ability to transport lipophilic endogenous substances (e.g. sex hormones) and exogenous drugs efficiently in the blood. This occurs via attachment to blood proteins in a 'protein bound' state, which is temporary and usually reversible. The affinity and position of protein binding can have important implications in the clinic. If a drug is highly protein bound, it can stay in the blood stream for months. If two drugs administered simultaneously, bind to the same site on a protein with different affinities, this can lead to problems. For example, aspirin and warfarin bind to the same binding sites, but aspirin binds with higher affinity. Hence, if taken together, aspirin will displace warfarin yielding a high concentration of free warfarin, which is potentially toxic. In kwashiorkor (dietary protein insufficiency), there may be insufficient blood proteins for transport, which can lead to higher free drug concentrations; this often occurs in burn victims or in chronic liver diseases. Conversely, many tumours secrete excess plasma proteins, which bind and therefore reduce free drug concentrations.

Body fluid compartments

Distribution relates to the spread of the drug throughout the body and this distribution can occur in a wide range of compartments in the body.

The apparent *volume of distribution* (Vd) is calculated according to the following equation:

$$Vd = Q/Cp$$

where Vd = apparent volume of distribution, Q = total amount of drug in body and Cp = plasma concentration.

A small Vd value indicates that a drug is present in the extracellular fluid or plasma and a large Vd indicates that the drug is concentrated in tissues (highly lipophilic drugs). A large number of factors can affect the distribution of a drug, including the plasma protein and tissue binding (see above), age, gender, blood flow, mass of body fat, size and lipophilicity of drug. A number of these factors can be affected in disease (e.g. liver and cardiovascular disease). There are a number of sites where drugs can redistribute, be excluded or accumulate. Thiopental delivered intravenously initially distributes to areas of highest blood flow (brain, liver, kidneys), and then *redistributes* over time to be stored in muscles and adipose tissue. There are some areas in the body that are relatively *inaccessible* (e.g. cerebrospinal, lymph, pleural, ocular and foetal fluids). Based on physico-chemical properties (see Henderson-Hasselbach equation), drugs can be *ion-trapped* in different environments. For example, weak organic base drugs can be trapped in acidic environments (stomach) and, conversely, weak organic acid drugs can be trapped in alkaline environments (intestine).

Drug metabolism or biotransformation

The primary goal of metabolism is enzyme-catalysed chemical modifications of drug molecules to inactivate and/or facilitate excretion. The liver is the main site of drug metabolism in the body, although other sites, such as the kidney, lung and gut, can contribute to the inactivation of drugs. There are two phases to drug metabolism, termed *Phase I* and *Phase II*. The products of the process are usually pharmacologically less active (but not always). The use of pro-drugs exploits the body's metabolism to convert the inactive drug form to the active metabolite (e.g. codeine, which is demethylated to morphine).

Phase 1 metabolism. The Phase 1 metabolism comprises *oxidation, reduction* and *hydrolysis* reactions that introduce functional groups, including $-NH_2$ and $-OH$, which ultimately increases the polarity of the drug.

Oxidation reactions are the most common, which are catalysed mainly by the microsomal, mixed-function oxidase system (cytochrome P450 enzymes), situated on the smooth endoplasmic reticulum. The hepatic cytochrome P450 system comprises a 'superfamily' of several hundred different isoenzymes, with extensive species and inter-individual variations. The enzyme is a haemoprotein that requires oxygen, reduced nicotinamide adenine dinucleotide (NADPH) and NADPH cytochrome P450 reductase for maximum activity.

Reduction reactions require microsomal enzymes, but are much less common (e.g. prednisone, which is a prodrug, is reduced to the active glucocorticoid prednisolone).

Hydrolysis occurs in many tissues, a good example is aspirin, which undergoes spontaneous hydrolysis to salicylic acid in the presence of moisture.

Phase 2 metabolism. Phase 1 'prepares' a drug molecule for conjugation. The drug is now susceptible to Phase 2 reactions, which involve conjugation of a large chemical group to the functional group on the drug molecule. The conjugation reaction, i.e. attachment of a substituent group, results in the drug being more hydrophilic (water-soluble), and, therefore, more amenable for excretion from the body. This phase again occurs mainly in the liver, but can also occur in a wide range of other tissues.

Common substituent groups include glutathione, glucuronyl (in ER), sulphate (in cytoplasm), methyl and acetyl. The conjugating enzymes again exist in many different isoforms, and display relative substrate and metabolite specificity. The resultant conjugate is usually pharmacologically inactive, one key exception being morphine, which is converted to morphine-6-glucuronide (M6G), which is an analgesic with an extended half-life.

It is notable that certain drugs can affect metabolising enzymes themselves. Some drugs increase the activity of certain P450 isoenzymes and, consequently, increase their own metabolism, as well as other drugs that may be taken simultaneously (e.g. barbiturates, ethanol and anti-convulsant drugs, such as phenytoin or carbamazepine). Conversely, some drugs inhibit microsomal enzyme activity, thus increasing their own activity as well as that of other drugs (e.g. cemetidine, MAO inhibitors).

Drug elimination or excretion

Excretion is the amount of drug and metabolites eliminated by any process per unit time. The clearance rate is the volume of plasma cleared of drug per unit time. Excretion can occur via various routes: by the kidneys into urine, by the gastrointestinal tract into bile and faeces and by the lungs through exhaled air. The most commonly used routes are via urine and faeces.

Drug *clearance* is the ability of the body to eliminate a drug by any elimination process; it is recorded as the volume of plasma cleared of drug in unit time.

Routes of drug (and metabolite) excretion

There are large differences in renal excretion rates between drugs, with Phase 1/ Phase 2 metabolites excreted more readily.

Kidney (renal route). The functional unit of the kidney is the nephron. The extent to which a drug is excreted via the kidney depends on *glomerular filtration rate*, *tubular reabsorption* and *tubular secretion*.

Glomerular Filtration. In the glomerulus, the capillaries permit the passage of molecules of low molecular weight (<20000) including drugs and drug metabolites out of the blood, leaving behind the plasma proteins. The glomerular filtration rate varies between individuals but in healthy individuals the normal range is 110 to 130 ml/min. More than 90% of the filtrate is reabsorbed. With a glomerular filtration rate of 120 ml/min this equates to 173 l/day, while normal urine output is much less than this, about 1 to 2 l/day.

Tubular Re-Absorption. In the distal tubule there is passive excretion and re-absorption of lipid-soluble drugs. Drugs, which are present in the glomerular filtrate, can be reabsorbed in the tubules. The membrane is readily permeable to lipids so filtered lipid-soluble substances are extensively reabsorbed. One reason for this is that much of the water, in the filtrate, has been reabsorbed and, therefore, the concentration gradient is now in the direction favouring re-absorption. Thus, if a drug is present in the non-ionised form it may be readily reabsorbed.

Many drugs are either weak bases or acids and, therefore, the pH of the filtrate can greatly influence the extent of tubular re-absorption. When urine is acidic, weak acid drugs tend to be reabsorbed. Alternatively when urine is more alkaline, weak bases are more extensively reabsorbed. These changes can be quite significant as urine pH can vary from 4.5 to 8.0 depending on the diet (e.g. a high meat content can cause a more acidic urine).

In the case of a drug overdose it is possible to increase the excretion of some drugs by suitable adjustment of urine pH. For example, in the case of pentobarbital overdose (a weak acid) it may be possible to increase drug excretion by making the urine more alkaline with sodium bicarbonate injection. The effect of pH change on tubular re-absorption can be predicted by consideration of drug pKa according to the Henderson-Hesselbalch equation (see previously).

Tubular Secretion. In the proximal tubule there is re-absorption of water and active secretion of some weak electrolytes but especially weak acids. As this process is an active secretion process it requires a carrier and a supply of energy. This may be a significant pathway for some compounds, such as the penicillin antibiotics. Because tubular secretion is an active process there may be competitive inhibition of the secretion of one compound by another (pharmacokinetic antagonism).

Individual variation

There are wide variations in an individual's pharmacokinetic characteristics, both in health and disease (e.g. liver disease, congestive heart failure and thyroid disease), which affects absorption, first-pass metabolism, volume of distribution and clearance. Furthermore, the age of the individual must be taken into account, with elderly individuals often taking polypharmacy (multiple drugs for a range of ailments), where drug–drug interactions may become a significant issue.

Furthermore, in terms of drug development, failure is predominantly due to adverse pharmacokinetics where a compound, although in terms of pharmacodynamics is highly potent and selective in vitro, becomes inactive and/or toxic in vivo (e.g. poor absorption, inability to cross blood–brain barrier, rapid/extensive metabolism, inactive metabolites, toxic metabolites or rapid excretion).

KEY POINTS

- The interaction of agonist and receptor is a multistage process
- Receptors may have more than one drug-binding site
- Drugs may have a reversible or irreversible action
- Dose–response curves help assess agonist and antagonist activity
- Drug transport within the body may interfere with other drugs
- Drug metabolism may influence the body's handling of other drugs

References

1. Arunlakshana O, Schild HO. Some quantitative uses of drug antagonists. *Br J Pharmacol Chemother* 1959; **14**(1): 48–58.
2. Mohler H. Benzodiazepine receptors: differential ligand interactions and purification of the receptor protein. *Adv Biochem Psychopharmacol* 1983; **38**: 47–56.

3. Bond RA, Ijzerman AP. Recent developments in constitutive receptor activity and inverse agonism, and their potential for GPCR drug discovery. *Trends Pharmacol Sci* 2006; **27**(2): 92–96.
4. Lefkowitz RJ. Historical review: a brief history and personal retrospective of seven-transmembrane receptors. *Trends Pharmacol Sci* 2004; **25**(8): 413–422.
5. Foster AC, Kemp JA. Glutamate- and GABA-based drugs: the next wave of CNS therapeutics? *Curr Opin Pharmacol* 2006; **6**(1): 5–6.
6. Moulin DE, Johnson NG, Murray-Parsons N et al. Subcutaneous narcotic infusions for cancer pain: treatment outcome and guidelines for use. *CMAJ* 1992; **146**(6): 891–897.
7. Nelson KA, Glare PA, Walsh D et al. A prospective, within-patient, crossover study of continuous intravenous and subcutaneous morphine for chronic cancer pain. *J Pain Symptom Manage* 1997; **13**(5): 262–267.

Further reading

Brody TM, Larner J, Minneman KP. *Human pharmacology, molecular to clinical*, 3rd edn. Publisher's details, 1998.

Carvey PM. *Drug action in the central nervous system*. Oxford University Press, 1998.

Golan DE, Tashjian AH, Armstrong EJ, Galanter JM, Armstrong AW, Arnaout RA, Rose HS. *Principles of pharmacology: the pathophysiological basis of drug therapy*. Lippincott, Williams and Wilkins, 2005.

Julien RM. *A primer of drug action*, 7th edn. WH Freeman and Co, 1995.

Katzung BJ. *Basic & clinical pharmacology*, 6th edn. McGraw-Hill Medical, 1995.

Mycek MJ, Harvey RA, Champ PC. *Lippincott's illustrated reviews*, 2nd edn. Churchill, 1996.

Neal MJ. *Medical pharmacology at a glance*, 2nd edn. Blackwell Science Ltd, 1992.

Page CP, Curtis MJ, Sutter MC, Walker MJA, Hoffman BB. *Integrated pharmacology*. Blackwell Science, 1997.

Rang HP, Dale MM. *Pharmacology*, 7th edn. Elsevier, 2007.

Websites

www.bphs.org.uk.
The British Pharmacological Society (BPS).
Other useful pages include: *www.bna.org.uk, www.biomednet.com, www.sciencedirect.com*.
IUPHAR Receptor Database *www.iuphar_db.org*.

Paul Farquhar-Smith

Peripheral mechanisms

Introduction

The primary afferent nociceptor is the first integral part of the pain pathway. It is clear that anatomical and biochemical specialisation is manifest at all levels of nociceptive processing. The complexity of the peripheral part of this system is reflected by the involvement of a plethora of chemical mediators that contribute and mediate changes in processing after inflammation or injury. The pain pathway is not 'hard wired', but is constantly modulated, a phenomenon often referred to as plasticity. Primary afferent nociceptor physiology manifests such plasticity.

Biochemical diversity and specialisation are important factors when considering peripheral pain mechanisms. This is exemplified by the division of nociceptive cells into classes based on specific trophic factor dependence and biochemical properties. Particular nociceptors may express different receptors or chemical mediators and project to separate pain-processing areas of the dorsal horn of the spinal cord.

Physiology of primary afferent nociceptors

Specialised detectors, *nociceptors*, respond to noxious stimuli from many modalities including: thermal, chemical and mechanical.

Somatic pain system

Somatic (i.e. from skin or muscle) nociceptors have been classified according to anatomical features and their physiological characteristics.

Mechanical, heat and chemical noxious stimuli are transduced to activate primary afferent nociceptors:

- Unmyelinated C-fibres are predominantly mechano-heat responsive and a lesser proportion solely mechanoreceptive.
- Thinly myelinated Aδ-fibres display mechano-heat sensitivity with high and low thresholds.

The process of transduction appears to be mediated by ion channels with individual nociceptor properties being determined by the relative expression of these transducing ion channels. These ion channels perform important pain processing functions and may become targets for analgesic medications.

Primary afferent nociceptors display specific nociceptive activity as well as intensity coding physiology. Specificity theory states that selective activation of a specific set of nerve fibres in the periphery leads to the activation of a specific group of spinal neurones that communicate with a specific site in the brain dedicated to pain.[1] In pain terms, these are also called *'nociceptor specific'* neurones and are common in somatic tissue innervation (Fig. 5.1).

Visceral pain system

Internal organs also utilise a pain system, referred to as the *'visceral pain system'*. There are several differences in pain processes compared to the somatic system. For instance, there appear to be few high-threshold visceral 'nociceptor specific' neurones that respond to stimuli only in the noxious range. Indeed, specific bladder nociceptors have been identified in rat bladder.[2] However, most visceral (and some somatic) mechanosensitive afferents exhibit linearity of response into the noxious range consistent with an *'intensity coding'* role.[3,4] For example, in the rat urinary bladder 70% of visceral sensory afferent neurones demonstrate 'intensity coding'. Evidence suggests a similar situation in other hollow viscera, such as the gut.[5]

One group of nociceptors does not appear to exhibit sensitivity to noxious stimuli. These *'silent'* nociceptors develop novel sensitivity usually after tissue injury or inflammation.[4] A proportion of visceral unmyelinated primary

Fig. 5.1 Nociceptor physiology: nociceptor specific and intensity coding neurones. Recordings from pelvic nerve of rat urinary bladder. In bladder, distension is the noxious stimulus. (A) Intensity coding. The response to the noxious stimulus (mean impulses/s) occurs at low levels and increases linearly with increasing distension. (B) Nociceptor specific. At lower levels of stimulus no firing occurs until a noxious threshold is reached. Reproduced from Sengupta and Gebhart,[2] with permission from the International Association for the Study of Pain® (IASP®)

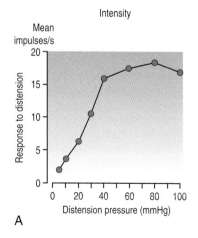

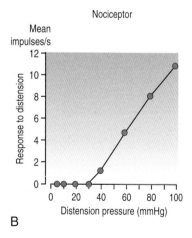

afferents are unresponsive to mechanical stimuli. For example, these are estimated to account for 50–90% of urinary bladder primary afferent neurones.[4,6] After inflammation, many of these 'silent afferents' become mechanosensitive and add to the resultant increased afferent barrage into the spinal cord.[4,7,8] Silent nociceptors have been well characterised in the visceral domain and there is some evidence supporting a somatic counterpart.[9]

Biochemical differentiation of primary afferent nociceptors

In the developing organism, innervated tissue produces a small but defined amount of neurotrophic substance. At a critical stage it binds to receptors, is internalised and undergoes retrograde transport to the cell bodies to mediate changes that are vital to the continuing survival of the cell.[10] The neurotrophin, nerve growth factor (NGF) is critical to this process. NGF knockout mice, in which the gene responsible for the production of NGF has been disrupted, do not develop small-to-medium-sized nerve cells (about 70% of cells) in the dorsal root ganglia (DRG) and display a marked reduction in pain sensitivity.[11] An analogous clinical situation exists in a rare congenital syndrome known as 'hereditary sensory and autonomic neuropathy IV' or congenital insensitivity to pain with anhidrosis.[12] These patients have a genetic abnormality of the high-affinity NGF receptor, tyrosine kinase A (trkA). They have insensitivity to pain and temperature and are deficient in thinly myelinated and unmyelinated nerve fibres.

Initially, 70–80% of developing DRG cells express the trkA receptor and these cells require NGF for survival during embryonic life. During development the situation changes as the proportion of neurones expressing trkA reduces to 40–45% in the adult.[13] The majority of these cells express the peptides, substance P (SP) and calcitonin gene-related peptide (CGRP).[14] These peptidergic, NGF-dependent primary afferent neurones project (have their primary synapses) to lamina I and II outer in the superficial dorsal horn of the spinal cord.[15] NGF regulates the functional properties of these neurones, including levels of neuropeptide expression and the nociceptive threshold.[16] The proportion of trkA expression is also related to the functional properties of DRG cells. There appears to be a higher degree of co-localisation of trkA with visceral primary afferent neurones (e.g. those that innervate the urinary bladder)[8] compared to somatic primary afferent neurones. The expression of other neurotrophin receptors differs markedly from that of trkA. A population of DRG cells do not express trkA in the adult, but have there own distinct immunocytochemistry.[15] These non-peptidergic cells express the adenosine triphosphate (ATP)-gated $P2X_3$ ion channel and project to lamina II inner of the superficial dorsal horn of the spinal cord. This biochemical division between peptidergic and non-peptidergic nociceptors has been postulated to have functional significance.[15]

In the resting state, noxious stimuli are transduced by nociceptors via ion channels (usually Na^+ and Ca^{2+}). Activation of these channels induces currents that depolarise the cell membrane. Voltage-gated ion channels are subsequently activated if the depolarisation is sufficient. Activation of these voltage-gated ion channels initiates action potentials. The intensity of the noxious stimuli determines the level of activation of transduction and is reflected by the duration and frequency of the nociceptor action potentials.[17] Voltage-gated sodium channels, such as $Na_V1.8$ and 1.9, which are selectively expressed by nociceptors, are involved in this acute pain mechanism. Non-selective local anaesthetics inhibit pain sensation by blocking these sodium channels, but also block sodium channels and nerve conduction in other sensory and motor neurones leading to potential numbness and weakness. A selective $Na_V1.8/9$ blocker could provide selective analgesia.

Inflammatory peripheral sensitisation

Inflammation: the drive to nociceptor activation and sensitisation

Inflammation is a major influence on the plastic changes in peripheral pain mechanisms. Inflammation is associated with a shift in the stimulus response function of primary afferent neurones (hyperalgesia; an increased response to a stimulus that is normally painful) and expansion of nociceptor receptive fields within the zone of tissue inflammation. Enhanced excitability of existing nociceptors (and in the visceral domain recruitment of silent nociceptors) contributes to the overall effect of increasing the total nociceptive afferent input to the spinal cord. This plasticity of the primary afferent nociceptor is also known as peripheral or 'primary sensitisation'. The increase afferent barrage to the spinal cord provokes multiple plastic changes that set up a state of enhanced excitability in spinal nociceptive neurones 'secondary hyperalgesia'. Furthermore, there is evidence suggesting that under certain circumstances, this state of hyperexcitability may become self-sustaining, so that pain continues to be perceived in the absence of on-going tissue injury, this is observed in some chronic pains.[18]

A myriad of substances are released by damaged tissue, immune cells are recruited and nerves themselves combine to create the potent proinflammatory and proalgesic 'inflammatory soup' that drives peripheral sensitisation. These mediators (such as H^+ ions, ATP and serotonin) can act directly and indirectly by interaction with nociceptors often via ion channels or by receptor-mediated second messenger action (for example bradykinin and NGF).[19]

Ion channels involved in nociception and peripheral sensitisation (Fig. 5.2)

Sodium channels

One family of channels has been the focus of a large body of research into the nature of modulation of nociceptor excitability: voltage-gated Na^+ currents (VGSCs) (Fig. 5.3). Evidence supports the role of VGSCs in controlling neuronal excitability and therapeutic compounds that block these channels may be effective in treating experimental hyperalgesia.[20] The Na^+ current evoked from sensory neurones is made up of activation of a number of distinct ion channels, which are divided into two types (tetrodotoxin TTX):

1. TTX-sensitive currents are present on all sensory neurones
2. TTX-resistant currents are largely restricted to neurones with nociceptive characteristics.[21]

Hyperalgesic inflammatory mediators increase the magnitude of TTX-resistant currents,[20] which may involve phosphorylation via protein kinase C (PKC)[21] or protein kinase A (PKA)[22] (Fig. 5.3). Furthermore, a sub-population of these channels are sensory nerve specific (SNS) and undergo increased expression in inflammation.[23] Mice in which the gene responsible for encoding

Fig. 5.2 A selection of components of the 'inflammatory soup' and the receptors at which they act. Bradykinin (BK) is released after tissue damage and is an agonist at B_1 and B_2 receptors. EP receptors are the target for prostaglandin E_2 (PGE_2) a product of cyclooxygenase metabolism. Peripheral glutamate acts on metabotropic glutamate receptors (mGlu). Acidity (protons, H^+) activates both acid-sensitive ion channels (ASICs) and the vanilloid receptor TRPV1 (formerly VR1), which is also an ion channel. Adenosine triphosphate (ATP) is present in the 'inflammatory soup' and acts at the sensory neurone specific purinergic receptor, $P2X_3$

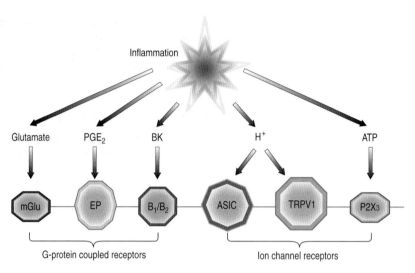

Fig. 5.3 Peripheral sensitisation by receptor phosphorylation. Activation of protein kinases A and C (PKA and PKC) by B_1/B_2 receptor activation or tyrosine kinase A (trkA), sensitises the nociceptor by phosphorylation (P+) of the vanilloid receptor TRPV1. Phosphorylation of the sensory neurone specific sodium channel ($Na_V1.8$) is also mediated by kinases, possibly including extracellular signal-related kinase (ERK). Inflammation-mediated (and after nerve damage) phosphorylation of $Na_V1.8$ induces increased excitability and lowered thresholds of nociceptors consistent with peripheral sensitisation

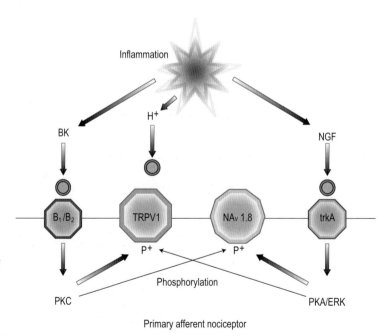

the SNS TTX-resistant channel has been disrupted, exhibited a pronounced analgesia to noxious mechanical stimuli and delayed development of inflammatory hyperalgesia.[24] After recent revision of sodium channel nomenclature, the SNS channel is now identified as $Na_V1.8$.[25] The $Na_V1.8$ is involved in nociceptor electrical function and central to inflammation-induced modification of excitability.

Heat-sensitive ion channels – TRPV1 receptors

Heat-sensitive ion channels on sensory neurones provide another possible candidate for a nociceptive specific channel and the key to direct peripheral sensitisation.

The capsaicin activated, vanilloid receptors or transient receptor potential channel 1 receptors (TRPV1, formerly VR1) are primarily expressed on unmyelinated and thinly myelinated neurones which are consistent with nociceptors.[26] Cells expressing TRPV1 are activated by sudden increases in temperature.[27] Capsaicin sensitivity correlates with heat sensitivity, which suggests that noxious heat and capsaicin both activate the TRPV1 receptor.[28] Mice lacking functional TRPV1 receptors demonstrate deficits in heat-evoked responses of dorsal root ganglion (DRG) cells and fail to develop inflammatory hyperalgesia.[29] TRPV1 receptors are also directly activated by protons (H^+ from low pH environments such as inflammation, Fig. 5.2) and indirectly activated by bradykinin and prostaglandins.[26] TRPV1 expression is increased in the first 24 hours after inflammation and is involved in the development of thermal sensitisation.[30]

In summary, the TRPV1 receptor is implicated in the mechanism of heat pain transduction and in the sensitisation secondary to acidity (H^+ ions) and bradykinin released in the 'inflammatory soup'. There is a separate family of ion channels that selectively respond to acidity (protons, H^+), acid-sensing ion channels (ASICs), some of which are expressed by sensory afferents and may be involved in acid-mediated changes in nociceptor sensitivity (Fig. 5.2).[31]

Purinergic receptors

Investigation into the recently characterised ATP-gated ion channels has re-fuelled interest into the role of ATP (also released in the inflammatory soup) and pain.[21] The large family of ion channels that are opened by ATP are called P2X purinoceptors, of which $P2X_3$ may be important in nociception, and may even be selectively expressed on nociceptors.[21]

Mediators of peripheral sensitisation
Cyclo-oxygenase and prostaglandins

Inflammation induces a cascade of events mediated by multiple components that contribute to the development of inflammatory hyperalgesia. Nociceptors may be activated directly, such as interaction with the ion channels described above. Nociceptors may also be sensitised indirectly via intracellular second-messenger systems. For example, the action of cyclo-oxygenase (COX) on arachidonic acid (AA) creates many pro-inflammatory products including prostaglandin E_2 (PGE_2) that causes peripheral sensitisation via a G-protein-coupled receptor (GPCR) resulting in increases in cyclic adenosine monophosphate (cAMP) within the nociceptor[32] (Fig. 5.2). Inflammation-induced hyperalgesia is associated with an increase in PGE_2, COX inhibition reduces levels of PGE_2 and the associated hyperalgesia.[33] Local administration of PGE_2 evokes hyperalgesia, mediated by an intracellular increase in cAMP.[34] PGE_2 also enhances sensitisation by other pro-inflammatory mediators, such as bradykinin.[32] The primary analgesic action of non-steroidal anti-inflammatory drugs (NSAIDs) is the inhibition of COX resulting in the reduction of peripheral prostaglandins, notably PGE_2.[32] More recently, a spinal and central role for prostaglandins in pain processing has been elucidated and is responsible for part of the efficacy of NSAIDs. The COX enzyme exists as two different isoforms. It has been suggested that inhibition of the COX-1 isoform results in side effects, such as gastric ulceration, whilst COX-2 inhibition mediates the analgesic effect. Although the introduction of COX-2-selective antagonists reduces gastric side effects, they also may have increased cardiac risk.

Peripheral neuropeptides and neurogenic inflammation

Part of the inflammatory process is mediated by neuropeptides released from sensory nerve endings. Neurogenic inflammation is responsible for the flare reaction following a scratch injury. Neurotransmitters (notably substance P and CGRP) are released from peripheral terminals, act via specific receptors inducing plasma extravasation and vasodilatation that helps sustain the inflammatory impetus.[35] Vasodilatation is mediated by both A and C polymodal nociceptors. Nociceptive activation of A- and C-fibres causes antidromic activation of adjacent chemosensitive fibres, these release neurotransmitters that act on the surrounding nociceptors. NGF increases the neuropeptide content of sensory nerves and increases local inflammation-induced release. These changes promote the recruitment of immune cells to the affected area and promote the development of oedema.

Neurotrophins: NGF and BDNF

Nerve growth factor (NGF) appears to be a key molecule in the orchestration of peripheral inflammation. NGF is released from many cells after tissue injury (including fibroblasts) and has several pro-inflammatory roles. In several inflammatory pain models it has been shown that local NGF tissue levels are raised.[36,37] Subcutaneous administration of carrageenan, another pro-inflammatory substance that provokes hyperalgesia, has been shown to increase NGF levels.[38] NGF also appears to be up-regulated in joint synovia of human patients with arthritis[39] and is found in increased levels in bladder tissue of patients suffering with interstitial cystitis.[40] Therefore, inflammation-induced increases of NGF are associated with hyperalgesia and human pain syndromes. Antagonism of these raised levels of NGF (using the trkA–IgG fusion molecule that blocks the NGF receptor) blocks thermal hyperalgesia,[41] suggesting that inflammation-induced peripheral NGF is an important endogenous mediator of hyperalgesia. NGF is also capable of direct and indirect sensitisation of nociceptors. Indeed, NGF occupies a commanding position in many pro-inflammatory processes, and is pivotal to the development of inflammatory hyperalgesia.

NGF has significant actions on the expression of another neurotrophin, brain-derived neurotrophic factor (BDNF).[42] Administration of exogenous NGF leads to up-regulation of BDNF in trkA-expressing sensory neurones and the BDNF protein was found to be antegradely transported to the periphery and centrally to CGRP containing terminals in the dorsal horn of the spinal cord.[43] Local administration of BDNF induces a thermal hyperalgesia and direct application of BDNF to the receptive field of C-fibres of skin-nerve in vitro preparations elicits increased sensitivity to noxious heat.[44] Moreover, peripheral inflammation increases BDNF mRNA levels in the DRG, especially in trkA-expressing cells and these increases were attenuated by co-administration of antibodies to NGF.[45] Thus, inflammation-induced release of NGF could induce augmentation of BDNF levels in the periphery and contribute to sensitisation and hyperalgesia.

Peripheral glutamate

Glutamate is a major excitatory neurotransmitter in the central and peripheral nervous systems. Glutamate in the spinal cord acts on α-amino-3-hydroxy-5-methyl-4-isozaxole (AMPA) receptors, N-methyl-D-aspartate (NMDA) receptors and the G-protein-coupled metabotropic glutamate (mGlu) receptors. The latter have been implicated in inflammation-induced peripheral sensitisation.[46] Glutamate is increased in inflamed skin and local injection causes pain behaviour in animals, as well as invoking electrophysiological changes of peripheral sensitisation. It is proposed that glutamate is released from peripheral C-fibre terminals and acts on peripheral mGlu receptors that in turn modulate ion channels and alter nociceptor sensitivity.[46] These processes identify a novel potential peripheral analgesic site for glutamate antagonists.

Mechanisms involving secondary messengers

Cyclic adenosine monophosphate and protein kinase A

Elevated levels of cAMP have been implicated as an important measure of nociceptive afferent sensitivity.[47] Stimulation of cAMP production or prevention of its breakdown prolongs hyperalgesia[48] and cAMP analogues can mimic the sensitising effects of PGE_2 (see above). A rise in cAMP activates a cAMP-dependent PKA that in turn heightens nociceptor sensitivity leading to thermal and mechanical hypersensitivity. Increased cAMP is required to induce inflammatory hyperalgesia, but activated PKA is required to maintain it.[49] Interestingly, the action of μ opioid agonists at peripheral opioid receptors reduce cAMP levels, which may contribute to the analgesic action of these agents.[50] One mechanism proposed to explain the action of cAMP on sensitisation is that cAMP causes changes in TTX-resistant sodium channels. Several inflammatory mediators (including PGE_2) activate cAMP-PKA receptors resulting in phosphorylation of TTX-resistant sodium channels (including $Na_V1.8$), which augments nociceptor excitability and lowers the activation thresholds consistent with peripheral sensitisation[22] (Fig. 5.3).

Bradykinin, protein kinase C and other kinases

The local cleavage of kinins from inactive precursors to the active compounds is a consequence of tissue injury. These kinins include bradykinin and its kinase I metabolite (des-Arg^9-bradykinin).[51] Bradykinin not only stimulates nociceptors directly, but also indirectly promotes sensitisation of primary afferents.[52] Bradykinin activates nociceptors via the G-protein-coupled B_2 receptor. This may also stimulate prostanoid, cytokine and nitric oxide (NO) production that mediate the sensitisation of nociceptors and in turn induce expression of the bradykinin B_1 receptor. The induction and subsequent function of B_1 receptors become more important in inflammation of longer duration.[52] Part of these actions is mediated via G-proteins to generate, amongst other substances, diacylglycerol. Diacylglycerol then activates protein kinase C (PKC) causing phosphorylation of various intracellular proteins that promote calcium mobilisation.[22] PKC activation has also been shown to potentiate TRPV1 activation[26] (Fig. 5.3) and mediate NGF-induced hyperalgesia.[22]

Phosphorylation of receptors and ion channels can have relatively fast modifying actions on pain sensitivity, they also instigate transcriptional changes that lead to longer-term modification and changes consistent with chronic pain.[19]

Other protein kinases have been implicated in the development of peripheral sensitisation.[53] For example, activation of mitogen-activated protein kinase (MAPK) increases TRPV1 levels in peripheral nociceptor terminals[30] and tumour necrosis factor α (TNFα)-induced hyperalgesia is mediated by MAPK.[51] Inhibitors of another kinase, extracellular signal-related kinase (ERK), block the development of capsaicin-induced hypersensitivity.[22] Thus, a number of protein kinases mediate the phosphorylation changes that modulate peripheral sensitisation.

Immune cells and cytokines involved in inflammation-induced activation and sensitisation

Neutrophils

Immune cells are recruited to the site and activated by inflammation (Fig. 5.4). These cells release compounds that directly or indirectly sensitise nociceptors. Neutrophils, macrophages and mast cells are important.

Leukotriene B4 (LTB4) and NGF promote neutrophil chemotaxis (attraction) to inflamed areas. Hyperalgesia induced by both LTB4 and NGF has been shown to be dependent upon neutrophils.[54,55]

Exogenous treatment with NGF induces a hyperalgesia that is reduced by removal of circulating neutrophils. Neutrophils accumulate in NGF-treated skin within 3 h of administration and this process is sensitive to 5-lipoxygenase (5-LOX) inhibition.[55] NGF-induced thermal hyperalgesia is associated with a rise in leukotriene B4 (LTB4), which is a powerful neutrophil chemoattractant. Hyperalgesia is diminished by administration of a 5-LOX inhibitor.[56] Indirect support of the importance of LTB4 and 5-LOX is offered by the

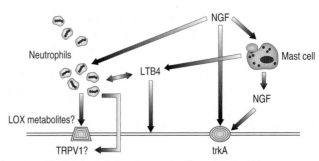

Fig. 5.4 Immune interactions contributing to inflammatory pain. The neurotrophin, nerve growth factor (NGF), can activate primary afferent nociceptors directly via its high affinity receptor tyrosine kinase A (trkA), but also is chemotactic to neutrophils both directly and by releasing the chemotactic leukotriene, leukotriene B4 (LTB4). Activated neutrophils can maintain sensitisation putatively by release of lipoxygenase (LOX) metabolites that act upon the TRPV1 receptor. NGF induces trkA-mediated mast cell degranulation that not only releases many pro-inflammatory mediators, but also liberates more NGF to amplify the process

observation that the COX inhibitor, indometacin, reduces prostaglandin E_2 production but does not alter NGF-induced hyperalgesia.[57]

Neutrophil accumulation could develop and maintain sensitisation by production of sensitising substances. Products of the action of lipoxygenase on arachidonic acid (generated by activated neutrophils), such as the dihydroxyeicosatetraenoic acids, are active at TRPV1 receptors and have been shown to have a direct activating effect on primary afferent nociceptors[58] (Fig. 5.4). Therefore, the production of endogenous vanilloid-like substance with agonist activity at the TRPV1 receptor may provide the link between neutrophils and hyperalgesia.[59]

Mast cells

Another peripheral cell type that expresses trkA and contributes to hyperalgesia is the mast cell. NGF induces inflammatory mediator release from mast cells via trkA activation.[60] Prior mast cell degranulation has been shown to delay and reduce the thermal hyperalgesia associated with systemic NGF administration.[61] NGF is also produced and released by mast cells.[62] Therefore, mast cell-released algogens (including NGF) could directly sensitise primary afferent neurones providing an indirect NGF-mediated, mast cell-dependent sensitisation. Cannabinoids reduce mast cell degranulation and neutrophil influx, which could, in part, account for their analgesic actions.[63]

Cytokines

Inflammation-driven release of cytokines from immune cells provokes hyperalgesia through stimulation and production of other pro-inflammatory agents. Interleukin-1β (IL-1β) and tumour necrosis factor α (TNFα) are the main stimulus to NGF release from connective tissue cells and are hyperalgesic when injected in animal pain models.[51] Clinically, TNFα levels correlate with pain and hyperalgesia in certain disease states, such as rheumatoid arthritis.[51] TNFα-induced hyperalgesia may itself be mediated by IL-1β release.[64] IL-1β prompts hyperalgesia in part by bradykinin B_1 receptor induction and prostaglandin activation.[51,65]

Numerous other chemokines, classified as CXC and CC groups, are elements of the inflammatory soup and either activate or modify nociceptor activity or direct immune cell chemotaxis and extravasation.[66] Chemokines can be neuromodulatory by modification of the sensitivity of other receptors and by recruitment of other pro-inflammatory cells.

Peripheral sensitisation of primary afferent nociceptors exists as an important component of inflammatory hyperalgesia and is a potential target for therapeutic intervention. However, increased peripheral input from sensitised nociceptors is instrumental in instigating activity-dependent changes in central processing that are responsible for central sensitisation.

Peripheral mechanisms of neuropathic pain

Neuropathic pain is defined as *'pain initiated or caused by a primary lesion or dysfunction in the nervous system'* or paraphrased as pain at a site of abnormal sensation. There are many causes for neuropathic pain and they are often considered together, however, different mechanisms may contribute to different neuropathic pain characteristics and influence treatment efficacy. Clinically, neuropathic pain is often expressed as burning or like electric shocks. It may also be associated with abnormal sensory processes manifest as *hyperalgesia* (painful stimulus perceived to be more painful) or *allodynia* (normally a non-noxious stimulus experienced as painful). Much of the research has examined animal models in which peripheral nerves have been selectively damaged by tying, cutting or constriction. However, in many clinical cases such neuronal destruction is rarely present. Other models have employed neuropathic agents to mimic specific diseases. For example, the administration of streptozotocin induces diabetes and consequently diabetic neuropathy. Administration of the chemotherapeutic agent, paclitaxel, induces peripheral neuropathy, as is observed clinically.

Although peripheral processes are integral and peripheral sensitisation occurs, there are important spinal and brain mechanisms that are involved with the induction and maintenance of neuropathic pain.

Abnormal electrophysiology and neuropathic pain

Many of the components of inflammation-induced peripheral sensitisation, including elements of the 'inflammatory soup' and immune cells, also play a role in the peripheral changes that are involved in neuropathic pain. Peripheral nerve injury induces biochemical and functional changes in both injured and uninjured parts of the nerve.

Peripheral changes after nerve damage:[67]

- Increase in spontaneous discharge
- Increase in ectopic discharge
- Alteration of ion channel and neuropeptide expression
- Collateral sprouting of primary afferent terminals
- Nociceptor sensitisation
- Sprouting of sympathetic nerves into DRGs.

Expression of many compounds is up- or down-regulated in both the injured and uninjured nerves, including inflammatory mediators and ion channels.

Afferent neurones increase ectopic and spontaneous firing after nerve damage. This has been confirmed in humans from recordings of post nerve injury neuromata. In animal models these 'ectopic' discharges have been recorded from both the DRGs and from the nerve itself.

Nerve injury increases the sub-threshold oscillations in the membrane potential that are usually present in the resting state and result in an increased probability of ectopic discharge. Furthermore, 'cross-talk' from neighbouring nerves (damaged or not) can augment this effect. This is also known as ephaptic conduction (activity of one nerve having an influence on the nerves surrounding it). The effect of this cross-talk is augmented by the increases in neuronal excitability after nerve damage and increases the likelihood of ectopic firing. Regeneration of axon terminals after nerve damage, which is NGF mediated, may enhance cross-talk, although the degree of sprouting does not correlate with the severity of pain behaviours.[68]

Alterations in ion channel expression

Abnormal electrophysiological function in damaged nerves, such as ectopic and spontaneous discharge, contributes to the development and maintenance of neuropathic pain.[69] However, changes in the neighbouring uninjured nerves can also develop sensitisation and ectopic activity and be part of the generation of pain.[70,71] The effect of their relative contributions is controversial, but injured and uninjured nerves are both implicated in neuropathic pain.[68] A possible mechanism is suggested by the observation of an increased density of membrane sodium channels after nerve damage. Nevertheless, different types of sodium channel undergo differing alterations in organisation and expression, often regulated by changes in expression of neurotrophic factors. For example, there is some evidence that the expression of the nociceptor specific $Na_V1.8$ is increased in injured nerves and blocking the $Na_V1.8$ reduces neuropathic pain behaviours.[44] However, the situation is complex since increased expression of voltage-gated sodium channels has been demonstrated in both injured and non-injured sensory afferents.[70] Indeed, other investigators observed that the expression of $Na_V1.8$ and $Na_V1.9$ were actually unchanged in uninjured nerves.[72] Nevertheless, the up- and downregulation, reorganisation and de novo synthesis of various voltage-gated sodium channels (including sensory neurone specific TTX-resistant channels) in injured and uninjured nerves, are likely to mediate electrical hyperexcitability and increased ectopic and spontaneous activity.[68]

Voltage-gated calcium channels are also altered following peripheral nerve injury and have been demonstrated to be involved in hyperalgesia and allodynia. The anti-neuropathic agent, gabapentin, is thought to act by inhibiting voltage-gated calcium channels by targeting a specific subunit of the channel. Like sodium channels there are many types of calcium channel, but blockade of the N-type calcium channel appears to have a locally mediated attenuation of neuropathic behaviours.[68] Mice lacking N-type calcium channels also develop less neuropathic pain.[67] In inflammatory pain, enhanced nociceptor excitability secondary to stimulation of TTX-resistant Na^+ channels may be mediated by T-type calcium channels. This could explain the efficacy of the T-type calcium channel blocker, ethosuxamide, in a chemotherapy model of neuropathic pain.[73]

The expression of the TRPV1 receptor is also influenced by nerve injury. Interestingly, after nerve damage, expression of TRPV1 (which is usually restricted to C-fibres) is increased in the uninjured DRGs of A-fibres.[74,75] However, the significance of these finding as regards neuropathic pain has been questioned.[76] TRPV1 may be involved in the nociceptor sensitisation observed after nerve injury.

Inflammatory processes in neuropathic pain

Inflammation has been suggested to be pivotal to the development of neuropathic pain as it is in inflammatory pain.[67] Changes occur in both B_1 and B_2 bradykinin receptor sub-types. After peripheral nerve injury, B_1 is synthesised de novo, and B_1 antagonists reduce neuropathic pain.[75] Theoretically, downstream activation of protein kinases would induce phosphorylation of ion channels and alter sensitivity, directly analogous to inflammatory pain. Cytokines, also released after nerve injury, are thought to induce up-regulation of B_1 expression.[67] Prostaglandins could also be involved, since COX inhibitors (e.g. NSAIDs) have been shown to reduce neuropathic pain in some animal models.[77] However, the general lack of efficacy of NSAIDs in human neuropathic pain may question the applicability of the animal models.

Similarly, immune cells have also been implicated in the development of neuropathic pain. Early depletion of neutrophils reduces neuropathic pain behaviour.[78] Moreover, other inflammatory mediators released from NGF-induced degranulation of mast cells have also been cited as contributing to neuropathic pain.[79] However, the same caveat of the degree of inflammation in animal models compared to human neuropathic pain must be applied.

The expression of peripheral peptides is also altered after nerve damage. The neuropeptides, substance P and calcitonin gene-related peptide (CGRP), are reduced, but others, including galanin and neuropeptide Y, are increased from normally low levels.[75] Although the actual role of these compounds is unclear, evidence suggests they influence both peripheral and central processes of neuropathic pain.

Sympathetic sprouting and sympathetic-sensory coupling

Sympathetic sprouting (new dendrite formation) and the subsequent coupling of the sensory and sympathetic nervous systems, has been postulated to increase the ectopic and spontaneous firing in injured (and perhaps uninjured) nerve fibres. This correlates with clinical observations that a small subset of patients demonstrate sympathetic nervous system-dependent neuropathic pain.[68] These patients may also exhibit pain sensitive to catecholamines. Several possible mechanisms of coupling have been postulated:

- Ephatic coupling
- Direct coupling in DRG
- Indirect coupling by sympathetic terminal releasing mediators that sensitise primary afferents.

Peripheral sympathetic sprouting of noradrenergic perivascular axons into DRGs has been described after ligation of the sciatic nerve. Large-diameter DRGs cells were encompassed by 'baskets' of sprouted sympathetic fibres, demonstrating a possible site for nociceptive-sympathetic coupling.[80] Similar sympathetic sprouting has been observed in other animal neuropathic pain models, but with differing times of development.[68] Increased expression of NGF at the level of the DRG is likely to be the key, but the cytokine leukaemia inhibitory factor (LIF) can also stimulate sympathetic sprouting. Although synapse-like structures exist between the DRG and the 'baskets' their function and significance is controversial. However, sympathetic stimulation has been shown to increase ectopic discharge from the DRG. Moreover, chemical or anatomical sympathectomy (procedures that temporarily or permanently stop sympathetic nerve activity) reduces hyperalgesia in animal neuropathic pain models. This reflects successful use of sympathetic blocks in some cases of human neuropathic pain.

Summary

Peripheral pain mechanisms display plasticity and undergo major changes in processing after inflammation and nerve damage. Pro-inflammatory compounds (elements of the 'inflammatory soup') act on receptors, ion channels and immune cells to generate and maintain nociceptor activation and sensitisation. Direct and indirect mechanisms are employed. Receptor phosphorylation by protein kinases is an important feature of nociceptor sensitisation. Peripheral nerve damage may induce similar mechanisms resulting in alterations of nociceptive function. However, up- and down-regulation and reorganisation of many pain-processing factors (especially ion channels) in damaged and undamaged nerve fibers contributes to peripheral neuropathic pain. In both cases the resulting increase in primary afferent input to the spinal cord is instrumental in inducing profound changes in pain processes known as secondary sensitisation.

KEY POINTS

- Primary afferent nociceptors demonstrate marked plasticity known as 'primary sensitisation'
- Nociceptive transduction is mediated in part by ion channels
- Different groups of nociceptor have different biochemical profiles, which may relate to their functional differences
- Silent nociceptors become active after tissue injury or inflammation. They are common in visceral processing but also exist in somatic systems
- Chemicals within the inflammatory soup act directly and indirectly on nociceptors via ion channels and receptor-mediated second messenger systems
- The effect of the peripheral sensitisation is to lower the activation threshold of nociceptors. Neuronal firing may become spontaneous
- Increased peripheral input from sensitised nociceptors is an important factor in central processing and sensitisation
- Bradykinin acts by directly stimulating nociceptors and by indirectly sensitising nociceptors
- Immune cells release compounds that directly or indirectly sensitise nociceptors

References

1. Ness TJ. Historical and clinical perspectives of visceral pain. In: Gebhart GF (ed.) *Visceral pain*. Seattle: IASP Press; 1995.
2. Sengupta JN, Gebhart GF. Mechanosensitive properties of pelvic nerve afferent fibers innervating the urinary bladder of the rat. *J Neurophysiol* 1994; **72**(5): 2420–2430.
3. Habler HJ, Janig W, Koltzenburg M. Myelinated primary afferents of the sacral spinal cord responding to slow filling and distension of the cat urinary bladder. *J Physiol* 1993; **463**: 449–460.
4. Koltzenburg M, McMahon SB. Mechanically insensitive primary afferents supplying the bladder. In: Gebhart GF (ed.) *Visceral pain*. Seattle: IASP Press; 1995.
5. Gebhart GF. Visceral pain – peripheral sensitisation. *Gut* 2000; **47**(Suppl 4): iv54–iv55.
6. Dmitrieva N, McMahon SB. Sensitisation of visceral afferents by nerve growth factor in the adult rat. *Pain* 1996; **66**(1): 87–97.
7. Habler HJ, Janig W, Koltzenburg M. Activation of unmyelinated afferents in chronically lesioned nerves by adrenaline and excitation of sympathetic efferents in the cat. *Neurosci Lett* 1987; **82**(1): 35–40.
8. McMahon SB, Armanini MP, Ling LH et al. Expression and coexpression of Trk receptors in subpopulations of adult primary sensory neurons projecting to identified peripheral targets. *Neuron* 1994; **12**(5): 1161–1171.
9. Xu GY, Huang LY, Zhao ZQ. Activation of silent mechanoreceptive cat C and Adelta sensory neurons and their substance P expression following peripheral inflammation. *J Physiol* 2000; **528**(Pt2): 339–348.
10. Bennett DL, McMahon SB, Rattray M et al. Nerve growth factor and sensory nerve function. In: Brain SD, Moore PK (eds). *Pain and neurogenic inflammation*. Basel: Birkhauser Verlag; 1999.
11. Crowley C, Spencer SD, Nishimura MC et al. Mice lacking nerve growth factor display perinatal loss of sensory and sympathetic neurons yet develop basal forebrain cholinergic neurons. *Cell* 1994; **76**(6): 1001–1011.
12. Indo Y, Tsuruta M, Hayashida Y et al. Mutations in the TRKA/NGF receptor gene in patients with congenital insensitivity to pain with anhidrosis. *Nat Genet* 1996; **13**(4): 485–488.

13. Molliver DC, Wright DE, Leitner ML et al. IB4-binding DRG neurons switch from NGF to GDNF dependence in early postnatal life. *Neuron* 1997; **19**(4): 849–861.

14. Averill S, McMahon SB, Clary DO et al. Immunocytochemical localization of trkA receptors in chemically identified subgroups of adult rat sensory neurons. *Eur J Neurosci* 1995; **7**(7): 1484–1494.

15. Snider WD, McMahon SB. Tackling pain at the source: new ideas about nociceptors. *Neuron* 1998; **20**(4): 629–632.

16. McMahon SB. NGF as a mediator of inflammatory pain. *Philos Trans R Soc Lond B Biol Sci* 1996; **351**(1338): 431–440.

17. Woolf CJ. Pain: moving from symptom control toward mechanism-specific pharmacologic management. *Ann Intern Med* 2004; **140**(6): 441–451.

18. Coderre TJ, Katz J, Vaccarino AL et al. Contribution of central neuroplasticity to pathological pain: review of clinical and experimental evidence. *Pain* 1993; **52**(3): 259–285.

19. Woolf CJ, Salter MW. Neuronal plasticity: increasing the gain in pain. *Science* 2000; **288**(5472): 1765–1769.

20. Gold MS, Reichling DB, Shuster MJ et al. Hyperalgesic agents increase a tetrodotoxin-resistant Na+ current in nociceptors. *Proc Natl Acad Sci USA* 1996; **93**(3): 1108–1112.

21. McCleskey EW, Gold MS. Ion channels of nociception. *Annu Rev Physiol* 1999; **61**: 835–856.

22. Bhave G, Gereau RW. Posttranslational mechanisms of peripheral sensitization. *J Neurobiol* 2004; **61**(1): 88–106.

23. Tanaka M, Cummins TR, Ishikawa K et al. SNS Na+ channel expression increases in dorsal root ganglion neurons in the carrageenan inflammatory pain model. *Neuroreport* 1998; **9**(6): 967–972.

24. Akopian AN, Souslova V, England S et al. The tetrodotoxin-resistant sodium channel SNS has a specialized function in pain pathways. *Nat Neurosci* 1999; **2**(6): 541–548.

25. Goldin AL, Barchi RL, Caldwell JH et al. Nomenclature of voltage-gated sodium channels. *Neuron* 2000; **28**(2): 365–368.

26. Cortright DN, Szallasi A. Biochemical pharmacology of the vanilloid receptor TRPV1. An update. *Eur J Biochem* 2004; **271**(10): 1814–1819.

27. Tominaga M, Caterina MJ, Malmbery AB et al. The cloned capsaicin receptor integrates multiple pain-producing stimuli. *Neuron* 1998; **21**(3): 531–543.

28. Nagy I, Rang H. Noxious heat activates all capsaicin-sensitive and also a sub-population of capsaicin-insensitive dorsal root ganglion neurons. *Neuroscience* 1999; **88**(4): 995–997.

29. Caterina MJ, Leffler A, Malmbery AB et al. Impaired nociception and pain sensation in mice lacking the capsaicin receptor. *Science* 2000; **288**(5464): 306–313.

30. Ji RR, Samad TA, Jin SX et al. p38 MAPK activation by NGF in primary sensory neurons after inflammation increases TRPV1 levels and maintains heat hyperalgesia. *Neuron* 2002; **36**(1): 57–68.

31. Kidd BL, Urban LA. Mechanisms of inflammatory pain. *Br J Anaesth* 2001; **87**(1): 3–11.

32. Levine JD, Reichling D. Peripheral mechanisms of inflammatory pain. In: Wall PD, Melzack R (eds) *Textbook of pain.* Edinburgh: Churchill Livingstone; 1999.

33. Zhang Y, Shaffer A, Portanova J et al. Inhibition of cyclooxygenase-2 rapidly reverses inflammatory hyperalgesia and prostaglandin E2 production. *J Pharmacol Exp Ther* 1997; **283**(3): 1069–1075.

34. Cunha FQ, Teixeira MM, Ferreira SH. Pharmacological modulation of secondary mediator systems-cyclic AMP and cyclic GMP – on inflammatory hyperalgesia. *Br J Pharmacol* 1999; **127**(3): 671–678.

35. Julius D, Basbaum AI. Molecular mechanisms of nociception. *Nature* 2001; **413**(6852): 203–210.

36. Woolf CJ, Safieh-Garabedium B, Ma Q et al. Nerve growth factor contributes to the generation of inflammatory sensory hypersensitivity. *Neuroscience* 1994; **62**: 327–331.

37. Safieh-Garabedian B, Poole S, Allchorne A et al. Contribution of interleukin-1 beta to the inflammation-induced increase in nerve growth factor levels and inflammatory hyperalgesia. *Br J Pharmacol* 1995; **115**(7): 1265–1275.
38. Aloe L, Tuveri MA, Levi-Montalcini R. Studies on carrageenan-induced arthritis in adult rats: presence of nerve growth factor and role of sympathetic innervation. *Rheumatol Int* 1992; **12**(5): 213–216.
39. Aloe L, Tuveri MA, Carcassi V et al. Nerve growth factor in the synovial fluid of patients with chronic arthritis. *Arthritis Rheum* 1992; **35**(3): 351–355.
40. Lowe EM, Anand P, Terenghi G et al. Increased nerve growth factor levels in the urinary bladder of women with idiopathic sensory urgency and interstitial cystitis. *Br J Urol* 1997; **79**(4): 572–577.
41. McMahon SB, Bennett DL, Priestley JV et al. The biological effects of endogenous nerve growth factor on adult sensory neurons revealed by a trkA-IgG fusion molecule. *Nat Med* 1995; **1**(8): 774–780.
42. Apfel SC, Wright DE, Wiiderman AM et al. Nerve growth factor regulates the expression of brain-derived neurotrophic factor mRNA in the peripheral nervous system. *Mol Cell Neurosci* 1996; **7**(2): 134–142.
43. Michael GJ, Averill S, Nitkunan A et al. Nerve growth factor treatment increases brain-derived neurotrophic factor selectively in TrkA-expressing dorsal root ganglion cells and in their central terminations within the spinal cord. *J Neurosci* 1997; **17**(21): 8476–8490.
44. Shu XQ, Mendell LM. Neurotrophins and hyperalgesia. *Proc Natl Acad Sci USA* 1999; **96**(14): 7693–7696.
45. Cho HJ, Kim SY, Park MJ et al. Expression of mRNA for brain-derived neurotrophic factor in the dorsal root ganglion following peripheral inflammation. *Brain Res* 1997; **749**(2): 358–362.
46. Karim F, Bhave G, Gereau RW. Metabotropic glutamate receptors on peripheral sensory neuron terminals as targets for the development of novel analgesics. *Mol Psychiatry* 2001; **6**(6): 615–617.
47. Taiwo YO, Levine JD. Further confirmation of the role of adenyl cyclase and of cAMP-dependent protein kinase in primary afferent hyperalgesia. *Neuroscience* 1991; **44**(1): 131–135.
48. Taiwo YO, Bjerknes LK, Goetzl EJ et al. Mediation of primary afferent peripheral hyperalgesia by the cAMP second messenger system. *Neuroscience* 1989; **32**(3): 577–580.
49. Aley KO, Levine JD. Role of protein kinase A in the maintenance of inflammatory pain. *J Neurosci* 1999; **19**(6): 2181–2186.
50. Levine JD, Taiwo YO. Involvement of the mu-opiate receptor in peripheral analgesia. *Neuroscience* 1989; **32**(3): 571–575.
51. Kress M. Role of inflammatory mediators and the response of primary afferents. In: Justins D (ed.) *Pain 2005 – an updated review: refresher course syllabus*. Seattle: IASP Press; 2005: 197–205.
52. Dray A, Perkins M. Bradykinin and inflammatory pain. *Trends Neurosci* 1993; **16**(3): 99–104.
53. Ji RR. Peripheral and central mechanisms of inflammatory pain, with emphasis on MAP kinases. *Curr Drug Targets Inflamm Allergy* 2004; **3**(3): 299–303.
54. Levine JD, Lan W, Kwiat G et al. Leukotriene B4 produces hyperalgesia that is dependent on polymorphonuclear leukocytes. *Science* 1984; **225**(4663): 743–745.
55. Bennett G, al-Rashid S, Hoult JR et al. Nerve growth factor induced hyperalgesia in the rat hind paw is dependent on circulating neutrophils. *Pain* 1998; **77**(3): 315–322.
56. Amann R, Schuligoi R, Lanz I et al. Effect of a 5-lipoxygenase inhibitor on nerve growth factor-induced thermal hyperalgesia in the rat. *Eur J Pharmacol* 1996; **306**(1–3): 89–91.
57. Amann R, Schuligoi R, Herzeg G et al. Intraplantar injection of nerve growth factor into the rat hind paw: local edema and effects on thermal nociceptive threshold. *Pain* 1996; **64**(2): 323–329.

58. Levine JD, Lam D, Taiwo YO et al. Hyperalgesic properties of 15-lipoxygenase products of arachidonic acid. *Proc Natl Acad Sci USA* 1986; **83**(14): 5331–5334.

59. Piomelli D. The ligand that came from within. *Trends Pharmacol Sci* 2001; **22**(1): 17–19.

60. Horigome K, Pryor JC, Bullock ED et al. Mediator release from mast cells by nerve growth factor. Neurotrophin specificity and receptor mediation. *J Biol Chem* 1993; **268**(20): 14881–14887.

61. Lewin GR, Rueff A, Mendell LM. Peripheral and central mechanisms of NGF-induced hyperalgesia. *Eur J Neurosci* 1994; **6**(12): 1903–1912.

62. Tam SY, Tsai M, Yamaguchi M et al. Expression of functional TrkA receptor tyrosine kinase in the HMC-1 human mast cell line and in human mast cells. *Blood* 1997; **90**(5): 1807–1820.

63. Rice AS, Farquhar-Smith W, Nagy I. Endocannabinoids and pain: spinal and peripheral analgesia in inflammation and neuropathy. *Prostaglandins Leukot Essent Fatty Acids* 2002; **66**(2–3): 243–256.

64. Watkins LR, Goehler LE, Relton J et al. Mechanisms of tumor necrosis factor-alpha (TNF-alpha) hyperalgesia. *Brain Res* 1995; **692**(1–2): 244–250.

65. Perkins MN, Kelly D, Davis AJ. Bradykinin B1 and B2 receptor mechanisms and cytokine-induced hyperalgesia in the rat. *Can J Physiol Pharmacol* 1995; **73**(7): 832–836.

66. Abbadie C. Chemokines, chemokine receptors and pain. *Trends Immunol* 2005; **26**(10): 529–534.

67. Ueda H. Molecular mechanisms of neuropathic pain – phenotypic switch and initiation mechanisms. *Pharmacol Ther* 2006; **109**(1–2): 57–77.

68. Bridges D, Thompson SW, Rice AS. Mechanisms of neuropathic pain. *Br J Anaesth* 2001; **87**(1): 12–26.

69. Gold MS. Spinal nerve ligation: what to blame for the pain and why. *Pain* 2000; **84**(2–3): 117–120.

70. Pertin M, Ji RR, Berta T et al. Upregulation of the voltage-gated sodium channel beta2 subunit in neuropathic pain models: characterization of expression in injured and non-injured primary sensory neurons. *J Neurosci* 2005; **25**(47): 10970–10980.

71. Shim B, Kim DW, Kim BH et al. Mechanical and heat sensitization of cutaneous nociceptors in rats with experimental peripheral neuropathy. *Neuroscience* 2005; **132**(1): 193–201.

72. Decosterd I, Ji RR, Abdi S et al. The pattern of expression of the voltage-gated sodium channels $Na(v)1.8$ and $Na(v)1.9$ does not change in uninjured primary sensory neurons in experimental neuropathic pain models. *Pain* 2002; **96**(3): 269–277.

73. Flatters SJ, Bennett GJ. Ethosuxamide reverses paclitaxel- and vincristine-induced painful peripheral neuropathy. *Pain* 2004; **109**(1–2): 150–161.

74. Hudson LJ, Bevan S, Wotherspoon G et al. VR1 protein expression increases in undamaged DRG neurons after partial nerve injury. *Eur J Neurosci* 2001; **13**(11): 2105–2114.

75. Ueda H, Rashid MH. Molecular mechanism of neuropathic pain. *Drug News Perspect* 2003; **16**(9): 605–613.

76. Di MV, Blumberg PM, Szallasi A. Endovanilloid signaling in pain. *Curr Opin Neurobiol* 2002; **12**(4): 372–379.

77. Syriatowicz J, Hu D, Walker JS et al. Hyperalgesia due to nerve injury: role of prostaglandins. *Neuroscience* 1999; **94**(2): 587–594.

78. Perkins NM, Tracey DJ. Hyperalgesia due to nerve injury: role of neutrophils. *Neuroscience* 2000; **101**(3): 745–757.

79. Theodosiou M, Rush RA, Zhou XF et al. Hyperalgesia due to nerve damage: role of nerve growth factor. *Pain* 1999; **81**(3): 245–255.

80. McLachlan EM, Rush RA, Zhou XF et al. Peripheral nerve injury triggers noradrenergic sprouting within dorsal root ganglia. *Nature* 1993; **363**(6429): 543–546.

Central mechanisms

Introduction

The central nervous system includes the spinal cord and brain. It is where the information from the peripheral nerves is integrated and modulated. Although there are pathways that are largely involved with specific roles, the system is not hard wired. With regard to pain modulation, there is a significant degree of plasticity that may be reversible, but in some situations becomes irreversible. This is significantly influenced by primary afferent nociceptive input, ion channels and second messenger systems.

Dorsal horn

The dorsal horn is no longer considered as a simple synaptic relay station. It is now known to play a key role in the modulation of pain and development of chronic pain states. The dorsal horn is an area in which there is convergence of primary afferent input and modulatory pathways; these act together to control the ongoing transmission of electrical activity within the pain pathways to supraspinal structures. Pain is only perceived if this electrical activity reaches the brain and, hence, any modulation or alteration within the dorsal horn can have profound effects on pain sensation.

The cell bodies of primary afferent neurones are located in the dorsal root ganglion. The cell body produces all of the materials required for that neurone to function properly. These cell bodies have a peripheral branch that innervates tissues and a central branch that enters the dorsal horn. It is important to recognise that these central branches have more than one synaptic end and have many dendrites. Therefore, one peripheral nerve has the potential to influence multiple central neurones.

Primary afferent neurones can be divided into Aβ (transmitting touch), Aδ (transmitting the fast component of pain) and C fibres (transmitting the slow component of pain). These fibres enter the dorsal horn and terminate in different Rexed lamina[1] (Table 6.1). Within the dorsal horn there is a body surface map; neighbouring peripheral receptive fields have neighbouring central terminals. There is also some collateralisation (i.e. to neighbouring spinal segments) of the central terminals via Lissauers tract. In health, these are silent, as the amount of membrane depolarisation in the collaterals is only ever enough to cause an end-plate postsynaptic potential that never reaches threshold for propagation of an action potential. Under conditions of increased primary afferent traffic, this may not hold true. If the amount of neurotransmitter released at the collaterals is enough then the degree of depolarisation will reach threshold and an EPSP will occur, resulting in an action potential. This may be one cause for how individual neurones can increase their receptive field under conditions of nerve injury. This is an example of where primary peripheral nerves have an influence on multiple central neurones.

Somatic input to the dorsal horn is via peripheral nerves. Visceral nociceptive input also involves Aδ and C fibres, travelling with the autonomic nervous systems.

In addition to the central terminals of primary afferent neurones, the dorsal horn contains propriospinal neurones, projecting neurones and local interneurones.[1]

Propriospinal neurones transfer inputs between segments at a local level within the dorsal horn. They have the potential to form multisynaptic pathways to the brainstem.

Projecting neurones, or *second-order neurones*, transmit sensory information from the dorsal horn, via the thalamus, to the brain. This onward transmission stimulates descending modulatory systems that can facilitate or inhibit nociceptive transmission within the dorsal horn. This occurs either directly or via descending nerves acting on local inhibitory or excitatory interneurones.

TABLE 6.1 Termination point of primary afferent neurones in the dorsal horn of the spinal cord as classified by the Rexed lamina

| Fibre type | Dorsal horn Rexed lamina termination | |
	Principal	*Weak*
Aβ fibres (touch)	III	
	IV	
	V	
Aδ fibres (fast pain)	I	II
		X
Cutaneous C-fibres (slow pain)	I	V
	II	X
Visceral C-fibres (visceral pain)	I	
	V/VI	
	X	

Adapted from Millan MJ. The induction of pain: an integrative review. Progress in Neurobiology 1999; 57:1–164

Second-order neurones

The majority of nociceptive projecting neurones are contained in the lateral part of the spinothalamic tract. Some projecting neurones are carried in other tracts such as the spinomesencephalic, spinoreticular, spinobulbar and post-synaptic dorsal column.[2]

Fibres of the spinothalamic tract originate from Rexed lamina I, IV, V, VII and VIII.

Lamina I

Lamina I contains predominantly *nociceptive-specific* (fusiform) cells that receive primary afferent input from Aδ and C fibres, as suggested by their name these cells receive individual pain modalities (mechanical, thermal or chemical). There are also *polymodal nociceptive cells* (responding to more than one nociceptive modality) receiving predominately C fibre input and *thermoreceptive-specific* (pyramidal) cells that respond to cold. Lamina I spinothalamic tract cells appear to transmit information to the thalamus that is specific for a particular modality, i.e. heat, cold, mechanical or chemical.

Lamina IV and V

Lamina IV and V contain the wide dynamic range (WDR) neurones. WDR neurones are innervated by Aβ touch fibres and also by Aδ and C pain fibres. They play an important role in the integration of stimulus intensity. WDR neurones receive primary afferent fibres from skin, muscle and viscera. As such they are implicated in viscero-somatic referral. This is where *referred pain* occurs at a site on the body wall innervated by the same spinal segment as that innervated by the viscera. The brain misinterprets information from the WDR neurones as coming from the body wall instead of the viscera itself. For example, irritation of the diaphragm often results in pain being felt in the shoulder tip on the affected side; this happens because primary afferents from the diaphragm enter the spinal cord at C3, C4 and C5, the same level as the somatic structures around the shoulder tip.

Under conditions of central sensitisation (discussed below) as well as referred pain being present, it is possible for there to be referred hyperalgesia (increased response to a stimulus which is normally painful) and referred allodynia (pain due to a stimulus that does not normally provoke pain) within somatic structures.[3]

Interneurones

Interneurones are cells with short axons that act at a very localised level within the dorsal horn. Interneurones play an important role in the 'tone' of the dorsal horn. At any one time it is highly likely that both inhibitory and excitatory interneurones are active at the same time and at the same synaptic clefts. This allows for a state of balance between facilitation and inhibition of onwards pain processing within the dorsal horn. The advantages of having dual controls are that the system becomes more sensitive and can be adjusted in either direction by altering either system. Descending modulatory control systems influence the interneurones and may be either inhibitory or excitatory.

Inhibitory interneurones

Inhibitory interneurones contain γ-aminobutyric acid (GABA) and glycine. Release of these neurotransmitters has both presynaptic and postsynaptic effects:

- Presynaptic receptor effects lead to a reduced amount of neurotransmitter being released from primary afferent neurones in response to depolarisation by an action potential.
- Postsynaptic receptor effects cause an inhibitory postsynaptic endplate potential (IPSP) that reduces the chances of an excitatory postsynaptic potential (EPSP) reaching the threshold for an action potential to be produced.

γ-aminobutyric acid

GABA acts via two different receptors:[4]

1. $GABA_A$ receptors are chloride-permeable ion channels that on activation generally hyperpolarise cells; therefore reducing the chance of threshold being reached by the influence of excitatory transmitters.
2. $GABA_B$ receptors are G-protein coupled receptors. Activation of these inhibits adenylyl cyclase, decreasing calcium currents and increasing potassium currents, thus hyperpolarising neurones and decreasing neurotransmitter release.

Glycine

Glycine acts via a chloride-permeable ion channel, activation of which hyperpolarises neurones in a similar way to $GABA_A$.[4]

This is in contrast to glycine's activity at N-methyl-D-aspartate (NMDA) receptors where it enhances the effect of the excitatory neurotransmitter glutamate. Glycine, therefore, has the potential to have both excitatory and inhibitory effects.

Excitatory interneurones

Excitatory interneurones act in a similar manner; their effects are mediated by glutamate as a neurotransmitter and increase the likelihood of a postsynaptic endplate potential reaching the threshold for production of an action potential.

Descending modulation

Descending modulatory control is bidirectional in nature. It may be either inhibitory or excitatory.[5] These descending control systems link the brain cortex, via a complicated network, to the dorsal horn, acting either directly on primary afferents, projecting neurones, or indirectly via inhibitory and excitatory interneurones, glial cells and immune cells, or at terminations of other descending modulatory pathways. The ability for modulatory control to act at both inhibitory and excitatory interneurones suggests either the presence of more than one neurotransmitter or there being more than one receptor subtype that results in opposing actions.

Study of the pathways of descending control suggests that the same supraspinal structures are involved in both descending inhibition (DI) and descending facilitation (DF). Indeed, it is possible that the same neurotransmitters are implicated in both DI and DF acting on different receptor subtypes.[6]

Descending modulatory control fibres tend to reach the dorsal horn in the dorsolateral and ventrolateral funiculi. It is unclear as to whether one carries DI and the other DF; it is, however, likely that they transmit both.

Supraspinal sites of origin

Hypothalamus

The hypothalamus plays a role in coordinating autonomic and sensory information. There are extensive links with the nucleus tractus solitarius (NTS), periaqueductal grey matter (PAG), rostroventral medulla (RVM) and with higher corticolimbic structures that are implicated in the affective and cognitive components of pain. The corticolimbic structures implicated are the somatosensory area of the postcentral gyrus, anterior cingulate cortex (ACC), the insular cortex and the medial prefrontal cortex.

Different nuclei within the hypothalamus have different roles. The medial preoptic nucleus projects to the PAG and RVM and has a role in the autonomic response to pain. Stimulation of this nucleus exerts descending inhibition. The anterior hypothalamus projects to wide dynamic range (WDR) neurones in the dorsal horn also causing descending inhibition. Stimulation of the lateral hypothalamus inhibits nociception through noradrenergic pathways via the PAG and RVM.[7]

The parabrachial nucleus appears to mimic the role of the hypothalamus with regards to pain, again coordinating autonomic and sensory information.

Nucleus tractus solitarius

Stimulation of the NTS leads to descending inhibition, but vagal stimulation of the NTS can trigger descending facilitation in the dorsal horn.

Dorsal reticular nucleus

The dorsal reticular nucleus of the medulla projects to both superficial and deep laminas of the dorsal horn. Stimulation of this nucleus leads to hyperalgesia via descending facilitation. This nucleus is involved in diffuse noxious inhibitory control: the process by which tissue damage and pain in one area elicits analgesia in other areas of the body. For example, when you next accidentally stub your toe try biting your lip or tongue.

Periaqueductal grey matter

The PAG appears to play a pivotal role in the modulation of nociceptive processing in the dorsal horn: GABAergic antagonists, cannabinoids and μ opioid agonists all initiate descending inhibition in the PAG via monoaminergic mechanisms. The PAG has direct and indirect input from the dorsal horn and is closely interconnected with all of the above structures and corticolimbic structures (frontal cortex and amygdala). Some PAG fibres project directly to the dorsal horn acting via substance P and cholecystokinin, but most fibres synapse with serotonergic and non-serotonergic neurones of the RVM and with the A7 noradrenergic nucleus of the medulla.[6]

Rostroventral medulla

The rostroventral medulla has been shown to contain different classes of neurones. There are 'OFF' cells that are excited by opioids and inhibited by nociceptive input: they are thought to contribute to the induction of descending inhibition. There are 'ON' cells that are inhibited by opioids and excited by nociceptive input: they are thought to trigger descending facilitation.[8]

Role of descending modulation

There is a critical balance between descending inhibition and facilitation within the dorsal horn. This can be rapidly altered according to both internal and external environments. Alterations tend to be reversible but can become irreversible under pathological conditions.[6]

The importance of descending inhibition is that it confines the extent of neuronal receptor fields. This has the effect of decreasing the likelihood of pain compromising performance under stressful or dangerous conditions. It also plays a role in the control of pain in circumstances where pain is anticipated. Descending facilitation on the other hand is protective and recuperative. The hyperalgesia promoted by DF leads to protection of the area of tissue damage and also normalises nociception following stressful or dangerous conditions.

Fear and anxiety have divergent effects on pain experience. Fear, as an immediate alarm system towards present threat, results in sympathetic arousal and inhibition of pain. Anxiety invokes hypervigilance towards bodily states and leads to increased attention towards pain.[9] In both animal and human studies fear leads to a reduced response to pain and anxiety to an increased response to pain.[10,11]

One hypothesis proposed for placebo analgesia is via descending modulation and is a route shared by opioid analgesia. Using positron emission tomography (PET) scanning researchers have shown that there is increased activity in the anterior cingulate cortex (ACC) during both these forms of analgesia.[12]

Under conditions of long-term noxious stimulation, descending inhibition is enhanced; this counterbalances the noxious stimulation. During pathological conditions, in which there may be irreversible changes in the dorsal horn, such as long-term potentiation, that enhance the excitability of nociceptive processing, the dorsal horn possibly becomes unresponsive to descending inhibition. Unfortunately, descending facilitation may continue to exert effects that promote nociceptive transmission.

Mechanisms of descending modulation

Descending modulatory neurotransmitters can be divided into:

- monoaminergic neurotransmitters: norepinephrine, dopamine and serotonin
- non-monoaminergic neurotransmitters: histamine, vasopressin, oxytocin, acetylcholine, GABA and glycine.

Norepinephrine

Norepinephrine, acting as an α_2-adrenergic receptor agonist leads to:

- inhibition of voltage-dependent calcium channels thus suppresses calcium ion currents
- activation of potassium ion currents
- inhibition of adenylyl cyclase, reducing intracellular (cAMP) levels.

All these actions lead to inhibition of the neurone. Presynaptic inhibition of primary afferent fibres, postsynaptic inhibition of projecting neurones or excitatory interneurones all lead to descending inhibition.

However, norepinephrine also acts as an α_1-adrenergic receptor agonist that has an excitatory influence through:

- activation of calcium currents
- activation of phospholipase C
- suppression of potassium currents.

This leads to presynaptic excitation of primary afferent fibres, postsynaptic excitation of projecting neurones or excitatory interneurones resulting in descending facilitation (Table 6.2). It should be noted that excitation of an inhibitory interneurone causes descending inhibition and inhibition of inhibitory interneurone causes descending facilitation.

This is an example of one neurotransmitter, in this case norepinephrine, having opposite effects, depending on which receptor and which cell it acts on. Dopamine and serotonin have similar actions, mediated by specific receptor subtypes that can lead to descending inhibition or facilitation.[6]

Non-monoaminergic neurotransmitters

Some of the non-monoaminergic neurotransmitters appear to be similar to norepinephrine, in that different receptor subtypes are involved in DI or DF. According to their mode of action at ionophores or how they are coupled (positively or negatively) to a particular enzyme (that if active may increase or decrease the excitability of neurones).

Other non-monoaminergic neurotransmitters, such as GABA, are solely inhibitory.

TABLE 6.2 Norepinephrine as an example of descending activity, having facilitatory or inhibitory effects in the dorsal horn of the spinal cord: opposing effects are due to its agonist affect at different receptors

Receptor	Site of action	Neurone type	Effect
α_2-adrenergic receptor agonist	Presynaptic inhibition Postsynaptic inhibition	Primary afferent Projecting neurones Excitatory interneurones	Descending inhibition
α_1-adrenergic receptor agonist	Presynaptic excitation Postsynaptic excitation	Primary afferent Projecting neurones Excitatory interneurones	Descending facilitation

Effects of nociceptor input

Under normal conditions, noxious stimulation of a nociceptor results in propagation of an action potential along $A\delta$- or C-fibres to the dorsal horn. The frequency of the afferent input at the dorsal horn is proportional to the magnitude of the noxious stimulus.[13] At this central synapse the action potential causes fusion of vesicles with the synaptic membrane that releases substance P and glutamate into the synaptic cleft. The amount of neurotransmitter released is proportional to the frequency of afferent input. These neurotransmitters activate neurokinin 1 (NK1) and α-amino-3-hydroxy-5-methyl-4-isoxazole propionic acid (AMPA) receptors respectively on the postsynaptic membrane. The activation of these receptors leads to an EPSP that is proportional to the amount of neurotransmitter released. Only if the EPSP reaches threshold will the dorsal horn neurone propagate an onward action potential. Hence, the magnitude of the response of a dorsal horn neurone is related to the magnitude of the evoking stimulus.

Substance P

Substance P is a neuropeptide neurotransmitter that activates NK1 receptors. The NK1 receptor is coupled to a G-protein, causing a slow depolarisation of second-order neurones by activation of phospholipase C. Activation of phospholipase C increases formation of inositol 1,4,5-triphosphate (IP_3). Calcium is released from IP_3-sensitive calcium stores leading to increased cytoplasmic calcium concentrations, resulting in depolarisation of the second-order neurone.[4] The increased cytoplasmic calcium concentrations are also responsible for activating phosphokinase C which increase the likelihood of phosphorylation of the NMDA receptor (as described below).[14]

Glutamate

Glutamate acts at three different classes of receptor:

- α-amino-3-hydroxy-5-methyl-4-isoxazole propionic acid (AMPA) receptors
- N-methyl-D-aspartate (NMDA) receptors
- Metabotropic receptors.

All these receptors have different subtypes and would be best described as families of receptors. More than one agent may have an influence on activating or inhibiting these receptors either directly or indirectly.

AMPA receptors

AMPA receptors are cation channels, their activation leads to a potent and fast depolarisation of second-order neurones and they are implicated in ongoing processing of nociception.

NMDA receptors

NMDA receptors are also cation channels. At resting membrane potential they are blocked by the presence of magnesium ions. They are important in central sensitisation and long-term potentiation and are discussed later.

Metabotropic receptors

Metabotropic receptors are G-protein-coupled receptors (GPCRs):

- Group I activate phospholipase C. This increases cytoplasmic calcium concentrations. In turn phosphokinase C is activated resulting in inhibition of potassium currents and activation of calcium channels, thereby enhancing neuronal excitability.
- Group II and III are negatively coupled to adenylyl cyclase, via inhibitory G-proteins, reducing cytoplasmic cAMP concentrations and cAMP-dependent protein kinase activation.[15]

WDR neurones

WDR neurones in Rexed lamina V are unusual in that they receive afferent input from Aβ and C fibres. Aβ fibre stimulation causes depolarisation of WDR neurones that is perceived as innocuous. It also causes a small depolarisation within primary afferent Aδ- and C-fibres. This occurs via presynaptic stimulation of local excitatory interneurones and is referred to as primary afferent depolarisation (PAD).[16] This depolarisation in Aδ- and C-fibres is not normally enough to initiate an EPSP reaching threshold. This may help explain the phenomena of allodynia where an innocuous stimulus results in pain being perceived. Under normal circumstances the PAD may have a presynaptic inhibitory effect on Aδ- and C-fibres and help explain the action of transcutaneous electrical nerve stimulation (TENS) and possibly dorsal column stimulation. This is an area that has not been fully elucidated.

Wind up

Repetitive stimulation by C-fibres (at a frequency of between 0.3 and 3 Hz) causes some WDR cells in the dorsal horn to augment their response. Thus, for a given input stimulus, the output is enhanced. This process is referred to as *wind up* and is very transient. If the evoking stimulus is withdrawn then the dorsal horn reverts to normal. Wind up is part of a process termed *central sensitisation*. Central sensitisation involves an increase in the receptive field of a nociceptor, an increase in the magnitude and duration of response to a noxious stimulus and a reduction in the threshold required to stimulate nociceptors.

Physiology of central sensitisation

NMDA receptors

Central sensitisation is triggered by C-fibre input and involves WDR neurones and NMDA receptors. NMDA receptors are unusual in two respects to other ligand-gated ion channels. First they require simultaneous binding of glutamate and glycine as a coagonist, for effective activation. Second, NMDA receptors, at resting membrane potentials, are blocked by the presence of a magnesium ion. When this block is present, glutamate, while binding to the receptor, is unable to cause opening of the channel.[17] The magnesium ion can only be removed under two circumstances (Fig. 6.1):

- Firstly, it will be removed as the membrane becomes progressively more depolarised
- Secondly, it will be removed if the NMDA receptor is phosphorylated. Phosphorylation occurs by activation of protein kinase C (PKC) or tyrosine kinases within the WDR neurone.

After the NMDA ion channel opens there is a rapid influx of calcium and sodium ions. PKC is calcium dependent (as is protein kinase A (PKA) and calcium-calmodulin-dependent protein kinase II). The influx of calcium and sodium ions leads to action potentials that reach threshold for propagation to the thalamus, but also increases the likelihood of phosphorylation of the NMDA receptor resulting in an ion channel that is more likely to open in response to glutamate (i.e. potentiation of synaptic strength). Thus a positive feedback loop develops.

Within the dorsal horn NMDA receptors are also found presynaptically on small-diameter nociceptive primary afferent fibres (PAF). Activation of these causes release of substance P from the PAF.[18] AMPA receptors are also phosphorylated by PKC and PKA resulting in potentiation of these receptors as well.

Repetitive electrical stimulation of both C- and Aδ-fibres leads to a potentiation of synaptic strength both *in vitro* and *in vivo*. This is often referred to as long-term potentiation (LTP).[19]

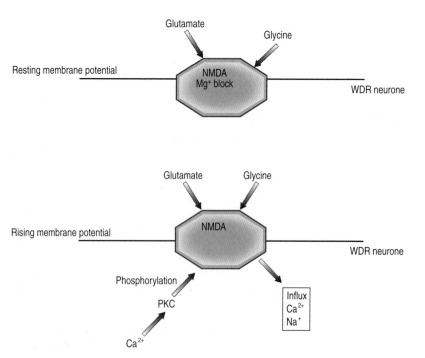

Fig. 6.1 NMDA receptors on wide dynamic range neurones (WDR). In the resting state the agonist glutamate and coagonist glycine have a limited effect on the membrane potential due to magnesium blocking the ion channel. Activation of the receptor is increased by a rising membrane potential or by phosphorylation of the receptor by protein kinase C (PKC) that is itself calcium dependent

Nitric oxide

Calcium also leads to induction of nitric oxide synthase, which catalyses the conversion of L-arginine into citruline and nitric oxide (NO). There are three isoforms of NO synthase:

- Type I and III are constitutive and calcium dependent
- Type II is an inducible form responsive to cytokines and also activated by calcium

NO is a highly diffusible molecule with a very short half-life and cannot be stored in vesicles like other neurotransmitters. NO may act within the cell that produced it, presynaptically or on other neighbouring cells. NO is very likely to be pro-nociceptive. Inhibitors of NO synthase have been shown to reduce hyperalgesia and allodynia associated with central sensitisation in a rat model.[20]

Researchers have shown that activation of NMDA receptors leads to NO production that then enhances the production of glutamate, i.e. a positive feedback.[21]

Long-term potentiation

Blockade of AMPA receptors, NMDA receptors and neurokinin receptors will prevent the induction of LTP in the dorsal horn, but only blockade of NMDA receptors will affect its maintenance in the dorsal horn. This shows that while other receptors are important in the initiation of LTP it is the NMDA receptor that is essential to maintain it.

LTP is involved in many neurological processes. It plays a role in learning within the hippocampus, leading to the ability for experiences to be turned into long-term memories.

LTP is a more prolonged response than wind up. It may start immediately, or take some time to develop after an initial noxious stimulus. It can last for hours, days or life (particularly in the case of memories).

Primary afferent depolarisation

As previously mentioned, there is collateralisation of central terminals of C-fibres via Lissauers tract. Under conditions of excess primary afferent traffic these synapses could be involved in nociceptive transmission, particularly if the dorsal horn cells they synapse with become sensitised (either by wind up or long-term potentiation).

In normal neurones, Aβ stimulation leads to PAD of nociceptive fibres that will not usually reach threshold. After an injury peripheral nociceptors at the injury site become sensitised. This leads to persistent afferent traffic within C-fibres resulting in sensitisation of the local dorsal horn interneurones. This sensitisation results in these excitatory interneurones becoming overtly responsive, such that a tactile stimulus transmitted along Aβ fibres leads to a more intense PAD that is strong enough to reach threshold for propagation within a nociceptive second-order neurone.[16] Thus, touch becomes painful, referred to as allodynia. A second potential mechanism for allodynia is that following nerve injury or ongoing peripheral inflammation, it is possible for Aβ fibres to switch on production of chemicals, such as substance P, that is conventionally confined to nociceptive fibres.[22] In essence, they switch their phenotype.

Effects of nerve injury

Following injury to nerves, or axotomy, it is well recognised both in animal models and humans that changes within the dorsal horn occur. These changes are possibly related to the maintenance of allodynia.

Anatomical changes

Anatomical changes include the loss of up to one-third of DRG cells, the loss of some synaptic connections and the development of some new abnormal synaptic connections. Damage to C-fibres appears to drive this process.

Following nerve damage:

- there is loss of synaptic connections from C-fibres within lamina II
- myelinated Aβ fibres sprout new dendrites that synapse within lamina II (which normally has no synapses from Aβ fibres)[23]
- additionally these large myelinated fibres that normally respond to innocuous stimuli start to express vanilloid 1 receptors (VR1) which are activated by capsaicin.[22]

Nerve growth factor

Nerve growth factor (NGF) is a neurotrophin that plays a key role in the development and maintenance of the nervous system. NGF acts by being a potent regulator of gene expression, for both receptor and ligand concentrations (including the tetrodotoxin (TTX)-resistant sodium channel subunit Na_v 1.8 and VR1 receptors). Nerve damage causes an interruption of retrograde transmission of NGF from the periphery to the dorsal horn[24] and it is recognised that administration of exogenous NGF can prevent these synaptic changes occurring. There are other important neurotrophic factors, such as NT3 (which supports large-diameter sensory neurones) and glial cell-line-derived neurotrophic factor (which supports small-diameter nociceptive neurones).

Autonomic nervous system

Activity in nociceptors leads to increases in sympathetic discharge. However, in 'normal' people the reverse is not true: activity in the sympathetic system does not lead to increases in nociception.

Following nerve injury it has been shown in humans and animal models that there is an abnormal connection between the sympathetic and the sensory nervous systems. Nociceptors start to express α-adrenergic receptors and become responsive to α-adrenergic agonists such as noradrenaline (norepinephrine) that is released from sympathetic nerve terminals. This leads to persistent afferent traffic that sensitises second-order neurones. A group of people following minor injury develop pain that is maintained by the sympathetic nervous system, referred to as sympathetically maintained pain (SMP). The mechanisms for this are complex and poorly understood.

Following peripheral nerve axotomy, there is increased expression of NGF in satellite cells (oligodendrocytes) surrounding the sensory neurone cell bodies in DRG.[25] This may be responsible for the sprouting of sympathetic fibres within the DRG that is observed following nerve injury[26] and leads to a 'basket' of sympathetic neurones within the DRG. Evidence supporting this includes:

- sympathetic neurones that sprout and form baskets express NGF receptors
- NGF causes sympathetic basket formation
- anti-NGF treatment reduces nerve-injury-induced basket formation.

Following partial nerve injury, nerve fibres start to express α_2-adrenergic receptors, in addition, large and medium diameter DRG cells start to express vanilloid receptors for capsaicin at the same time as up-regulating their expression of α_2-adrenergic receptors.[27] These changes mean that damaged neurones become more responsive to α-adrenergic agonists such as noradrenaline (norepinephrine). The normal release of noradrenaline (norepinephrine) from efferent sympathetic nerve terminals, and possibly the sprouted baskets, now influences nociceptive neuronal fibres in the DRG. There are two α-adrenergic receptors involved in SMP; α_1-adrenergic receptors on nociceptors (postsynaptic) lead to excitation, while α_2-adrenergic receptors present on sympathetic nerve terminals (presynaptic) inhibit the release of noradrenaline (norepinephrine).

Immune cells and chronic pain

Immune and glial cells may also have a role in maintaining chronic pain states. Within the central nervous system there are approximately 10^{11} neurones and 10–50 times as many glial cells.[28] These cells become activated, hypertrophied and swollen after both central and peripheral nerve injury. They become activated by glutamate, substance P and calcitonin gene-related peptide (CGRP) released from the central terminals of nociceptive primary afferent fibres. Activation of glial cells leads to: production of pro-inflammatory cytokines, ATP and neurotrophic factors, such as NGF; the up-regulation of cyclo-oxygenase 2 (COX-2), resulting in increasing amounts of prostanoids; and also the up-regulation of nitric oxide synthase, leading to increasing amounts of NO. These actions are probably mediated by calcium currents. However, all these mediators are also produced by neuronal cells and it is difficult to be clear what proportion is due to activation of glial cells. What is clear, though, is that these mediators are all implicated in the maintenance of chronic pain.[29,30]

Genetics and pain

The variability in pain sensitivity both in different genders and in different ethnic groups suggests a role for genetics in pain. The role of these genes is then modified by environmental factors to create major differences in pain sensitivity. Examining the role of genetics is a challenge for many reasons. There are likely to be a multitude of genes involved, all with different interactions and, additionally, environmental, social, psychological, physiological and developmental factors all contribute to variability in pain perception and tolerance. Pain perception is different among different ethnic groups[31] and there are genetic factors involved in gender differences to pain.[32] Rarely, gene mutations can lead to decreased pain sensitivity, as in hereditary sensory and autonomic neuropathy (HSAN), these mutations lead to frequent injuries. Much more commonly, genetic variation is due to small differences in numerous genes. Recent findings in chronic lower back pain have suggested that there may be a genetic contribution involved; a single-nucleotide polymorphism of the endogenous interleukin-1 receptor antagonist may be associated with increased pain levels.

With regards to analgesics, it is well recognised that some people are poor metabolisers of codeine. In this subset of the population there is a mutation in a cytochrome P450 gene resulting in the reduced ability to metabolise codeine to morphine. In the cytochrome P450 family there are also poor and ultra-fast metabolisers of nortriptyline.

KEY POINTS

- The central nervous system has significant plasticity, with changes being both reversible and irreversible
- The dorsal horn is a point of convergence for peripheral afferent information integration prior to ascending transmission to supraspinal structures
- There is descending modulation of spinal nociceptive activity that may be facilitatory or inhibitory
- The same neurotransmitter can have opposing effects depending on which receptors it act on (e.g. noradrenaline (norepinephrine) on α_1- and α_2-adrenoreceptors or glycine on chloride channels and NMDA receptors)
- NMDA receptors require glutamate as an agonist and glycine as a coagonist
- Wind up is a transient central augmentation of afferent activity increasing the patients' awareness of C-fibre activity; it reverts to normal on withdrawal of the stimulus
- Central sensitisation involves an increase in the receptive field of a nociceptor, an increase in the magnitude and duration of response to a noxious stimulus and a reduction in the threshold required to stimulate nociceptors; this may not be reversible
- Nerve injury has anatomical and physiological consequences that influence central changes and central sensitisation; these include new dendrite formation, new connections with the sympathetic nervous system as well as altered receptor expression

---

References

1. Millan MJ. The induction of pain: an integrative review. *Prog Neurobiol* 1999; **57**(1): 1–164.
2. Craig AD, Dostrovsky JO. Medulla to thalamus. In: Wall PD, Melzack R (eds). *Textbook of pain*. London: Churchill Livingstone; 1999: 183–214.
3. Giamberardino MA. Visceral pain. In: *Pain Clinical Updates*. Seattle: IASP; 2005: 1–6.
4. Ganong WF. Synaptic and junctional transmission. In: Ganong WF (ed.) *Review of Medical Physiology*. New York: Lange Medical Books/McGraw–Hill; 2005: 85–120.
5. Ren K, Dubner R. Descending modulation in persistent pain: an update. *Pain* 2002; **100**(1–2): 1–6.
6. Millan MJ. Descending control of pain. *Prog Neurobiol* 2002; **66**(6): 355–474.
7. Fields HL, Basbaum AI. Central nervous system mechanisms of pain modulation. In: Wall PD, Melzack R (eds). *Textbook of pain*. London: Churchill Livingstone; 1999: 309–329.

8. Fields HL, Heinricher MM, Mason P. Neurotransmitters in nociceptive modulatory circuits. *Annu Rev Neurosci* 1991; **14**: 219–245.

9. Barlow DH, Chorpita BF, Turovsky J. Fear, panic, anxiety, and disorders of emotion. In: Hope DA (ed.) *Nebraska symposium on motivation, 1995: perspectives on anxiety, panic, and fear. Current theory and research in motivation.* Lincoln, NE: University of Nebraska Press; 1996: 251–328.

10. Lichtman AH, Fanselow MS. Cats produce analgesia in rats on the tail-flick test: naltrexone sensitivity is determined by the nociceptive test stimulus. *Brain Res* 1990; **533**(1): 91–94.

11. Rhudy JL, Meagher MW. Fear and anxiety: divergent effects on human pain thresholds. *Pain* 2000; **84**(1): 65–75.

12. Petrovic P, Kalso E, Peterson ICM et al. Placebo and opioid analgesia – imaging a shared neuronal network. *Science* 2002; **295**(5560): 1737–1740.

13. Guyton AC. Sensory receptors; neuronal circuits for processing information. In: Guyton AC (ed.) *Textbook of medical physiology.* Philedelphia, PA: W.B. Saunders; 1991: 495–506.

14. Yaksh TL. Molecular biology of pain. In: Warfield CA, Bajwa ZH (eds). *Principles and practice of pain medicine.* New York: McGraw-Hill; 2004: 13–27.

15. Neugebauer V. Metabotropic glutamate receptors – important modulators of nociception and pain behavior. *Pain* 2002; **98**(1–2): 1–8.

16. Cervero F, Laird JM. Mechanisms of touch-evoked pain (allodynia): a new model. *Pain* 1996; **68**(1): 13–23.

17. Petrenko AB, Yamakura T, Bata H et al. The role of N-methyl-D-aspartate (NMDA) receptors in pain: a review. *Anaesth Analg* 2003; **97**: 1108–1116.

18. Liu H, Mantyh PW, Basbaum AI. NMDA-receptor regulation of substance P release from primary afferent nociceptors. *Nature* 1997; **386**: 721–724.

19. Sandkühler J. Learning and memory in pain pathways. *Pain* 2000; **88**: 113–118.

20. Wu J, Fang L, Lin Q et al. Nitric oxide synthase in spinal cord central sensitization following intradermal injection of capsaicin. *Pain* 2001; **94**: 47–58.

21. Sorkin LS. NMDA evokes an L-NAME sensitive spinal release of glutamate and citrulline. *Neuroreport* 1993; **4**: 479–482.

22. Rashid MH, Inone M, Kondo S et al. Novel expression of vanilloid receptor 1 on capsaicin-insensitive fibers accounts for the analgesic effect of capsaicin cream in neuropathic pain. *J Pharmacol Exp Ther* 2003; **304**: 940–948.

23. Cameron AA, Cliffer KD, Dougharty A et al. Time course of degenerative and regenerative changes in the dorsal horn in a rat model of peripheral neuropathy. *J Comp Neurol* 1997; **397**: 428–442.

24. Raivich G, Hellweg R, Kreutzberg GW. NGF receptor-mediated reduction in axonal NGF uptake and retrograde transport following sciatic nerve injury and during regeneration. *Neurone* 1991; **7**: 151–164.

25. Zhou XF, Dong YS, Xian CJ et al. Neurotrophins from dorsal root ganglia trigger allodynia after spinal nerve injury in rats. *Eur J Neuroscience* 2000; **12**: 100–105.

26. Ramer MS, Thompson SW, McMahon SB. Causes and consequences of sympathetic basket formation in dorsal root ganglia. *Pain Supplement* 1999; **6**: S111–S120.

27. Ma W, Zhang Y, Bantel C et al. Medium and large injured dorsal root ganglion cells increase TRPV-1, accompanied by increased alpha2C-adrenoceptor co-expression and functional inhibition by clonidine. *Pain* 2005; **113**(3): 386–394.

28. Ganong WF. Excitable tissue: nerve. In: Ganong WF (ed.) *Review of medical physiology.* New York: Lange Medical Books/McGraw-Hill; 2005: 51–84.

29. McMahon SB, Cafferty WBJ, Marchand F. Immune and glial cell factors as pain mediators and modulators. *Experimental Neurology* 2005; **192**: 444–462.

30. Hansson E. Could chronic pain and spread of pain sensation be induced and maintained by glial activation. *Acta Physiologica* 2006; **187**: 321–327.

31. Lasch KE. Culture and pain. In: *Pain clinical updates.* Seattle: IASP; 2002.

32. Kim H, Dionne RA. Genetics, pain and analgesia. In: *Pain clinical updates.* Seattle: IASP; 2005: *XIII*(3).

Allistair Dodds

Non-pharmacological interventions

Introduction

Pain is usually a symptom of an underlying pathology. It represents increased electrical activity in the peripheral nerves, spinal cord and brain.

Melzack and Wall (1965) published the 'gate theory' of pain;[1] in essence this states that the central nervous system is capable of modulating its response to incoming electrical activity from pain nerves. As a result of filtering, the perception of pain in the higher centres of the brain is amplified or reduced according to the prevailing environmental and emotional context. A consequence of the gate theory, is that pain is susceptible to the placebo effect.

A conflict may arise as a consequence of our training to judge efficacy based on controlled trial data and the recognition that, on a humanitarian level, the use of non-pharmacological treatments may reduce suffering and pain, despite the fact they may not be proven to have an effect greater than placebo. This leads to a tension between non-pharmacological treatments and evidence-based medicine. If pain is an electrical entity within the brain of patients that can be modified by endogenous means (e.g. the placebo effect),[2] we must ask ourselves if it is reasonable to withhold such treatments.

A second important issue is the use of population statistics for what is a very personal subjective experience. If a purely symptomatic treatment for an individual is helping, should they be denied this opportunity because other patients within the cohort fail to benefit from the same treatment? If we are to use a pragmatic, rather than evidence-based approach, we should factor in the exceptionally low side effect profile of most of the following treatments and remember that the outcome for the patient is usually improved by a reduction of pain (e.g. less suffering, improved compliance with physiotherapy or other rehabilitation protocols). Modern medicines' desire to eradicate treatments that are not proven to be better than placebo may in fact be counterproductive for certain individuals, assuming that they do not suffer from significant side effects.

There are insufficient data from underpowered trials regarding non-pharmacological treatments for pain. The use of meta-analysis is hampered by difficulties with producing a control arm in the trial and widely differing protocols. (Think about it: how do you produce an effective, believable, sham arm for TENS?) It is often tempting to regard no evidence as a negative association with respect to any given treatment rather then a wake-up call that large well-controlled studies of sufficient power are urgently needed.

This chapter will review the commonly used non-pharmacological treatments of pain:

- Cold
- Heat
- Support and immobilisation
- TENS
- Acupuncture
- Homeopathy.

Cold

The application of cold (or ice) to an acutely inflamed or injured tissue is usually done as part of the RICE protocol (rest, ice, compression, elevation). Together with simple analgesia this forms the backbone of management of most minor injuries within the Accident and Emergency Department. In the acute phase, immediately after injury, it is preferable to the application of heat. Cooling the injured tissue reduces the inflammatory response, which in turn may attenuate pain.

Mode of action

The application of ice (in a protective coat) can:

- reduce histamine release
- promote vasoconstriction
- decrease muscle spindle activity, which may help to reduce 'protective' muscle spasm further, reducing pain and disability.[3]

Although a wide variety of delivery systems are available both commercially and home made, it is important that ice is not directly applied to the injury – it is both messy and can lead to damage to the skin. It is normal to wrap the frozen material (or ice) in a cloth (e.g. tea towel) before application. Whilst commercially available gel packs are often more convenient, they are obviously more expensive and less likely to be immediately available within the home.

Cautions

The application of cold is not suitable for all injuries. A history should be taken to exclude Raynauds disease, paroxysmal cryoglobulinaemia and cold haemoglobinuria. Great care should be taken in those with arterial insufficiency or sickle cell disease. It is also important not to contaminate open wounds.

The underlying injury should be regularly inspected for new skin damage. A normal application time might be 10–20 min subject to visual assessment.

Heat

The application of heat has long been used to relieve pain and expedite physiotherapy. It is used after the acute inflammatory response has subsided.

Modes of action

- Vasodilation – may inhibit the accumulation of inflammatory mediators. Tends to make oedema and ecchymoses worse
- Muscle relaxation (subjective) – reduction in reported muscle spasm despite a tendency to facilitate afferent nerve conduction
- Central mechanism – modulation of spinal cord activity reducing pain transmission and perception.

Two types of heat therapy are commonly used, conductive heat therapy and radiant heat therapy.

Conductive heat therapy

This involves the direct application of heat to the damaged tissue. Often an inexpensive and convenient option, this is familiar to patients and requires little expertise to administer safely. A variety of gel-filled pockets are available, together with those containing beads. They can be quickly and conveniently warmed by a microwave oven. Alternatively a hot water bottle can be used; the specific heat capacity of water makes it useful for extended use, but care must be taken to provide an insulating layer to prevent direct thermal injury. The temperature of the tissues can be raised by several degrees celcius by this method. It is very important that the patient does not feel the area to be 'uncomfortably hot'.

Radiant heat

This involves the indirect application of heat (e.g. from a heat lamp). Infrared energy can be used as a surface heating agent in those patients unable to tolerate direct contact of the heater with the skin. This method may be better tolerated in the presence of sensitive skin (e.g. allodynia). The equipment is often less convenient to use and requires a higher degree of skill to avoid a thermal burn.

Indications

- Analgesia
- Reduce muscle spasm
- Increase mobility.

Contraindications

The largest drawback of heat application is the potential for inducing thermal injury to the underlying tissues. The provision of feedback from the patient is the key to avoiding a burn. Clearly anything that impedes this process is a relative contraindication:

- Insensitive skin – nerve damage, local anaesthesia
- Decreased level of consciousness or communication difficulties
- There is a tendency to increase oedema and bruising
- Heat therapy is contraindicated in the presence of a burn.

Support and immobilisation

The immobilisation of damaged tissues can minimise pain from secondary hyperalgesia (the pain associated with the inflammatory response). It can be provided in a number of ways:

- Plaster of Paris
- 'Soft' and 'hard' collars
- Corsets
- Bandages (elastic and crepe)
- Splints (e.g. Thomas, Zimmer, Box)
- Direct traction (e.g. Steinman pins).

Immobilisation represents an effective analgesic strategy with minimal systemic side effects. It can, however, cause local problems such as:

- Stiffness
- Loss of muscle power and bulk
- Deep vein thrombosis.

The need for immobilisation and support must be regularly reviewed. The short-term use of splinting devices in association with physiotherapy often facilitates a good recovery, simultaneously limiting the need for analgesic use.

When used in a chronic setting, the stiffness and restriction of movement can be counterproductive leading to a significant diminution of function (e.g. tendon shortening) and must be used with great care.

TENS (transcutaneous electrical nerve stimulation)

TENS machines are in common use both in the hospital and home environments. Its lack of systemic side effects has bolstered its popularity despite the data suggesting that it has limited efficacy.[4]

The mechanism of action of TENS is not well understood. Electrical stimulation of cutaneous structures at the segmental level of the injured tissues may, via the gate-control theory, reduce onward transmission of nociceptive pain information from the spinal cord to the brain.

There are two variants of TENS in terms of mode of action:

1. High-intensity, low-frequency stimulation of cutaneous structures (acupuncture-type TENS) produces analgesia that is antagonised by naloxone (an opioid receptor antagonist). Its effects are thought to be

mediated by the endogenous opioids, the endorphins and enkephalins. It tends to give slow-onset, long-duration analgesia.

2. Low-intensity, high-frequency (conventional TENS) probably works through the direct stimulation of large-diameter myelinated sensory skin fibres (Aβ). This results in analgesia when applied at the spinal segmental level associated with the area of tissue injury. The effect of this type of TENS is not altered by naloxone and may operate through GABAergic mechanisms.

Indications

Most trials of TENS are small, low-powered and suffer from difficulties in providing a convincing placebo for comparison. Meta-analysis of the trials is fraught with difficulties as the mode, intensity and duration of stimulation often varies greatly between trials.

What little evidence there is, suggests that TENS should, at most, be used as an adjunct in acute pain (consistently less effective than licensed pharmaceutical agents).[4]

TENS appears to influence the severity of labour pain very little.[5] In this context TENS may be behaving as a (useful) placebo.

There are some positive studies in chronic pain (above cautions not withstanding).

Some motivated individuals find TENS a useful adjunct to their overall pain management plans.

Contraindications

- Electrodes should not be placed over the anterior aspect of the glottis. Stimulation of the neural or muscular tissues could potentially occlude the airway whilst stimulation of the carotid sinus may lead to detrimental cardiovascular changes.
- The electrodes should only be placed on skin with intact sensation (to improve efficacy and minimise the risk of electrical burns to the skin).
- Open wounds and healing skin should be avoided to reduce the risk of infection.
- In today's medico-legal climate, stimulation over the pregnant uterus is ill advised. Although any premature contractions or spontaneous abortion is likely to be coincidental, most manufacturers recommend against this practice despite a lack of incriminating evidence.
- Implantable devices, such as pacemakers, dorsal column stimulators and intrathecal delivery systems may be vulnerable to interference from a TENS unit. Any attempt to use a TENS in these circumstances should be referred to the physician with overall responsibility for the implant.
- TENS should not be used in situations where the electrodes could short circuit (e.g. bathing).
- TENS should not be used whilst driving or operating machinery. A device malfunction or short-circuit could distract the patient resulting in accidental injury.
- TENS is less well tolerated by those at the extremes of age. Children often find the stimulation uncomfortable or intolerable. The elderly and patients with cognitive impairment may find the use of TENS intimidating or confusing. They are at increased risk of electrical burns.

Use of TENS

Consent for TENS should include a description of the parasthesias produced by the unit (often described as pins and needles, prickling or burning). The patient should be warned that prolonged or excessive use might burn underlying skin; occasionally it causes an increase in pain severity. TENS is generally used as an adjunct to analgesia rather than replacement therapy.

Pads

Two types of pads are commonly used:

1. Self-adhesive electrodes are more convenient, less messy and easier to apply. They should be replaced on the supplied plastic strip and can be used repeatedly. Placing them in a refrigerator between treatments can extend their adhesive properties.
2. Carbonised rubber electrodes and conducting gel are fiddly and less convenient to use, but have the advantage of being more economical. These pads are preferred in those patients who are allergic to self-adhesive electrodes, because of the availability of a wide range of conducting gels that may be used with the inert carbon rubber.

Placement of pads

TENS pads can be placed in two general ways:

- Associated with peripheral nerve innervation; generally placed longitudinally along the course of the nerve. This can produce helpful parasthesia in the affected area.
- In the territory associated with a spinal segment serving the injured tissue. This may not provide paraesthesia in the territory of the wound but can help to influence pain control (modulation) at a spinal segmental level.

The pads should never touch, to prevent short-circuiting. Multiple electrode channels may be needed to stimulate large areas of skin as the current required to produce adequate stimulation increases the further the electrodes are apart.

The placement of pads requires a degree of dexterity that has to be considered before trailing TENS. A patient's carer may be able to assist in electrode placement. Manual dexterity often limits the potential use of this technique.

Connection to the TENS unit

The electrodes are connected to the stimulator via leads, usually marked positive and negative. When multiple channels (commonly 2) are used it is important to attach the leads to electrode pairs in conjunction with the guidelines above.

TENS unit (pulse generator)

Despite numerous trials, no single pattern of stimulation has proven to be the most effective. In general terms TENS stimulation can be divided into:

1. High-frequency, low-amplitude (conventional TENS).
2. Low-frequency, high-intensity type (acupuncture type).

Patients should be encouraged to experiment with their settings, altering the frequency and pulse width to find an effective strategy.

TENS manufacturers often include additional features such as ramped, random and burst modes. They are aimed at reducing tolerance in experienced users by modulating the signal.

Conventional TENS

Apply the pads as described above. Attach the electrode cables between the pads and pulse generator, ensuring it is switched off. Select a moderately high frequency (100 Hz) and a pulse width of about 100 ms. Allow the patient to switch the device on and increase the amplitude until a 'strong but comfortable' feeling is achieved in the affected area. Allow time for the patient to acclimatise to the stimulus (equivalent to tachyphylaxis) and increase the amplitude as necessary. The patient is instructed to administer the treatment for 20–30 min three times daily. The unit should be switched off prior to disconnecting the pads.

Acupuncture-type TENS

Using the same approach as above, but a low frequency of 1–10 Hz is selected, with a longer pulse width of 200–250 ms. The amplitude is increased until strong stimulation is perceived. Muscle twitching is normal (even desirable), but the stimulation should be below the threshold for pain. The duration of this treatment should again be approximately 30 min.

Characteristics of different modes of TENS

Conventional
- More immediate pain relief
- Effect often stops shortly after unit is switched off.

Acupuncture type
- Slower onset of analgesia
- May need repeated stimulations to achieve effect
- Once endogenous opioid production is stimulated, effect is often prolonged.

Complications

- *Electrical burns* often associated with skin that does not have normal innervation or when the current amplitude is too high.
- *Allergic reactions*: consider switching electrode manufacturer if using disposable pads, or switching to carbonised rubber paddles and conducting gel.
- *Inflamed skin*: ensure the position of the electrodes is changed regularly, the electrodes are not worn when not in use and that a high level of hygiene is maintained.
- *Tolerance to effect*: consider changing stimulation frequencies, trying additional modes, such as random or burst, or using a TENS holiday (temporarily stop using the machine).

Acupuncture

The origins of acupuncture are obscure. It is known to have been practised in the Far East before the birth of Christ. The discovery of the tattooed body of 'Oetzi', the Tyrolean 'iceman' has led to speculation that some of the tattoos on his body signify acupuncture points. If this is the case, the first evidence for acupuncture is, therefore, from Central Europe around 3300 BC.

Mode of action

Chinese medicine has a complex and elaborate structure to describe ill health. The aim of acupuncture is to harmonise the flow of Qi (Chi) (life energy) to restore balance within the individual and heal disease.

Western medicine's explanation of the pain relief resulting from acupuncture uses the concept of neuromodulation. This is the complex interaction of electrical signals and chemical neurotransmitters, which modify the behaviour of neural tissue.

Acupuncture can often be antagonised by naloxone (an opioid antagonist), leading to the assumption that endogenous opioids such as enkephalin and endorphin are produced in response to this treatment. The increased expression of these chemicals leads to a partial closure of the 'pain gate' and consequently pain relief.

Traditional Chinese vs. Western medical traditions

Relatively recently healthcare professionals in the West have become interested in acupuncture. They have tended to dispense with the traditional practises of 'pulse and tongue diagnosis' in favour of a more conventional approach. A standard approach of history, examination and investigation is used. Acupuncture may be used to support conventional treatment (e.g. combined with physiotherapy), or as a primary treatment where the patient requires only symptom control.

Point location

Traditional Chinese medicine takes many years to master and has an elaborate system for the identification of acupuncture points. The Western medical variant is greatly simplified and, consequently, introductory sessions can be completed in a weekend for health professionals.

The acupuncture site should have normal innervation; changes are unlikely to occur at spinal-cord level if the stimulus cannot be perceived. Sites showing signs of infection are not suitable for needling.

In the Western medical variant needles may be used as follows:

- Direct needling of myofascial trigger points (areas of knotted muscle palpated by the practitioner).
- 'Local' acupuncture points in the vicinity of the injury.
- Myotomal points – acupuncture points within a muscle to stimulate the appropriate level within the spinal cord.
- Sclerotomal points: as above but stimulation of bony structures.
- Distant points: borrowed from traditional Chinese acupuncture.

Complications

Acupuncture is an extremely safe technique, but complications do exist. The following factors must be considered before embarking on treatment:

- There is a risk of haemorrhage in patients with a bleeding diathesis, e.g. haemophilia or use of warfarin.
- In pregnant patients certain points are associated with miscarriage. It must be borne in mind that coincidental occurrences may be blamed on acupuncture.
- Transmission of blood-borne viruses or infection: this can be minimised by the use of single-use needles, which is preferable to autoclaving and reusing needles. This should be supplemented by a high standard of hand hygiene.
- Vulnerability of implanted devices (e.g. pacemakers and dorsal column stimulators) to electrical interference from electro-acupuncture.
- Patients who respond very strongly may be unable to drive home safely due to excessive sedation.
- Vasovagal responses due to a psychological response to needles. Patients should be positioned to minimise this problem.
- Underlying structures may be damaged with aggressive needle techniques; for example, it is possible to penetrate pleura or renal tissue. The needles are of a very small diameter, much smaller than biopsy needles used by conventional medicine, and serious organ damage is very rare.

Treatment sessions

Like all biological reactions, the increased production of opioids can take some time. Often it is necessary to give four to six sessions of acupuncture before evaluating the efficacy of the treatment. If successful, the treatment may need to be consolidated with many more sessions.

The use of myofascial trigger points is often associated with a virtually instantaneous improvement in pain. The mechanism of action in this case is local to the muscle.

Augmentation of acupuncture

Sometimes it is necessary to use methods to give very high levels of stimulation. This may be necessary in the context of chronic pain. The commonest techniques are:

- *manual stimulation*: where the needle is rotated or moved by hand
- *electro-acupuncture*: the use of an alternating current between adjacent acupuncture needles, which often leads to muscle contractions causing the needles to oscillate. Vasovagal responses are more common. Electro-acupuncture can interfere with pacemakers and implanted devices (e.g. dorsal column stimulators)
- *moxibustion*: the rolled leaves (moxa) of the herb *Artemisia vulgaris* can be attached to an implanted acupuncture needle and ignited. There is a risk that the needle will transmit sufficient heat to damage cutaneous and deep structures. The technique is only suitable for experienced practitioners with sufficient anatomical knowledge to prevent damage to peripheral nerves.

Indirect and direct moxibustion are the techniques of holding a burning roll of *Artemisia vulgaris* near to an acupuncture point or direct burning of the skin respectively. Occasionally practitioners may deliberately leave the burning cone of moxa on the site to cause a burn and consequential scarring.

Efficacy

Of all the complementary-type medicines acupuncture is the best studied using validated scientific tools. The beginning of a consensus for the efficacy of acupuncture is appearing in chronic and acute back pain,[6] headache[7] and osteoarthritis of the knee[8] amongst others.

Homeopathy

In recent years homeopathy has gained considerable favour with the general public, yet many 'mainstream' medical practitioners remain sceptical. Homeopathy is a system originally developed by Samuel Hahnemann, based upon the principle of similars. This states that an undiluted agent causing certain symptomatology in a healthy individual can be used in a potentiated form to heal similar symptoms in the sick. Potentiation is the serial dilution and vigorous shaking (*succussion*) of the agent.

A thorough unhurried history is taken (the clinician often having superior interpersonal communication skills) and after a diagnosis is made, a remedy is prescribed. Single or multiple agents are used. *Arnica, hypericum* and *staphisagria* are commonly prescribed remedies for the treatment of pain.

The art of potentiation brings the system into conflict with the laws of chemistry and pharmacokinetics as the potentiated solutions are felt to be more beneficial as the dilution increases. Dilutions can be centile (C) or decile (D) and refer to 100-fold and 10-fold dilutions respectively. The integer following the dilution factor represents the number of serial dilutions (e.g. D2 represents two 10-fold dilutions). Common remedies can be so dilute that it is questionable if any active ingredient remains at greater that C12/D24 dilutions. Exponents of the art of homeopathy refer to imprinting of the solvent by the active ingredient, which may no longer be physically present; it is not clear what this represents in pharmacological terms.

There are many published trials of homeopathic remedies, some positive, others negative; it is not clear where the truth lies.[9,10] Confounding factors for the analysis of data include:

- Much of the trial data are widely heterogeneous and meta-analysis is often inappropriate
- Publication bias is often cited by sceptics as an explanation of the many positive trials
- Weak trial methodology
- Small sample size
- Publication in 'alternative journals'.

The questions raised by homeopathy are unlikely to be answered until a systematic research effort is made using high-quality trials of sufficient power with clear, focused clinical objectives.

KEY POINTS

- Some non-pharmacological interventions are simple to institute with few complications
- The evidence base for non-pharmacological interventions is weak and studies often poorly designed
- A balance has to be reached over individual patient benefit and the broader statistics for low-risk interventions. It may be that an individual who gains a good response (possibly placebo) with few risks should not be denied such interventions
- Support and immobilisation have a greater role in acute pain situations
- TENS has significant popularity despite the weak evidence base; this is an area where further research is required
- Acupuncture has some good evidence developing with a role in musculoskeletal pain
- Homeopathy has significant popular appeal, but the absence of adequate studies leaves many questions unanswered

---

References

1. Melzack R, Wall PD. Pain mechanisms: a new theory. *Science* 1965; **150**(699): 971–979.
2. Petrovic P, Kalso E, Petersson K. Placebo and opioid analgesia – imaging a shared neuronal network. *Science* 2002; **295**(5560): 1737–1740.
3. Eldred E, Lindsley DF, Buchwald JS. The effect of cooling on mammalian muscle spindles. *Exp Neurol* 1960; **2**:144–157.
4. Carroll D, Tramer M, McQuay H et al. Randomization is important in studies with pain outcomes: systematic review of transcutaneous electrical nerve stimulation in acute postoperative pain. *Br J Anaesth* 1996; **77**(6): 798–803.
5. Carroll D, Tramer M, McQuay H et al. Transcutaneous electrical nerve stimulation in labour pain: a systematic review. *Br J Obstet Gynaecol* 1997; **104**(2): 169–175.
6. Furlan AD, van Tulder MW, Cherign DC et al. Acupuncture and dry-needling for low back pain. *Cochrane Database Syst Rev 2005*; (1): CD001351.
7. Melchart D, Linde K, Berman B et al. Acupuncture for idiopathic headache. *Cochrane Database Syst Rev 2001*; (1): CD001218.
8. Berman BM, Lao L, Langenberg P et al. Effectiveness of acupuncture as adjunctive therapy in osteoarthritis of the knee: a randomized, controlled trial. *Ann Intern Med* 2004; **141**(12): 901–910.
9. Kleijnen J, Knipschild P, ter Riet G. Trials of homeopathy. *BMJ* 1991; **302**(6782): 960.
10. Lokken P, Straumshiem P, Tveiten D et al. Effect of homoeopathy on pain and other events after acute trauma: placebo controlled trial with bilateral oral surgery. *BMJ* 1995; **310**(6992): 1439–1442.

Andrew Lloyd

Non-steroidal anti-inflammatory drugs and paracetamol

Introduction

The lowest rung on the World Health Organization (WHO) analgesic ladder for cancer pain management consists of non-opioid, simple analgesics.[1] The main members of this drug group are the non-steroidal anti-inflammatory drugs (NSAIDs) and paracetamol. Despite the term 'simple' they are very effective in treating mild-to-moderate somatic pain, cancer pain and acute pain. Their use perioperatively has consistently demonstrated an opioid-sparing effect. Treating the inflammatory component of chronic musculoskeletal conditions constitutes their greatest use worldwide with over 100 million people taking NSAIDs regularly.[2]

NSAIDs work as anti-inflammatory analgesic agents by blocking the production of prostaglandins and the prostaglandin-mediated sensitisation of peripheral tissues to noxious stimuli. They also exhibit an anti-pyretic action. The widespread nature and complexity of the prostaglandin system has resulted in difficulty targeting NSAID actions purely to those of analgesia. The term 'simple' belies the fact that these drugs (some available as over-the-counter medications) have both minor and major side effects, even at recommended dosage.[3] Significant gastro-intestinal, renal and coagulation systems effects have been documented over the years. Increased pharmacovigilance following the recent introduction of the Coxib class of NSAIDs has led to greater awareness and understanding of the associated cardiovascular risks.

Paracetamol, although having no demonstrable peripheral anti-inflammatory action, is thought to have a central anti-inflammatory effect and is discussed with the NSAIDs.

Prostaglandins

'Eicosanoid' is an umbrella term referring collectively to locally acting, lipid mediators that have been derived from the 20-carbon unsaturated fatty acid arachidonic acid.

Subdivided into:

- prostanoids (prostaglandins, prostacyclin and thromboxanes)
- leukotrienes.

These agents are traditionally viewed as playing an important role in initiating, sustaining and resolving inflammatory processes with effects on platelets, vascular smooth muscle and mast cells. Prostaglandins (PGs) are involved in the control of a wide range of the body's systems and processes.

Prostaglandins originally extracted from the prostate gland (hence the name), are, in fact, ubiquitous throughout the body. They play a variety of 'housekeeping' roles, such as temperature control, maintenance of gastric mucosal integrity and renal perfusion, in addition to their effects on immune and inflammatory processes.

From a pain perspective, they are believed to be involved in the sensitisation of tissues to inflammatory mediators and also to affect neurotransmitter release in the central nervous system.

Prostaglandin actions are localised to the vicinity of the cell in which they are produced, but their widespread nature leads to significant effects throughout the body. Although not stored in cells, various stimuli can significantly increase prostaglandin production.

Prostaglandin synthesis

An enzymatic chain of reactions is involved in the conversion of phospholipids within cell membranes into active prostaglandins (Fig. 8.1).

There are three main steps:

1. The production of arachidonic acid by the action of phospholipase on membrane phospholipid.
2. The enzyme cyclo-oxygenase (COX) catalyses the conversion of arachidonic acid into the cyclic endoperoxides (PGG_2 and PGH_2).
3. Cyclic endoperoxides are then converted into a variety of tissue-specific prostaglandins.

Steroids inhibit the first step (by increased production or activation of the inhibitor protein lipocortin).

NSAIDs inhibit the second step by acting on the COX enzymes.

The prostaglandin nomenclature appears confusing. For example, PGD_2 and PGE_2 cause bronchoconstriction whereas PGI_2 is responsible for bronchodilatation. PGA_2, PGE_2 and PGI_2 cause arteriolar vasodilatation and thromboxane A_2 vasoconstriction, but PGF_{2a} can cause vasoconstriction or vasodilatation, depending on the vascular bed involved. PGE_2 and PGI_2 have the majority of effects on pain mechanisms, with PGD_2 having little or no pain activity.

Fig. 8.1 The production of prostaglandins

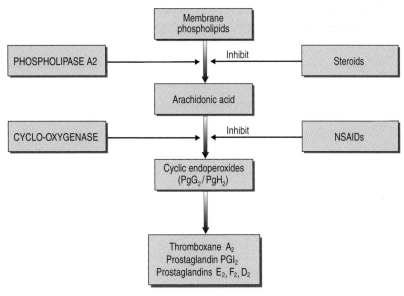

Prostaglandin-mediated pain

Tissue injury results in the release of a multitude of chemical substances that mediate the inflammatory process. Some are thought to directly activate nociceptors, while others act indirectly on mast cells, macrophages and other inflammatory cells to enhance the release of substances, such as bradykinin, serotonin and histamine. Other mediators produce a hyperalgesic effect by modifying nociceptor action, sensitising the response to both noxious (chemical, thermal and mechanical) and normally innocuous stimuli.

A variety of receptors have been identified in the dorsal root ganglia and more distally in peripheral nociceptive nerve fibres. These include specific receptors for PGE_2, PGD_2 and PGI_2, with the coupling of each receptor to a particular G-protein determining the effects of activation.

The enzymes regulating prostaglandin synthesis, COX, are expressed in inflammatory cells, dorsal root ganglia and in the spinal cord itself.[4] Animal models have shown up-regulation of the enzyme and hence increased levels of prostaglandins, both peripherally and centrally, following peripheral injury.

Although NSAIDs have no significant effect on normal pain thresholds, they do attenuate the pain experienced with inflammatory conditions. There is evidence to support the theory that NSAIDs work centrally as well as peripherally (e.g. intrathecal administration of a COX inhibitor suppresses experimentally induced inflammatory hyperalgesia).

Cyclo-oxygenase

Prostaglandins were first discovered in the 1930s as substances within seminal fluid capable of causing smooth muscle contraction and changes in vasomotor tone. It was in the 1970s that Nobel Prize winning work by Sir John Vane[5] led to the discovery of the rate-limiting enzyme responsible for catalysing the first steps of prostaglandin synthesis: cyclooxygenase. Further work in the early 1990s by Needleman[6] led to the realisation that there were in fact two isoenzymes, COX-1 and COX-2.

COX-1 (constitutive)

This form of the enzyme mediates normal cellular processes. It controls the production of prostaglandins that affect homeostatic physiological functions such as temperature control, protection of the gastric mucosa, maintenance of platelet function and renal vascular tone.

COX-2 (inducible)

This form of the enzyme is predominantly involved with the body's inflammatory response, being induced by tissue damage. Increased expression in macrophages, monocytes, synoviocytes, chondrocytes, fibroblasts and endothelial cells, amongst others, leads to a rise of up to 20 times the basal level. There is also some constitutive expression in the brain, reproductive tract and kidney.

COX-2 selectivity and the development of Coxibs

Scientific work established that the noxious, painful effects of inflammation were mediated in part by prostaglandins synthesised by COX-2 and that the adverse gastrointestinal effects of NSAIDs were attributable to inhibition of COX-1. This led to what is now realised to be an overly simple hypothesis that preferential or exclusive inhibition of COX-2 would provide analgesia without the harmful effects on normal physiological processes mediated by COX-1 inhibition. As detailed below there have been benefits with the introduction of specific COX-2 inhibitors, but associated disadvantages have also come to light.

COX-3 (splice variant of COX-1)

A third form of COX has more recently been described and is found predominantly in the brain (and heart).[7] It is a variant of COX-1 that is especially sensitive to paracetamol and its related compounds. It is suggested that this may be responsible for a central mechanism of decreasing pain and fever. The COX-1 and COX-2 models do not explain paracetamol's characteristics of being anti-pyretic and analgesic without demonstrable peripheral anti-inflammatory activity.

Earlier work showed that paracetamol inhibited COX activity in dog brain homogenate more than the COX activity in splenic homogenate and thus is a potential site of action for paracetamol.[8]

Structure of COX-1 and COX-2

Targeting of specific enzymes required an advance in understanding of COX enzyme structure and was provided by X-ray crystallography. COX-1 and COX-2 were found to be structurally very similar with 65% amino acid homology. Both are membrane bound and consist of a long, narrow hydrophobic channel into which free arachidonic acid could enter. At the end of the channel is a hairpin bend around which arachidonic acid needed to be manipulated during the process of creating the prostanoid precursors.

The enzymes were found to be particularly similar around the active enzyme site. However, a single amino acid difference close to this site was found to be responsible for a slightly wider channel opening in COX-2 with a small gap in the wall of the channel allowing access to a side-pocket (Fig. 8.2).

Traditional NSAIDs were shown to block COX-1 (and COX-2) approximately half way down the main channel of the enzyme by way of a hydrogen bond developing with an arginine molecule at position 120. The presence of valine rather than isoleucine at position 523 in the COX-2 enzyme allowed the side pocket of the enzyme to be targeted for selective drug binding (COX-2). A new class of NSAID drugs was developed with a structure that is capable of making conformational changes or covalent bonds in the side-pocket to inhibit the COX-2 enzyme. These drugs, the selective COX-2 inhibitors, are termed the 'Coxibs'.

COX assays and selectivity

Measurement of NSAIDs' ability to inhibit COX-1 or COX-2 has become important when assessing their relative specificity. Most of the traditional NSAIDs block both forms of the COX isoenzyme non-selectively (Table 8.1).

While diclofenac and nimesulide have a tendency towards COX-1 inhibition, meloxicam appears to show a degree of preferential COX-2 inhibition (range 3–70-fold). Preferential does not equate with specific and at therapeutic drug levels there is still considerable COX-1 inhibitory activity. In comparison, the truly specific COX-2 drugs have inhibition ratios of the order of several hundred and negligible effects on platelets. They are so much more selective that the problem of loss of selectivity at higher doses is not a concern.

COX-1 enzyme activity is estimated from the platelet synthesis of thromboxane during clotting and that of COX-2 from the amount of PGE_2 synthesised in monocytes exposed to lipopolysaccharide. COX-2 selectivity is quoted as the

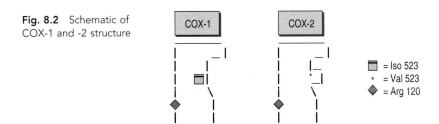

Fig. 8.2 Schematic of COX-1 and -2 structure

■ = Iso 523
* = Val 523
◆ = Arg 120

TABLE 8.1 Selectivity of COX inhibition	
Non-specific	Aspirin, diclofenac, ibuprofen, indometacin, ketorolac, mefanamic acid, naproxen phenylbutazone
Preferential	Meloxicam
Selective COX-2	Celecoxib, etodolac, etoricoxib, lumaricoxib, parecoxib

ratio COX-2 IC_{50}:COX-1 IC_{50} so that the more selective the COX-2 inhibition, the larger the quoted ratio (IC_{50} = half maximal inhibitory concentration). For example aspirin has no selectivity with a ratio of 0.26 and etodolac has a specificity ratio of 23.3. The assays used quote differences in selectivity for each drug, but they can vary 10-fold (dependent on the specific assay used). These are in vitro assays and do not necessarily predict in vivo selectivity. There is a general acceptance that a high ratio represents a lower COX-1 inhibition and a reduced overall side effect profile.

Introduction of the Coxibs

The selective COX-2 inhibitors were introduced from the late 1990s. Based on pre- and post-marketing claims, there were high hopes of reducing the risk of gastrointestinal toxicity. There was some reduction in symptoms of dyspepsia and visualisation of gastric ulcers on endoscopy, but over the longer term a significant difference in the incidence of serious gastrointestinal complications failed to be established. This was despite highly selective COX-2 suppression (e.g. celecoxib up to 375-fold).

Various explanations were postulated, including inadequate COX-2 suppression, the more frequent use of the agents in patients susceptible to gastrointestinal complications or a possible constitutive role for COX-2 within the gastrointestinal tract involving the healing of ulcers. It was subsequently demonstrated that the COX system was more complex than originally thought with COX-2 having a far greater distribution in the body. For example, high expression (of COX-2) was found in the female reproductive tract, parts of the brain and in the bowel. The role of the enzyme in these regions was not understood and several novel trials of COX-2 inhibitors as potential treatments in prevention of colorectal adenomas and Alzheimer's disease were initiated.

Increased pharmacovigilance associated with the launch of these new drugs led to an awareness of an unexpected increase in cardiovascular complications. Further evidence confirmed this increased cardiovascular risk as a class effect of the selective COX-2 inhibitors. A worldwide review followed leading to the withdrawal of several agents from the market. The cardiovascular risks of using traditional NSAIDs have also come under increasing scrutiny.

There has been significant interest and altered clinical practice as a result of a series of trials and voluntary reporting of the effects of Coxibs over recent years. The discussion below demonstrates some of the issues around research and its limitations and gives an understanding of the current situation with regard to NSAIDs use.

Selective COX-2 inhibitors

Given the vast worldwide market for the use of NSAIDs, and the high incidence of gastric side effects, the pharmaceutical companies invested heavily in developing 'safer' NSAIDs as the financial and clinical benefits were potentially huge. A series of 'Coxib' drugs were released into the marketplace in the late 1990s. Several pre-marketing randomised trials had demonstrated equivalent analgesic efficacy to the traditional NSAIDs (number needed to treat [NNT] for a 50% reduction in pain of 1.9 for 50 mg rofecoxib and 2.8 for 200 mg celecoxib), but what was the evidence that they were safer in clinical practice?

Some of these trials are briefly reviewed below to give an understanding of the issues surrounding current NSAID use and the effect of introducing the Coxibs into the market.

Vioxx GI Outcomes Research Study

The VIGOR[9] study randomised over 8000 patients with rheumatoid arthritis to receive rofecoxib (COX-2) or naproxen (traditional NSAID) for 9 months and looked at the rate of gastroduodenal perforation, symptomatic ulcer and upper gastrointestinal bleeding. The occurrence of these primary outcomes was significantly lower (50%) in the rofecoxib than the naproxen group (2.1 vs. 4.5 per 100 patient years). The corresponding NNT (i.e. the number of patients needing to be treated to prevent one major gastrointestinal event) was 42. It should be remembered that NNTs for prophylaxis (rather than treatment) will tend to be large as the relatively small number of patients affected in a large study population will result in a small difference between treatment and control groups. Patients taking aspirin were excluded from the trial.

Celecoxib Long-term Arthritis Safety Study

The CLASS[10] study randomised over 8000 patients (with either osteo- or rheumatoid arthritis) to receive celecoxib, ibuprofen or diclofenac. Originally designed to run for 12 to 15 months, the first 6 months of preliminary data were extrapolated to give a predicted rate for symptomatic ulcers and ulcer complications (bleeding/perforation/obstruction) at 1 year. The extrapolated results suggested no significant difference in the groups overall or in patients taking low-dose aspirin (20% total) for the primary outcome measure of ulcer complications. There was a suggested significant reduction in risk in the celecoxib group (2.08 vs. 3.54 per 100 patient years) for the secondary outcome of confirmed symptomatic ulcers *and* ulcer complications with an NNT of 68. Actual results from 12 months were even less impressive.

Therapeutic COX-189 Arthritis Research and Gastrointestinal Event Trial

The TARGET[11] trial enrolled 18 325 osteoarthritis patients. They took lumiracoxib, ibuprofen or naproxen for 1 year. The primary outcome was the difference in time to definite (or probable) upper gastrointestinal ulcer complication (as assessed by an independent board of experts). Lumiracoxib patients experienced significantly fewer ulcer complications overall (0.32% vs. 0.91%) and in those not also taking aspirin (0.20% vs. 0.92%). There was no significant difference in complications in patients receiving additional aspirin therapy (approximately 25%).

The randomisation process was criticised. There was a fourfold reduction in relative risk of ulcer complications, but the absolute reduction was small with approximately 120 patients requiring treatment with lumiracoxib for 1 year to avoid one ulcer complication. Ibuprofen was used in the study at a full anti-inflammatory dose of 800 mg tds, which is higher than typical clinical practice. It was noted that 2.5% of patients taking lumiracoxib had a transient rise of more than three times the baseline level in their transaminases compared to controls.

In summary, there was little conclusive evidence that patients taking Coxibs had a significant reduction in serious gastrointestinal events.

There was little insight into risk reduction in patients with a past history of ulcer complications. The only trial to show a sustained reduction in severe gastrointestinal bleeding was that involving rofecoxib, which was withdrawn from the market for cardiovascular complications.

Cardiovascular safety concerns of Coxibs

Before rofecoxib or celecoxib were approved for use in 1998, over 500 patients at low risk of cardiovascular disease had received the drug in a series of small, short trials. These studies were powered to look at pain relief, with cardiovascular events being self-reported. The US Food and Drug Administration (FDA) picked up a signal suggesting a possible increase in rates of cardiovascular events, but general release was still granted.

Subjects with recent cardiovascular events or those taking aspirin were excluded in the VIGOR trial.[9] There was no standardised procedure for collecting cardiovascular data and there was no cardiologist on the drug-safety monitoring board. These omissions have been criticised, particularly as the drug company's own scientists had discovered a significant reduction in urinary prostacyclin metabolites and raised concerns that rofecoxib might have a harmful effect on vascular endothelium.

Concerns about the cardiovascular effects of Coxibs did enter the public domain in 2000 when the VIGOR study revealed a significantly higher incidence of myocardial infarction (0.4% vs. 0.1%) in patients treated with rofecoxib than naproxen. The company voluntarily withdrew the drug from worldwide use in September 2004. This followed the release of further evidence from the APPROVE[12] trial that confirmed the findings of VIGOR that Coxibs were associated with a small increased risk of cardiovascular thrombotic events.

Adenomatous Polyp Prevention on Vioxx (APPROVE) Trial[12]

This trial enrolled 2586 patients and was randomised, placebo-controlled over 3 years looking at rofecoxib as a drug to prevent recurrence of colorectal polyps. Of the 1287 rofecoxib patients, 46 had thrombotic events (1.50 events per 100 patient years) versus 26 in the 1299 placebo patients (0.78 events per 100 patient years), a relative risk of 1.92 for myocardial infarction (MI) and cerebrovascular accident (CVA) for patients taking the drug for longer than 18 months (on reviewing the data the risk occurs earlier at 4–6 months).[13] This equates to an extra MI or CVA for every 133 patient years of treatment. This is significant when considering the number of patients worldwide taking these drugs, a market worth US $2.5 billion. In the UK alone, several hundred-thousand patients were being prescribed the drug at the time of its withdrawal.

Adenoma Prevention with Celecoxib (APC) Study[14]

In this trial, sponsored by the US National Cancer Institute, celecoxib was used in an attempt to prevent colon cancer, involving 2400 patients over a period averaging 33 months. Celecoxib was associated with an almost tripling of risk of cardiovascular events compared to placebo.

Prevention of Spontaneous Adenomatous Polyps (PRESP) Trial[15]

This pharmaceutical-company-supported trial using celecoxib was similar to the APC study in design. Using the same total daily dose of celecoxib in one dose (divided in the APC trial), the results did not show a greater risk of cardiovascular events in patients taking celecoxib compared to placebo.

Valdecoxib/parecoxib in Coronary Artery Bypass Grafting Trial

There are no long-term randomised trials looking at the use of valdecoxib or parecoxib (the pro-drug of valdecoxib) with respect to placebo or traditional NSAIDs. Two short-term, placebo-controlled studies evaluated the safety of intravenous parecoxib followed by oral valdecoxib for postoperative pain following coronary artery bypass grafting surgery (CABG).[16] Both showed higher (almost double) rates of serious cardiovascular thrombotic events in the treatment versus placebo groups. A similar study in the non-vascular general surgical setting showed no significant difference in rates of cardiovascular adverse events.

Preliminary cardiovascular conclusions

The strongest evidence for cardiovascular events is for rofecoxib. In addition to epidemiological studies suggesting a link between rofecoxib and cardiovascular events, the VIGOR trial also showed an increased risk compared to a traditional NSAID. It is estimated that between 88 000 and 140 000 cases of acute MI or sudden cardiac death occurred in the USA before it was withdrawn from the market.

For celecoxib the data were less clear. Epidemiological studies failed to link celecoxib with cardiovascular events in the same way that they had with rofecoxib. The CLASS trial found no difference in cardiovascular event rates when celecoxib was compared to the traditional NSAIDs (ibuprofen and diclofenac), but it was not powered to look at cardiovascular events and was relatively short in duration.

Conflicting trial data for the remaining COX-2 drugs made it difficult to assess if there was a true class effect. Having reviewed the data, the drug regulating authorities decided that there was sufficient evidence to confirm that the Coxibs were responsible for a small increased risk of cardiovascular thrombotic events vs. placebo, approximately 1.4-fold. Though difficult to quantify or give relative risk between the Coxibs, it was estimated to equate to no more than one extra MI or CVA for every 100 patients treated for 1 year.

The concern was that traditional NSAIDs, by inhibiting COX-2 (non-selectively) also had an increased risk of cardiovascular thrombotic events. Previous trials looked at pain relief and long-term placebo-controlled trials were not done. The long marketing history could not be equated to safety as cardiovascular events are common in the general population and drug-related events are impossible to detect from the others by means of spontaneous reporting. VIGOR had shown an increased risk for rofecoxib versus naproxen, but there was no placebo arm so the possibility remained that chronic naproxen use may also have an increased risk.

Cardiovascular safety and national agencies

In the USA the FDA[17] set up an advisory panel following rofecoxib's withdrawal. It did not recommend the withdrawn of all Coxib drugs. It was assumed that the increased cardiovascular risk with valdecoxib was similar to the other Coxibs, combined with an increased risk of serious skin conditions; valdecoxib was withdrawn from the market. The remaining NSAIDs, both Coxib and traditional, were to be contraindicated for use immediately post coronary-bypass surgery and had to carry 'black box' warnings on their packaging to indicate the increased risk of serious cardiovascular events.

A review by the European Medicines Agency[18] was also undertaken. They contraindicated the use of selective COX-2 inhibitors in patients with established ischaemic heart disease, cerebrovascular disease, peripheral vascular disease and moderate-to-severe heart failure. Patients already taking Coxibs were to be switched to an alternative. Patients with risk factors (i.e. hypertension, hyperlipidaemia, diabetes and smoking) required careful consideration including patient-specific gastrointestinal or cardiovascular risk factors and whether or not aspirin was being co-prescribed before being prescribed a Coxib.

This advice had a major impact on the management of patients with chronic pain syndromes as many of those dependent on Coxibs for management of their pain also had established ischaemic heart disease or risk factors for its development. While some pain physicians chose to use a traditional NSAID (+/− additional gastric protection medication for higher-risk patients), regular full-dose paracetamol or even opioids as an alternative; others questioned the legitimacy of the advice as the evidence seemed to point to an increased risk for all the NSAIDs, not just the Coxibs. In 2005 there were insufficient data to make firm conclusions about their safety. Evidence from trials with clinically relevant doses of traditional NSAIDs taken for long enough and powered to look accurately at cardiovascular events were awaited.

Cardiovascular safety and NSAIDs

Trials of traditional NSAIDs looking at cardiovascular risk were needed to assess their risk compared to the Coxibs.

Alzheimer's Disease Anti-inflammatory Prevention Trial (ADAPT)[19]

Epidemiological studies suggested that NSAIDs might delay or prevent the onset of Alzheimer's disease. This trial was designed to look for any effect of celecoxib on the prevention of cognitive decline. Though not specifically looking at cardiovascular events, it was the first randomised study to compare a traditional NSAID (naproxen) and placebo to long-term Coxib use. Over 2500 participants were enrolled (aged over 70 years) from 2001; the trial was halted for safety reasons in 2004 following the release of the APC trial data (showing increased cardiovascular risks with celecoxib treatment). In 2006 the safety data were published. It showed no significant difference compared to placebo in terms of the composite end-point of death, MI or CVA. This conflicted with previous studies suggesting that naproxen had a lower cardiovascular risk compared to the Coxibs, if not a protective effect similar to aspirin. These data required careful interpretation, as it was not designed to detect differences in cardiovascular and cerebrovascular risks. It was limited by the low trial mortality and small number of cardiovascular events. These results, however, did add some weight to the theory that all NSAIDs have a degree of cardiovascular risk.

MEDAL programme

This was a group of three studies (EDGE,[20] EDGE II and MEDAL[21]) looking at etoricoxib in arthritis patients around the world. Enrolling more than 34 000 patients in 38 countries, it was the largest and longest running comparison of a selective COX-2 inhibitor to a traditional NSAID. They were the first studies to have cardiovascular safety as the primary end-point.

EDGE[20] (etoricoxib vs. diclofenac sodium gastrointestinal tolerability and effectiveness trial) enrolled 7111 patients to receive etoricoxib or diclofenac with an average 9 months follow-up. The number of cardiovascular events was small with a higher incidence in patients taking etoricoxib, but did not reach statistical significance.

MEDAL[21] ran from 2002 to 2006 and was the largest component of the programme with over 23 000 patients. Etoricoxib was compared with diclofenac in treating osteo- and rheumatoid arthritis. The rate of confirmed thrombotic cardiovascular events was similar between diclofenac and etoricoxib with rates of 1.24 and 1.30 per 100 patient years respectively (approximately four extra cardiovascular events for every 1000 patients treated for 1 year). More patients in the etoricoxib groups discontinued therapy due to hypertension, but only the higher dose was associated with oedema and a trend towards increased cases of cardiac failure. The higher discontinuation rate for adverse gastrointestinal events was in patients taking diclofenac (9.1% vs. 7.1%), though the rate for upper gastrointestinal perforation/ulceration/bleeding was similar for both drugs.

Pharmacokinetics of NSAIDs

NSAIDs are most commonly taken orally in tablet or capsule form. There are formulations available for sublingual, im, intravenous, rectal or topical administration. Being weak acids with a pKa 3–5, they are rapidly absorbed via the stomach and small bowel mucosa. NSAIDs are more than 95% protein-bound restricting their volume of distribution to approximately that of the plasma volume and putting other highly protein-bound drugs at risk of having their action potentiated by being displaced (e.g. warfarin).

Metabolism is predominantly in the liver, by oxygenation and conjugation, to produce inactive metabolites that are typically excreted in urine; some are partially excreted in bile. There are variations in half lives (e.g. ibuprofen and diclofenac 2–3 hours, piroxicam 20 hours) that influence the dosing interval for individual drugs.

Adverse effects of NSAIDs (Table 8.2)

NSAIDs are generally well tolerated; however, the widespread distribution of prostaglandins and the inability to accurately target effects results in the

TABLE 8.2 Side effects of NSAIDs

Nausea
Diarrhoea
Vomiting
Drowsiness
Headache
Anxiety
Bronchospasm
Dizziness
Vertigo
Tinnitus
Photosensitivity
Haematuria
Blood disorders
Hypersensitivity reactions:
    rashes, angioedema

potential for adverse reactions. Some are made use of (e.g. aspirin's anti-platelet effect in arteriopaths), most are unwanted and harmful, and some are potentially life threatening.

Gastrointestinal

By far the commonest side effect of the NSAIDs is gastric intolerance. They directly irritate the gastrointestinal tract due to their acidic nature. NSAIDs also act indirectly, by disrupting the role prostaglandins play in the protection of the gastrointestinal tract from peptic acid and enzymes. Symptoms of nausea, dyspepsia, abdominal pain or diarrhoea may be experienced by up to one-third of patients commenced on NSAIDs. This may lead to withdraw of therapy (approximately 10%).

Life-threatening gastric perforation and haemorrhage requiring emergency surgery may occur; sometimes without prodromal symptoms or signs on endoscopy. The morbidity and mortality associated with NSAID use is significant, with upwards of 10 000 upper-gastrointestinal-related emergency admissions and 2000 deaths annually in the UK. For every 1200 patients taking NSAIDs for at least 2 months, one death will occur.[22] Factors placing patients at particular risk include: old age, alcohol excess, smoking, steroid or anticoagulant use and prolonged NSAID use. It should be noted that endoscopic findings of gastric ulceration do not necessarily correlate with symptoms of dyspepsia or with progression to perforation.

Different NSAIDs cause differing degrees of gastric iritability and complications with ibuprofen being traditionally thought of as best tolerated and aza-propazone (no longer available) as least well tolerated with the others in a spectrum between.[23] Ideally, the lowest effective dose should be used for the shortest period of time, as duration of use relates to risk of side effects. Rectal formulations, and even topical formulations, still put the upper gastrointestinal tract at risk of injury as the inhibitory effects on prostaglandins occur as a systemic effect following absorption.

Respiratory

NSAIDs precipitate acute asthma in 10–20% of asthmatics, patients with chronic airway disease may also be affected.[24] Typically, bronchospasm is accompanied by rhinitis and facial flushing, with onset usually within 1–3 hours of ingestion of aspirin or other NSAID and can be fatal (rarely). Cross sensitivity can occur between the structurally different groups of NSAIDs.

Frequently these patients are not atopic, but have increased basal levels of leukotrienes. If the COX-mediated conversion of arachidonic acid to cyclic endoperoxides is blocked by an NSAID, there will be greater production of the leukotriene inflammatory mediators by the parallel, unblocked lipoxygenase pathway. The leukotrienes act on the airways producing a degree of bronchospasm. The reaction is more likely to occur in adults than children, but all asthmatic patients should be asked before being prescribed NSAIDs if they have noted a worsening of respiratory symptoms whenever they have taken NSAIDs in the past. Particular caution should be exercised when there is an associated history of chronic rhinitis or nasal polyps.

Renal

COX-related NSAID effects on the renal system range from simple salt and water retention to acute renal impairment to rarer conditions of renal papillary necrosis, nephrotic syndrome and interstitial nephritis.

Renal function is only partially dependent on cyclo-oxygenase-derived prostaglandins. Under normal conditions these prostaglandins do not significantly affect renal physiology.[25] Under conditions of compromised renal blood flow with high levels of circulating vasoconstrictors (e.g. volume depletion), prostaglandins (PGE_2 and to a lesser extent PGD_2) play an important role in dilating the renal vascular bed to maintain blood flow. PGI_2 principally affects renal homeostatic mechanisms and PGE_2 in the thick ascending limb of the loop of Henle also promotes diuresis and natriuresis.

A reduction of PGI_2 and PGE_2 (by using NSAIDs) can predispose to renal impairment. A spectrum of effects from a non-significant rise in serum creatinine to oedema and weight gain or hypertension, and sometimes hyperkalaemia and acute renal failure may occur.

The rise in blood pressure is usually of the order of 5 mmHg. A sustained rise in diastolic pressure of this magnitude has been associated with an increased risk for both CVA and coronary heart disease (CHD). Patients with congestive cardiac failure (CCF), liver disease, pre-existing renal impairment and those on treatment for hypertension need to be observed closely. Particular caution should be exercised when co-prescribing angiotensin converting enzyme (ACE) inhibitors or diuretics in addition to NSAIDs.[26] Acute renal failure may occur within 24 hours of treatment, but is usually reversible.

Cardiovascular

Traditional NSAIDs have long been known as a risk factor for hypertension and cardiac failure, predominantly secondary to their renal effects. More recently an increased risk in cardiovascular thrombotic events, MI and CVA has emerged, initially with the use of the newer Coxib class of NSAID and latterly with the more traditional NSAIDs.[27] These risks, postulated mechanisms and the continuing debate regarding risk–benefit analysis, are discussed in detail above.

Coagulation

Thromboxane A_2 enhances platelet aggregation and, therefore, diminished levels reduce platelet aggregation, inhibiting haemostasis. This potentially increases perioperative blood loss (though there are limited data showing a direct correlation) or can exacerbate any gastrointestinal bleeding. Aspirin inhibits platelet COX irreversibly (see below). Platelet effects with the other NSAIDs are reversible and short lived depending on the half-life of the agent in question.

Bone

When bone fractures occur, an initial inflammatory phase is followed by osteoclast-driven bone resorption and subsequently osteoblast-mediated new bone formation. Prostaglandins play an important role in both this process of bone repair and in bone homeostasis. NSAIDs, though effective at treating the inflammatory pain of acute musculoskeletal injuries, may impair fracture healing. Several animal and in vitro studies have confirmed this in the experimental situation but few have shown this to be a significant effect in clinical practice. The published studies have usually been of low quality and retrospective, producing inconclusive results.[28]

Hepatic

NSAIDs can cause a small rise in liver enzymes (in approximately 10% of patients); a small minority of patients (approximately 1%) experience a more significant rise. These patients, and any others with signs or symptoms of impaired hepatic function, need close monitoring. Rarely, severe hepatic reactions occur, resulting in hepatic failure.

Skin

Most reactions occur at the start of treatment, usually within 2 weeks of commencing the drug. They are usually mild and self-limiting, but this is not always the case. Post marketing surveillance identified valdecoxib as responsible for several life-threatening serious skin reactions before being withdrawn from use. The European Medicines Evaluation Agency has issued a public statement on parecoxib (valdecoxib's prodrug) highlighting an increased risk of serious skin conditions such as Stevens-Johnson syndrome, toxic epidermal necrolysis, erythema multiforme and exfoliative dermatitis. Discontinuation of therapy should be considered at the first sign of a rash or mucosal lesion developing. Previous sulphonamide allergy is an associated risk factor.

Photosensitivity reactions have also been reported with most of the NSAIDs, but particularly with azopropazone.

Rare adverse events

There are several case reports of acute temporary visual disturbance associated with NSAID use. Exacerbations of neuro-psychiatric conditions such as depression, hallucinations and anxiety have also been recorded. These reactions can mimic naturally occurring disease in the elderly (e.g. dementia) and withdrawal of drug should be considered.

Drug interactions

NSAIDs can increase the effect of warfarin resulting in severe, potentially fatal, haemorrhage. The mechanism is not fully understood but is probably due to the displacement of warfarin from protein-binding sites. NSAID anti-platelet action will have an additive effect to warfarin's anti-coagulant effect. Close monitoring is recommended, particularly at the start of therapy and in the elderly.

Phenytoin levels can become elevated due to displacement from protein-binding sites, particularly when prescribed with high-dose ibuprofen or aspirin.

All the antihypertensive medications (β-blockers, ACE inhibitors, vasodilators and diuretics) will have their effects antagonised to some degree. Potassium levels should be monitored when using ACE inhibitors or potassium-sparing diuretics.

Reduced renal clearance due to NSAIDs can lead to toxic levels of lithium, digoxin and methotrexate.

Pregnancy

No evidence of a direct teratogenic risk exists, but NSAIDs should ideally be avoided in pregnancy, particularly in the later stages because their inhibitory action on prostaglandin synthesis may cause premature closure of the ductus arteriosus. They are sometimes used under specialist supervision on obstetric units to delay onset or prolong labour. Aspirin is sometimes used in the treatment of the pregnant patient with thrombophilia.

NSAIDs do enter breast milk with the concentration being of the order of 1–2% of maternal plasma levels. Their use in breastfeeding mothers is not recommended.

Clinical use of NSAIDs

General considerations

There are over 20 NSAIDs listed in the British National Formulary.[29] Anecdotally, inter-individual variation in the effectiveness of each NSAID can occur and in the past rotation through a series of NSAIDs would often be tried. The latest reviews on the use of NSAIDs suggest there is no evidence to support this practice. A range of NSAIDs are available in the case of poor tolerability or patient contraindication. Good prescribing practice would suggest building up experience in using a limited number of each class of drug. The lowest effective dose of a drug should also be used for the shortest possible time.

Gastrointestinal protection

The National Institute for Health and Clinical Excellence (NICE) recommended against the routine use of COX-2s in patients with osteoarthritis when it carried out its last review of the subject.[30] The Coxibs retain a role, though, in patients without cardiovascular disease and at high risk of developing serious gastrointestinal adverse events. These include those: aged 65 or over, taking concomitant medication known to increase the likelihood of upper-gastrointestinal adverse events, or requiring prolonged treatment with maximum doses of traditional NSAIDs.

The benefit–risk balance remains positive for COX-2s in patients at low risk of cardiovascular events if prescribed in accordance with the guidelines. Improved patient tolerability is a valid reason to use a Coxib rather than cheaper traditional NSAIDs. There is no gastrointestinal benefit in using a COX-2 drug for patients already taking aspirin.

For the patient at high risk of gastrointestinal injury, where Coxibs are contraindicated, several options remain. Regular, full-dose paracetamol has a good safety profile, is well tolerated and is surprisingly effective. The alternative is to combine a traditional NSAID with an additional agent:

- Misoprostol, the prostaglandin analogue, has been proven to be effective in reducing adverse gastrointestinal events. Its use is limited by cost and diarrhoea; this may be less of a problem in elderly patients.
- Ranitidine and other H2 antagonists reduce duodenal ulceration, but have not been shown to prevent NSAID-induced gastric ulcers. They may increase the probability of a serious adverse gastrointestinal event by suppressing warning symptoms, thus providing a false sense of security.
- Proton pump inhibitors such as omeprazole are effective in treating NSAID-related ulcers, but remain unproven in terms of primary prevention.

The duration of use of a Coxib, or traditional NSAID, should be reassessed periodically and modified accordingly.

The concomitant use of aspirin (or other antiplatelet drugs) increases the risk of adverse gastrointestinal events. It should only be co-prescribed if absolutely necessary, and usually with additional gastric protection (e.g. a proton pump inhibitor).

Cardiovascular safety advice

A review of the use of traditional NSAIDs undertaken by The European Medicines Agency (Oct 2006)[17] including the most up-to-date research findings considered the drugs diclofenac, etodolac, ibuprofen, ketoprofen, ketorolac, meloxicam, nabumetone, naproxen, nimesulide and piroxicam, came out in favour of their continued use. Although it was accepted that they were associated (at high doses and long term) with a small increased risk for cardiovascular thrombotic events, the risk–benefit balance was felt to remain favourable as these drugs are an important treatment modality for painful conditions such as arthritis.

Musculoskeletal conditions

There has been a move away from the first line use of NSAIDs in the management of chronic musculo-skeletal conditions in patients with, or at risk of, ischaemic heart disease. Consideration should be given to non-drug interventions and paracetamol before using NSAIDs.

Rheumatoid arthritis

Joint damage occurs early in the course of this systemic inflammatory disease and the general consensus of opinion is to use potent disease-modifying and anti-inflammatory drugs earlier to try to prevent further joint damage.

Acute pain

The above guidelines apply to chronic treatment with NSAIDs. A considerable proportion of NSAID use in the general population is over the counter, short-term treatment of acutely painful conditions and it is difficult to apply the long-term trial findings to the acute setting. No rise in cardiovascular risk has been seen with short-term use, particularly as it is usually low dose and intermittent.

The contraindication of parecoxib in coronary heart surgery led to questions regarding the cardiovascular safety of its short-term use in the perioperative period for other types of surgery. A meta-analysis of 4000 patients who received parecoxib perioperatively found no significant difference from placebo with regards to the incidence of cardiovascular events.[31] The cardiovascular risk for short-term use of these drugs perioperatively is assumed to be very small and NSAIDs continue to have a role within balanced analgesia techniques by reducing opioid requirements and improving the quality of postoperative recovery.

Aspirin (acetylsalicylic acid)

The use of plant-derived salicylates to treat pain and fever can be traced back to the earliest civilisations. The Reverand Edmond Stone from Chipping Norton in Oxfordshire published the first description of the use of willow bark to reduce fever in 1763. Salicylic acid was identified as the active component in 1828, 40 years later it was successfully synthesised.

Bayer, a German pharmaceutical company coined 'aspirin' as a trade name in 1899. Named partly on the plant genus from which it is derived, or one of the scientists who isolated the active substance (depending on which version of the story one believes), the rights to the trade name were lost by the company at the end of the First World War. The drug and name were being copied by various manufacturers, leading to the acceptance of aspirin as a generic term. Although used for over 100 years to treat minor aches and pains, aspirin's mechanism of action was not understood until 1971, when Vane[5] showed that it inhibited the synthesis of prostaglandins.

Mechanism of action

Aspirin is classified as a NSAID because of its prostaglandin inhibitory effect, but there are several features that set it apart from the other members of the class and deserve special consideration. Aspirin irreversibly inhibits cyclo-oxygenase with a covalent bond between an acetyl group and a serine residue at the active site of the COX enzyme.

Indications

In the prophylaxis of cardiovascular disease, the inhibition of COX-mediated thromboxane-A_2 production within platelets reduces platelet aggregation and thus thrombus formation. The lack of DNA within platelets means that re-synthesis of COX is impossible and the inhibition persists for the lifetime of each platelet. This contrasts with other NSAIDs, which are reversible inhibitors. Seventy-five milligrams per day have been shown to effectively reduce the incidence of cardiovascular thrombotic events and primary or secondary prevention of such events is the most common indication for use. Three-hundred milligrams are given to patients with evidence of an acute coronary syndrome, again for the anti-platelet effect. Much larger doses (up to 4 g per day) may be used in the treatment of inflammatory and arthritic conditions. Enteric-coated preparations of aspirin are available, but have slower onset of action.

Contraindications

The use of aspirin is contraindicated in children and adolescents under the age of 16. Epidemiological studies revealed an association between aspirin use in children and Reye's syndrome; a potentially fatal metabolic condition characterised by raised intracranial pressure, cerebral oedema and an extensive fatty liver process. Though occasional cases have been recorded in adults,[32] it is predominantly seen in childhood and generally occurs during the recovery period following a viral infection. The mechanism remains unclear. Aspirin is occasionally prescribed in children, but only under specialist supervision for the treatment of severe juvenile rheumatoid arthritis (Still's disease) or Kawasaki disease.

Overdose

Aspirin overdose has several unusual features. Mild toxicity generally results in symptoms of gastrointestinal upset, abdominal pain, tinnitus and dizziness. More significant overdoses produce symptoms of hyperthermia, hypoglycaemia, and tachypnoea.

The mechanism involves uncoupling of oxidative phosphorylation within cell mitochondria resulting in increasing oxygen consumption and carbon dioxide production, with an associated rise in minute volume. Arterial blood gas analysis reveals a picture of respiratory alkalosis with underlying metabolic acidosis. Very high aspirin levels are associated with additional direct respiratory centre stimulation. Pulmonary oedema, seizures and cerebral oedema can result in death.

In children, high levels of aspirin depress the respiratory centre so that a mixed respiratory and metabolic acidosis may be seen.

Treatment of overdose

Treatment of aspirin overdose involves the use of activated charcoal to adsorb aspirin within the gastrointestinal tract, monitoring of blood drug, glucose and electrolyte levels, arterial blood gases and attempted correction of any significant derangements.

Unlike paracetamol poisoning, there is no specific antidote. Alkalinisation of urine may be used to try to increase salicylate elimination. Haemodialysis is reserved for the most serious cases, to reduce salicylate levels, and in managing acidosis, pulmonary oedema and renal failure.

Paracetamol (acetaminophen)

The analgesic efficacy of paracetamol and its potential toxicity tend to be underestimated, perhaps because it can be bought cheaply over the counter. When taken regularly and at full dose, paracetamol is a useful component in the armoury to treat chronic pain.[33] In the perioperative period, like the traditional NSAIDs, it has a significant opiate-sparing effect. The intravenous preparation of paracetamol gives the option of an alternative, convenient route of administration with predictable bioavailability. Adding paracetamol to NSAIDs or opioids may have an additional benefit.[34]

Mechanism of action

The use of paracetamol as an antipyretic and analgesic is well established, the exact mechanism of action remains to be fully elucidated. There is no significant demonstrable peripheral anti-inflammatory effect via cyclo-oxygenase and several theories for a central action have been postulated. These include a central or spinal effect on 5HT3 (5-hydroxytryptamine receptor type 3), but paracetamol has not been shown to actually bind to 5HT3 receptors. The most popular theory is a central COX-3 inhibitory effect (see COX-3 above). As such, it is grouped with the NSAIDs, but has a number of characteristics that set it apart.

Administration

Paracetamol has long been available for use in oral and rectal forms, more recently an intravenous formulation has been licensed (in the UK). The suggested maximal adult daily dose is 4 g, whatever the chosen route of administration. There is no direct correlation between blood levels and analgesic effect.[34]

Oral

Oral paracetamol is well tolerated, producing no gastric irritation. It is available as a dispersible or plain tablet (or capsule) or as an oral suspension (with or without sugar) for young children. Rapid absorption from the gastrointestinal tract with only limited hepatic first-pass metabolism gives a systemic bioavailability of over 70%, with peak plasma levels achieved within 1–2 hours of ingestion.

The usual oral dose in adults is 10–15 mg/kg every 4–6 hours, to a daily maximum of 4 g. Paracetamol (1 g) has a NNT (for a 50% reduction in pain score) of 4.6 against 2.7 for ibuprofen in acute pain.[35]

Rectal

Rectal paracetamol has been a popular route of administration in the perioperative period, particularly in paediatric practice and when the oral route is contraindicated (e.g. bowel obstruction or following upper gastrointestinal surgery). The bioavailability is unpredictable with a large range quoted. Variations in the suppository composition can affect the time taken for it to dissolve and be absorbed, as can using more than one suppository at a time.

Whatever the formulation, peak plasma levels are reached more slowly than with oral preparations (several hours) and absorption may be variable.

Initial rectal doses of up to 40 mg/kg have been recommended, followed by regular oral doses to the maximum of 90 mg/kg/day.

Younger children (under 6 years) seem to be less susceptible to toxicity, possibly due to the slightly shorter half life (1.5 hours vs. 2 hours) or increased activity of detoxifying mechanisms. However, critically ill children may be at increased risk of toxicity, particularly with repeated dosing.

Intravenous

Propacetamol is a pro-drug of paracetamol that has been available for use as a parenteral agent in continental Europe (though not in the UK) for many years. Following intravenous injection, it is completely hydrolysed within 6 min, with 1 g of propacetamol yielding 500 mg of paracetamol. Its use is associated with pain and irritation at the injection site and contact dermatitis in medical staff handling the drug during its reconstitution into a solution.

A solubilised formulation of paracetamol for intravenous use has now been developed. It is free of apparent side effects, of similar cost to the suppository formulation (in the UK) and with a 2-year shelf life. It is presented in glass vials for slow infusion and is used for the short-term treatment of moderate pain (e.g. following surgery) and fever. The onset of action is within 5 to 10 min with a peak effect at 1 hour making it ideal for relatively short surgical procedures. Its duration of effect is 4 to 6 hours. The daily maximum dose remains the same at 4 g/day for adults.

Metabolism

Conjugation with cysteine and glucuronic and sulphuric acids in the liver accounts for 98% of paracetamol metabolism with the conjugates subsequently being excreted in the urine.

The remaining 2% is metabolised by an alternative mechanism, involving N-hydroxylation by the cytochrome P450 enzyme system to produce N-acetyl-p-amino-benzoquinoneimine (NAPQ1). Sulphydryl groups present in the liver's stores of glutathione are used to combine with and inactivate the otherwise toxic NAPQ1.

Side effects

Paracetamol is extremely well tolerated with minimal side effects. Only rarely have cases of skin rashes and blood dyscrasias been reported in the medical literature.

Caution is required when prescribing paracetamol in cases of severe renal insufficiency as the elimination time is prolonged, requiring an increase in the minimum dosing interval to 6 hours.

Significant liver disease, chronic alcoholism, malnutrition and dehydration all require increased vigilance.[36]

Overdose

The main complications arise with overdose, either intentional or accidental. Twenty to 30, 500 mg tablets (10–15 g) are enough to produce hepatocellular damage and even death if not treated. Fifteen tablets (7.5 g), can lead to hepatic damage in patients with hepatic enzyme induction (e.g. anti-convulsant therapy or alcoholic liver disease).[32]

Saturation of the normal conjugation pathways result in a diversion of paracetamol metabolism into the alternative, cytochrome P450-mediated metabolism (see Fig. 8.3). Hepatic stores of glutathione (sulphydryl donor) are rapidly depleted in the neutralisation of the toxic metabolite NAPQ1. Unmetabolised NAPQ1 react with sulphydryl groups found in hepatic proteins, leading to the development of irreversible centilobular hepatic necrosis (with peri-portal sparing).

The early symptoms from a significant overdose are mild. There may be no symptoms, mild gastrointestinal upset or vague abdominal discomfort and patients may not seek medical attention, resulting in a significant mortality rate ($\approx$5%). Despite a lack of initial symptoms, hepatotoxicity continues unless glutathione levels are quickly replenished artificially. Abnormal liver function tests occur from 24 hours; it is usually not until the third or fourth day that the symptoms and signs of jaundice, haemorrhage and CNS impairment herald the onset of fulminant hepatic failure. By this stage, the only treatment options available are supportive or transplantation.[37]

Treatment of overdose

Once basic resuscitation has been initiated and any gastric-emptying measures performed, attempts to increase glutathione levels in the liver are required. Glutathione precursors can be provided by treatment with oral methionine or intravenous N-acetylcysteine ('Parvolex'). Traditionally, treatment needed to be commenced within 15 hours of any overdose, but more recent work suggests benefit beyond this time limit. Therapy is guided by measuring the plasma paracetamol concentration (at least 4 hours after ingestion) and plotting it on a treatment nomogram.

Fig. 8.3 Paracetamol metabolism

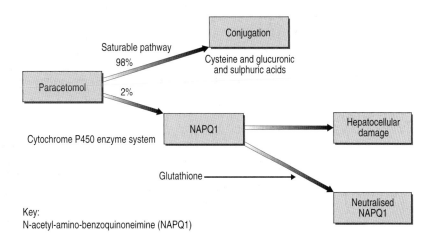

Key:
N-acetyl-amino-benzoquinoneimine (NAPQ1)

Drug interactions

In comparison to most other drugs, there are very few interactions. The most commonly quoted interaction is with the uricosuric anti-gout medication, probenecid. By inhibiting paracetamol's conjugation with glucuronic acid, it reduces the clearance rate twofold.

The prolonged, regular use of paracetamol possibly enhances warfarin's anti-coagulant effect. Cholestyramine reduces paracetamol absorption and metoclopramide increases paracetamol absorption. Liver-enzyme-inducing drugs increase the risk of toxicity as described above.

Pregnancy

As with all drugs, paracetamol should only be used in pregnancy if really necessary. However, it can be taken safe in the knowledge that no teratogenic effects have been detected in many years of clinical use or in animal-based studies. In addition, there are no documented harmful effects on breast-feeding infants from the excretion of small quantities of paracetamol into breast milk (Table 8.3).

TABLE 8.3 NSAIDs in clinical practice: information from various sources including the British National Formulary

Drug	Indications	Formulation	Dose	Comment
Traditional NSAIDs				
Diclofenac	Rheumatic disease Musculo-skeletal disorders Acute gout Postoperative pain	Tablets Slow release tablets Suppositories Combined with misoprostol Intravenous (iv) infusion	Maximum 150 mg/day Children 1–3 mg/kg	Good efficacy Relatively low incidence of side effects Rectal formulation useful perioperatively Similar risk of cardiovascular events as some COX-2s
Ibuprofen	Rheumatic disease Musculo-skeletal disorders Dysmenorrhoea Postoperative pain Fever and pain in children	Tablets Oral suspension Topical gel	*Adults:* 400–600 mg tds *Children:* over 5 kg, 20–30 mg/kg in divided doses 3–6 months: 50 mg tds 6 months–1 year: 50 mg qds 1–3 yrs: 100 mg tds 4–6 yrs: 150 mg tds 7–9 yrs: 200 mg tds 10–12 yrs: 300 mg tds	Good safety profile Cheap Weakest anti-inflammatory effect, therefore, unsuitable in predominantly inflammatory conditions (e.g. acute gout)
Indometacin	Pain and moderate-to-severe inflammation in rheumatic disease Acute gout (closure of ductus arteriosus)	Capsules Suppositories	*Oral:* 50–200 mg in divided doses, with food *Rectal:* 100 mg bd	Poor side effect profile Not recommended for children

Ketorolac	Short-term treatment of moderate-to-severe acute postoperative pain	Tablets iv/ intramuscular (im) injection	Iv or im: 10 mg initially, then 10–30 mg 4–6 hourly to max. 90 mg daily In the elderly under 50 kg, max. 60 mg daily Not recommended in children	Useful perioperatively when oral route restricted Only licensed for 5 days use perioperatively Increased risk GI or postoperative bleeding in patients over 75 years of age
Mefenamic acid	Mild-to-moderate pain in rheumatoid arthritis (RhA) and osteoarthritis (OA) Dysmenorrhoea	Capsules Paediatric suspension	*Adults:* 500 mg tds after food *Children:* 25 mg/kg daily in divided doses	Well tolerated Effective in dysmenorrhoea Occasionally causes diarrhoea Rarely, associated with haemolytic anaemia
Meloxicam	Long-term treatment RhA (including juvenile) Exacerbations OA (short-term) Ankylosing spondylitis	Tablets Suppositories	7.5–15 mg, once daily (with food)	Preferential COX-2 inhibitor with probably more favourable gastrointesintal (GI) profile than diclofenac or piroxicam Only short-term GI studies Limited data on cardiovascular risks
Naproxen	RhA (including juvenile) Other musculo-skeletal disorders Dysmenorrhoea Acute gout	Tablets standard or enteric coated	*RhA:* 500 mg–1 g daily in divided doses *Musculoskeletal pain and dysmenorrhoea:* 500 mg initially then 250 mg tds *Gout:* 750 mg initially then 250 mg tds	Generally well tolerated with good efficacy Lowest rate of cardiovascular thrombotic events (other than aspirin) Not as well tolerated as ibuprofen
Piroxicam	RhA (including juvenile) Other musculoskeletal conditions Acute gout (postoperative pain is not a listed indication)	Tablets Capsules Dispersible tablet (on tongue) Deep im injection (gluteal)	*RhA:* Initially 20 mg daily, 10–30 mg maintenance *Acute musculoskeletal pain:* 40 mg × 2 days then 20 mg daily × 7–14 days *Acute gout:* 40 mg daily for 1 week	Dispersible formulation useful in the postoperative recovery room Pain at injection site Rectal irritation from suppositories
Selective COX-2 inhibitors				
Celecoxib	OA RhA	Capsules	*OA:* 200 mg in 1–2 divided doses, increased if inadequate response to max. 200 mg bd *RA:* 200–400 mg daily in 2 divided doses *Elderly:* Caution if <50 kg	Well tolerated Once-daily dosing possible Only to be used in preference to traditional, non-selective NSAIDs when high risk of GI complications Expensive Contraindicated in children <16 years

(Continued)

TABLE 8.3 NSAIDs in clinical practice: information from various sources including the British National Formulary—cont'd

Drug	Indications	Formulation	Dose	Comment
			Half dose if moderate liver impairment (limited experience with mild-moderate renal impairment)	
Etoricoxib	OA RhA Acute gout	Tablets	*OA:* 60 mg od *RhA:* 90 mg od *Acute gout:* 120 mg od	Better tolerated than diclofenac Cardiovascular risks similar to diclofenac No significant reduction of major GI events Expensive Increased risk hypertension
Lumiracoxib	OA symptomatic relief Acute pain Short-term relief of moderate-to-severe pain Dysmenorrhoea	Tablets	*OA:* 100 mg od *Postoperative pain:* 400 mg od × max. 5 days *Dysmenorrhoea:* 200 mg od, max. 3 days/cycle	Good GI profile Similar efficacy as celecoxib for treating OA and naproxen for orthopaedic pain Cardiovascular risks similar to those of ibuprofen Perioperative use only Limited study data for use >1 year Any GI benefit negated by concurrent aspirin
Parecoxib	Short-term treatment of postoperative pain	Powder in vial (for reconstitution) for iv or im injection	40 mg iv or im followed every 6–12 h by 20 mg or 40 mg as required, not to exceed 80 mg/day If patient weight <50 kg, half the dose, max. 40 mg/day Moderate hepatic impairment, half the dose	Iv bolus can be given rapidly and easily intraoperatively No dosage adjustment necessary with elderly or mild-to-moderate renal impairment or mild hepatic impairment No effect on platelet aggregation or bleeding time Expensive Metabolism requires caution with concurrent fluconazole or omeprazole use Limited experience in use >3 days Contraindicated <18 years as not studied in this population Severe hepatic impairment as no experience in use

Data from British Medical Association & Royal Pharmaceutical Society of Great Britain. Non-steroidal anti-inflammatory drugs. *British National Formulary (BNF)* 2007; (10.1.1.)

KEY POINTS

- NSAIDs are anti-inflammatory, antipyretic analgesics with a clinical role in managing acute and some chronic painful conditions
- NSAIDs have an opioid-sparing effect
- NSAIDs act by inhibiting cyclo-oxygenase enzymes and reducing levels of thromboxanes, prostacyclins and prostaglandins
- Thromboxanes, prostacyclins and prostaglandins have a wide variety of physiological roles that account for many of the side effects of NSAIDs
- Gastrointestinal side effects are common and may be fatal
- Coxibs were introduced to reduce the side effects of traditional NSAIDs but have been shown to have thrombotic cardiovascular complications in some patients
- Caution is required in using NSAIDs but the risk is relatively low with appropriate patient selection, dosing and timing of administration
- Paracetamol is an antipyretic analgesic with benefit in acute and chronic pain and can be used safely at full dose
- Overdose of paracetamol may lead to hepatic failure and caution is required in severe renal insufficiency, liver damage and alcoholic liver disease
- Paracetamol is opioid sparing and has few interactions

References

1. World Health Organization. National cancer control programmes: policies and managerial guidelines. Geneva: World Health Organization; 2002.
2. Berd CB, Rowbotham MC. COX-2 inhibitors: a status report. Technical Corner from IASP Newsletter. Seattle: IASP; 1998.
3. Gallelli L et al. Retrospective evaluation of adverse drug reactions induced by nonsteroidal anti-inflammatory drugs. *Clin Drug Investig* 2007; **27**(2): 115–122.
4. Lipsky LP et al. The classification of cyclooxygenase inhibitors. *J Rheumatol* 1998; **25**(12): 2298–2303.
5. Vane JR. Inhibition of prostaglandin synthesis as a mechanism of action for aspirin-like drugs. *Nat New Biol* 1971; **231**(25): 232–235.
6. Needleman P, Isakson PC. The discovery and function of COX–2. *J Rheumatol Suppl* 1997; **49**: 6–8.
7. Simmons DL. Variants of cyclooxygenase-1 and their roles in medicine. *Thromb Res* 2003; **110**(5–6): 265–268.
8. Flower RJ, Vane JR. Inhibition of prostaglandin synthetase in brain explains the anti-pyretic activity of paracetamol. *Nature* 1972; **240**: 410–411.
9. Bombardier C et al. Comparison of upper gastrointestinal toxicity of rofecoxib and naproxen in patients with rheumatoid arthritis. VIGOR Study Group. *N Engl J Med* 2000; **343**(21): 1520–1528.
10. Silverstein FE et al. Gastrointestinal toxicity with celecoxib vs nonsteroidal anti-inflammatory drugs for osteoarthritis and rheumatoid arthritis: The CLASS Study. A randomized controlled trial. *JAMA* 2000; **284**(10): 1247–1255.
11. Schnitzer TJ et al. Comparison of lumiracoxib with naproxen and ibuprofen in the Therapeutic Arthritis Research and Gastrointestinal Event Trial (TARGET), reduction in ulcer complications: randomised controlled trial. *Lancet* 2004; **364**(9435): 665–674.
12. Bresalier RS et al. Cardiovascular events associated with rofecoxib in a colorectal adenoma chemoprevention trial. *N Engl J Med* 2005; **352**(11): 1092–1102.

13. Lagakos SW. Time-to-event analyses for long-term treatments – the APPROVe trial. *N Engl J Med* 2006; **355**(2): 113–117.
14. Bertagnolli MM et al. Celecoxib for the prevention of sporadic colorectal adenomas. *N Engl J Med* 2006; **355**(9): 873–884.
15. Arber N et al. Celecoxib for the prevention of colorectal adenomatous polyps. *N Engl J Med* 2006; **355**(9): 885–895.
16. Nussmeier NA et al. Complications of the COX-2 inhibitors parecoxib and valdecoxib after cardiac surgery. *N Engl J Med* 2005; **352**(11): 1081–1091.
17. Jenkins JK, Seligman PJ. Analysis and recommendations for agency action regarding non-steroidal anti-inflammatory drugs and cardiovascular risk. Available from: *http://www.fda.gov/cder/drug/infopage/COX2/NSAIDdecisionMemo.pdf* Cited 2005.
18. Opinion of the committee for medicinal products for human use prsuant to article 5 (3) of regulation (EC) No 726/2004, for non-selective non steroidal anti-inflammatory drugs (NSAIDs). Available from:*http://www.emea.europa.eu/pdfs/human/opiniongen/nsaids.pdf* Cited 2006.
19. Cardiovascular and Cerebrovascular Events in the Randomized Controlled Alzheimer's Disease Anti-Inflammatory Prevention Trial (ADAPT). *PLoS Clin Trials* 2006; **1**(7): e33.
20. Baraf HS et al. Gastrointestinal side effects of etoricoxib in patients with osteoarthritis: results of the Etoricoxib versus Diclofenac Sodium Gastrointestinal Tolerability and Effectiveness (EDGE) trial. *J Rheumatol* 2007; **34**(2): 408–420.
21. Cannon CP et al. Cardiovascular outcomes with etoricoxib and diclofenac in patients with osteoarthritis and rheumatoid arthritis in the Multinational Etoricoxib and Diclofenac Arthritis Long-term (MEDAL) programme: a randomised comparison. *Lancet* 2006; **368**(9549): 1771–1781.
22. Tramer MR et al. Quantitative estimation of rare adverse events which follow a biological progression: a new model applied to chronic NSAID use. *Pain* 2000; **85**: 169–182.
23. Henry D et al. Variability in risk of gastrointestinal complications with individual non-steroidal anti-inflammatory drugs: results of a collaborative meta-analysis. *BMJ* 1996; **312**: 1563–1566.
24. Sturtevant J. NSAID-induced bronchospasm – a common and serious problem. A report from MEDSAFE, the New Zealand Medicines and Medical Devices Safety Authority. *NZ Dental J* 1999; **95**(421): 84.
25. Murray MD, Brater DC. Effects of NSAIDs on the kidney. *Prog Drug Res* 1997; **49**: 155–171.
26. Stuart R, Rodger C. Analgesic-induced renal damage. *Prescribers' Journal* 2000; **40**(2): 151–164.
27. Hernandez-Diaz S, Varas–Lorenzo C, Garcia Rodriguez LA. Non-steroidal anti-inflammatory drugs and the risk of acute myocardial infarction. *Basic & Clinical Pharmacology & Toxicology* 2006; **98**(3): 266–274.
28. Gerstenfeld LC, Einhorn TA. COX inhibitors and their effects on bone healing. *Expert Opin Drug Saf* 2004; **3**(2): 131–136.
29. British Medical Association & Royal Pharmaceutical Society of Great Britain. Non-steroidal anti-inflammatory drugs. *British National Formulary (BNF)* 2007; 2007(10.1.1.).
30. National Institute for Health and Clinical Excellence. Osteoarthritis and rheumatoid arthritis-cox II inhibitors: guidance. Osteoarthritis and rheumatoid arthritis – cox II inhibitors: guidance. 2001: TA27.
31. White PF. Changing role of COX-2 inhibitors in the perioperative period: is parecoxib really the answer? *Anesth Analg* 2005; **100**(5): 1306–1308.
32. Benson GD. Hepatotoxicity following the therapeutic use of antipyretic analgesics. *Am J Med* 1983; **75**(5A): 85–93.
33. Nikles CJ et al. The role of paracetamol in chronic pain: an evidence-based approach. *Am J Ther* 2005; **12**(1): 80–91.
34. Bannwarth B, Pehourcq F. Pharmacologic basis for using paracetamol: pharmacokinetic and pharmacodynamic issues. *Drugs* 2003; **63 Spec No 2**: 5–13.

35. Hyllested M et al. Comparative effect of paracetamol, NSAIDs or their combination in postoperative pain management: a qualitative review. *Br J Anaesth* 2002; **88**(2): 199–214.
36. Forrest JA et al. Paracetamol metabolism in chronic liver disease. *Eur J Clin Pharmacol* 1979; **15**(6): 427–431.
37. Larson AM et al. Acetaminophen-induced acute liver failure: results of a United States multicenter, prospective study. *Hepatology* 2005; **42**(6): 1364–1372.

Amit Kumar

Local anaesthetics: other membrane stabilisers

Introduction

Local anaesthetics produce a membrane-stabilising action by blocking sodium channels in excitable tissues. These sodium ion conducting channels open in response to membrane depolarisation and are called voltage-gated sodium channels (VGSC). VGSCs are responsible for the initiation and propagation of action potentials in both nerve and muscle cells. Local anaesthetics are, therefore, able to produce a conduction blockade in nerve fibres by inhibiting the propagation of a nerve impulse. A nerve impulse is essentially a wave of depolarisation that is carried forward by the successive activation of sodium channels. Upon activation, they open transiently to allow sodium ions to enter the cell. The intracellular passage of sodium ions produces a flow of current, which causes further depolarisation and activation of nearby sodium channels. Hence, the conduction of a nerve impulse occurs. The blockade produced is reversible and terminates when the local anaesthetic dissociates from the sodium channels and is metabolised. The duration of the block depends upon the drug characteristics, the rate of washout from the tissues concerned and additives added to the local anaesthetic solution. Following a regional block procedure (the deposition of local anaesthetic in close proximity to a nerve) the conduction of autonomic, sensory and motor impulses are inhibited at that site, thereby, respectively producing an autonomic blockade, sensory anaesthesia and skeletal muscle paralysis. These actions are to some extent concentration dependent and this property can be exploited in pain management.

History of local anaesthetics use

The first compound to be discovered with local anaesthetic properties was cocaine. It was isolated from the coca leaves (*Erythroxylon coca*) in 1860 by Albert Niemann. These leaves were brought to Germany from South America by German and Austrian explorers who noticed the natives of Peru chewing them for their intoxicating properties. The natives were aware of their lips and tongue going numb in the process of chewing the leaves, but it hadn't been put to any medicinal use. Carl Koller, a German doctor, in 1884 first documented cocaine's use as a local anaesthetic for topical anaesthesia of the cornea.[1] Soon cocaine was being used for a variety of blocks and 1885 saw the first spinal being performed, with James Leonard Corning using cocaine through a hypodermic needle to demonstrate a reversible spinal block.[2]

Dibucaine was the first amide local anaesthetic to be discovered and introduced into clinical practice in the 1930s. However, being too toxic, its use was mainly limited to spinal blocks where only a small dose of the drug is required. Lignocaine was discovered and demonstrated as an excellent local anaesthetic for digital nerve blocks of the fingers and toes in 1948, and to date it continues to be used worldwide as a safe local anaesthetic. The newer amides are purified selective isomers such as levobupivacaine and ropivacaine. Separating the stereoisomers into its purified optical isomer components, i.e. the dextro and levo subtypes, allows us to use the subtype, which has a safer clinical profile. Thus, levobupivacaine exhibits less cardiac toxicity than its counterpart dextro-bupivacaine or the racemic mixture bupivacaine.[3]

Over the last few decades, conduction blockades using injected local anaesthetics have been employed not only for every conceivable peripheral nerve, but also for tissue infiltration, field blocks, intravenous regional anaesthesia and topical anaesthesia.

Pharmacology

Pharmacodynamics

Mechanism of action

The VGSCs open transiently to allow sodium ion inflow and then close very rapidly to an inactive, resting state. Electrophysiological experiments have shown that local anaesthetics block VGSCs in their open state. It is hypothesised that local anaesthetics bind to the intracellular element of the VGSC molecule.

The VGSC is a complex long protein chain molecule embedded in the phospholipid matrix of the cell membrane.[4] The long protein chain is folded upon itself several times to form a transmembranous channel pore (Fig. 9.1). There are amino acid sequences in the protein chain that regulate the ion-pore by functioning as activation and inactivation gates. The VGSC protein molecule is folded into four similar groups called domains, each consisting of six segments. The amino acids comprising these segments contribute to the formation of binding sites for various drugs and hormones. One such receptor site is located on the sixth segment of the fourth domain, on the intracellular surface, and binds to local anaesthetics.[5] VGSCs in different organs like the brain, spinal cord, peripheral nerves, heart and muscles, differ minutely in their amino acid sequence and are further classified into various subtypes.[6] However, structurally they are similar and respond similarly to local anaesthetics, which explains the widespread systemic side effects.

Fig. 9.1 Schematic drawing of the voltage gated sodium channel. Four homologous domains consisting of six segments, each are wrapped around, surrounding an ion pore. Sequences in the long amino acid chain contribute to the formation of activation gate, inactivation gate and receptor sites. Reproduced from CPD Anaesthesia 2003; 5(2): 72–75

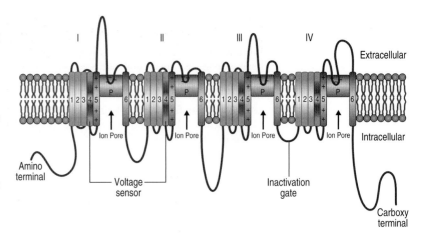

Chemistry

Chemically, local anaesthetics are molecules with a hydrophilic portion and a lipophilic portion linked with a hydrocarbon chain. The lipophilic end is an aromatic ring, while the hydrophilic end is an amine (Fig. 9.2). The linking chain joining the two could be an ester or amide (Table 9.1).

Clinical effect

As the VGSC binding site for local anaesthetics is intracellular, the local anaesthetics have to enter the cell to produce a blockade. An organic drug stays in equilibrium between two fractions, the ionised form and the non-ionised form. It is only possible for the non-ionised fraction of the local anaesthetic to enter the cell, while it is the ionised fraction that is active and binds to the receptor. The relative proportions of the two fractions vary with the pH

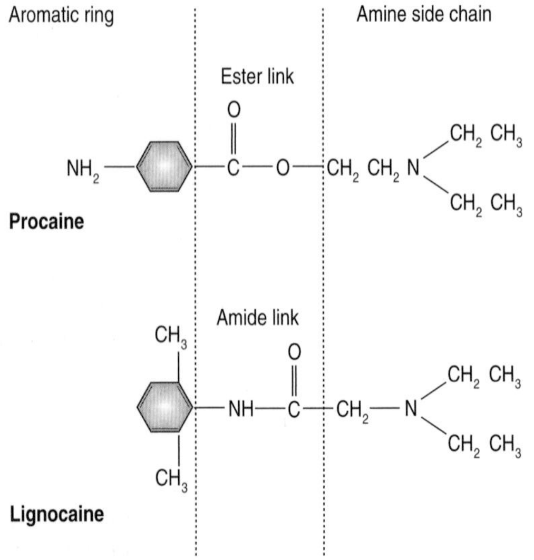

Fig. 9.2 Chemical structure of two common local anaesthetics demonstrating the ester or amide links between the aromatic and amine ends

Aromatic ring

Amine side chain

Ester link

Procaine

Amide link

Lignocaine

TABLE 9.1 Classification of local anaesthetics based on their molecular structure

Esters	Amides
Cocaine	Lignocaine
Procaine	Mepivacaine
Chlorprocaine	Bupivacaine
Tetracaine	Etidocaine
Benzocaine	Prilocaine
	Ropivacaine
	Dibucaine

of the ambient solution. The pH at which the two fractions are in equal proportions is called the pKa of the drug. A drug with a low pKa will dissociate into a higher proportion of the non-ionised form compared to a drug with a high pKa. Hence, a greater proportion of lignocaine with a pKa of 7.9 is in the non-ionised form than of bupivacaine with a pKa of 8.1. At the extracellular pH of 7.4, about 76% of lignocaine is in the ionised state and 24% in the non-ionised state. However, upon diffusion into the cell at a pH of 7.1, the lignocaine shifts to 86% in the active ionised state, hence lignocaine exhibits a quicker onset of action than bupivacaine.

Nerve fibres show varying susceptibility to blockade depending upon their cross-sectional diameter, presence of a myelin sheath and concentration of the local anaesthetic. This also reflects the fact that the receptor site for binding local anaesthetics is intracellular. Upon inactivation, the VGSCs stop the conduction of the depolarisation wave. Fast-conducting, myelinated nerve fibres, like the A-fibres, carrying proprioception, touch, pressure sensation and somatic motor impulses are more resistant to blockade as the depolarisation wave jumps from one node of Ranvier to the next. It is known that sodium channels are densely concentrated at the nodes of Ranvier. The relatively slower conducting C-fibres are unmyelinated and easily susceptible to a local anaesthetic blockade. They carry the sensation of pain, temperature and some reflex responses. A differential block can thus be produced to the patient's advantage by using a weaker concentration of local anaesthetic. An example would be the walking epidural for analgesia during labour, where a 0.1% solution of bupivacaine is administered epidurally either as an infusion or small boluses, produces autonomic and sensory blockade, but very little motor blockade. This can provide an excellent form of pain relief during labour contractions, without immobilising the expectant mother. The same principle is used to provide postoperative analgesia using an epidural infusion, following a surgical procedure. It allows the patient to mobilise, tolerate physiotherapy and make a good recovery with a shorter hospital stay.

Drugs with a higher degree of protein binding demonstrate a higher affinity for membrane proteins and a prolonged duration of action. Thus, bupivacaine, which is 96% protein bound, has a longer duration of action than lignocaine, which is 64% protein bound.

Pharmacokinetics

Metabolism

Amino-esters are rapidly metabolised in the circulation by the plasma cholinesterase enzyme, while the amino-amides are metabolised by microsomal enzymes located primarily in the liver. The clearance of amino-amides is slower and an accumulation more likely to occur and the risk of systemic toxicity greater.

Allergic reactions are more likely to be encountered with esters than amides.

Lignocaine is metabolised in the liver by microsomal oxidases and amidases. The N-dealkylation and hydrolysis produces metabolites that are excreted in the urine. Bupivacaine undergoes similar N-dealkylation to produce renally excreted metabolites. Prilocaine is metabolised in the liver, lungs and kidney to O-toluidine and then to hydroxytoluidine. Significantly high systemic absorption of prilocaine produces methaemoglobinaemia (Table 9.2).

Systemic toxicity

Local anaesthetics are likely to manifest central nervous system (CNS) toxicity before cardiovascular system (CVS) toxicity. Cardiovascular depression occurs less frequently, but is more resistant to treatment. The ratio of the dose required to produce severe cardiac toxicity to the dose that produces convulsions is lower for bupivacaine and etidocaine when compared to lignocaine. This makes it safer to use lignocaine for systemic administration in pain management.

The difference between half-maximal effective dose (ED_{50}) and the half-maximum lethal dose (LD_{50}) is known as the 'therapeutic window'. The larger the therapeutic window of a drug, the safer it is to administer the drug systemically. Lignocaine has a larger therapeutic window than bupivacaine. The maximum dose of lignocaine generally accepted as a safe limit for administration for a regional block procedure is 5 mg/kg body weight, while that for bupivacaine is 2 mg/kg. Lignocaine can be administered systemically with relative safety in the management of some painful conditions. For systemic administration, lignocaine is given by infusion over half an hour up to a maximum of 5 mg/kg lean body weight. Bupivacaine is considered too toxic for systemic use, as it is very slow to dissociate from the myocardium and the cardiac complications usually end with fatal consequences.

Systemic absorption

When used for regional procedures, there are various factors that determine the rate of systemic absorption and hence risk of developing systemic toxicity:

- *Site of injection*: Some tissues have a high vascularity. Systemic absorption of local anaesthetic is rapid in these conditions producing higher plasma

TABLE 9.2 Classification of local anaesthetics by their duration of action		
Short (30–60 min)	Intermediate (1–2 h)	Long (>2 h)
Cocaine	Lignocaine	Bupivacaine
Chlorprocaine	Prilocaine	Levobupivacaine
Benzocaine	Mepivacaine	Ropivacaine
	Tetracaine	Etidocaine
		Dibucaine

concentrations. Intercostal blocks are an example that can lead to high plasma concentration of local anaesthetics especially when performed at multiple levels.

- *Mass of drug*: Blocks requiring high volumes of local anaesthetic can eventually lead to high plasma concentrations. Three-in-one blocks for the lower limb aim to block femoral, obturator and lateral cutaneous nerve of thigh and requires 30 ml of solution. The drug concentration should be appropriately diluted to compensate for the larger volume required whilst remaining within the upper safe dose for that agent. Multiple nerve blocks performed at the same time can also involve significant volumes of the local anaesthetic drug.
- *Addition of vasoconstrictors*: Adding adrenaline (epinephrine) produces vasoconstriction in the local tissues and can slow the rate of absorption of the local anaesthetic into the systemic circulation. It is extremely important not to add a vasoconstrictor in a block for the digits or the penis, as ischaemic necrosis may result due to a total loss of circulation.
- *Alkalisation*: The addition of bicarbonate solution to the local anaesthetic raises the ambient pH, thereby increasing the non-ionised fraction, which diffuses rapidly through the nerve membrane producing a quicker onset of nerve block. Hence, it may be possible to produce a satisfactory block using smaller volumes of local anaesthetic.

CNS toxicity

Circulating local anaesthetic initially produces excitation features of CNS toxicity by selective blockade of inhibitory pathways in the cerebral cortex.[7] With increasing blood levels of local anaesthetics, both inhibitory and facilitatory pathways are blocked resulting in CNS depression. The clinical manifestations include numbness of the tongue with associated slurring of speech followed by a feeling of light headedness and visual or auditory disturbances. The worrying signs of drowsiness, tremor and facial twitchiness are soon followed by convulsions before a generalised state of CNS depression produces coma and respiratory arrest.

CVS toxicity

CVS toxicity is a result of blockade of cardiac sodium channels and manifests as depression of myocardial contractility and rhythm abnormalities, namely bradycardia, atrio-ventricular dissociation, sinus arrest, ventricular arrhythmias and often, fatal ventricular fibrillation.

Prilocaine

A unique systemic side effect of prilocaine, usually in doses in excess of 600 mg, is methaemoglobinaemia.[8] It is believed to be due to the metabolism of prilocaine to O-toluidine in the liver which oxidises the ferrous iron of the haem in haemoglobin to ferric iron producing methaemoglobinaemia. Clinically this is seen as cyanosis with a pulse oximeter reading shifted towards 85%. This is a relatively benign side effect, reverses spontaneously and has little clinical significance in patients with normal oxygen-carrying capacity.

Role in pain management

Regional blocks

Regional blocks are commonly used for acute pain management in the peri-operative period. The nervous system can be blocked at various levels by the application of local anaesthetics.

Neuroaxial blockade

Central or neuroaxial blockade is produced by placing local anaesthetic at the spinal cord level by the following means.

Intrathecal injection

This is the injection of local anaesthetic into the cerebrospinal fluid (CSF). The spinal cord ends at the level of the first lumbar vertebra in an adult, although the dural sheath continues down to the sacral level. It is, therefore, safe to perform this procedure below the level of the second lumbar vertebra to avoid needle trauma to the spinal cord. The spinal cord extends lower down in children and may reach the third lumbar vertebra in infants.

Epidural injection

This involves injection of local anaesthetic outside the dural membranes sur-rounding the spinal cord. There is a potential space outside the dura, normally filled with loose connective tissue, fat and a venous plexus. An injection per-formed into this space allows the local anaesthetic to spread over a large area depending upon the volume of solution injected. The local anaesthetic blocks the nerve roots as they exit from the intervertebral foramina and some drug also diffuses through the dura to act directly upon the spinal cord receptors. This procedure can be performed at any level of the spine from the cervical level down to the caudal–sacral level.

Paravertebral block[9]

This is where a mass of local anaesthetic drug is deposited in a potential space (the paravertebral space), about 5 cm lateral to the spinous process, deep to the erector spinae muscles. The nerve roots, sympathetic chain and the dorsal root ganglion lie in this space and specific segments can be blocked by this technique. The procedure is commonly performed at the thoracic level for postoperative analgesia following thoracic surgery or for analgesia after fractured ribs.

Selective nerve root block

This procedure is often performed to relieve radicular pain (pain radiating along a dermatomal distribution). The nerve root in question is blocked under image intensifier (X-ray) guidance by depositing a small volume (approxi-mately 2 ml) of local anaesthetic in close proximity to the nerve.

Peripheral nerve blocks

Moving away from the spinal cord, regional blocks may be performed along the route of peripheral nerves at several sites, such as those mentioned below. These regional procedures can be made more effective by using confirmation techniques, for example, visualisation under CT scan, ultrasound or by the use of a nerve stimulator. The aim is to ensure the needle tip is as close to the nerve as possible without actually damaging it.

Plexus blocks

The anterior primary rami of nerve roots form plexuses before dividing again into various peripheral nerves that have both sensory and motor components. Several plexuses (e.g. cervical, lumbar and sacral plexuses) can be blocked using a large volume (about 25 ml) of local anaesthetic solution.

Peripheral nerve blocks

Nerves can be blocked anywhere along their route, but the sites chosen are usually next to bony landmarks or prominent arterial pulsation, where the nerve position can be reliably predicted (e.g. the ulnar nerve at the elbow, femoral nerve in the groin).

Field block/ring block

Local anaesthetic solution is infiltrated into the loose subcutaneous connective tissue plane where it spreads and blocks any nerves that are around.

Bier's block

Also known as *intravenous regional anaesthesia*. The limb to be blocked is exsanguinated and isolated by inflating a double cuff tourniquet. A large volume (about 25 ml) of local anaesthetic solution is then injected into a vein of the exsanguinated limb. The local anaesthetic diffuses out of the veins into the tissues and blocks all the nerve endings in the limb.

Third space instillation

Local anaesthetic solutions can be injected into an intra-articular space, peritoneal space or interpleural space, where it produces analgesia by blocking nerve endings.

Usually, a long-acting amide like bupivacaine or ropivacaine is chosen to prolong the effects of a procedure (see Table 9.2). In some situations, it may be advantageous to use a short-acting, rapidly metabolised, local anaesthetic. For example, prilocaine in Bier's blocks is used for short surgical procedures of the limb that are not expected to be particularly painful afterwards.

Chronic pain management

Long-term local-anaesthetic blocks

The reversible nature of a local anaesthetic block limits its use in most chronic pain conditions. Techniques such as placement of an intrapleural, intrathecal or a nerve block catheter can all be connected to an infusion device delivering a concentrated local anaesthetic solution at a rate that can be titrated. An opioid may be added to the solution for synergistic analgesia. These procedures may be prolonged in special circumstances, such as palliative care for the terminally ill.

A few practical concerns have to be kept in mind for an intrathecal infusion system to be effectively used in chronic pain conditions. There is a risk of infection spreading to the central nervous system and the most likely port of entry for organisms would be the catheter's entry site through the skin. This risk is reduced by tunnelling the catheter subcutaneously to the flank (away from the epidural site) and bringing it through the skin for a continuous infusion to be attached. Such a procedure is often usefully employed for palliative pain relief in terminally ill patients, typically malignancies with painful metastasis. In patients suffering from chronic pain conditions, but having a longer life expectancy, an intrathecal catheter can be placed and tunnelled subcutaneously across to the front of the abdomen and an infusion pump placed within a pocket created in the subcutaneous tissues. Thus, the entire infusion system is implanted, similar to an implanted internal cardiac pacemaker device. These specialised pumps are small, have a long battery life and can be refilled as well as reprogrammed. However, because of the constraints of the pump's reservoir volume, it is more practical to use opioids rather than local anaesthetics to obtain satisfactory analgesia at relatively low infusion volume rates.

Systemic administration

In certain painful conditions, which are generalised or of a neuropathic nature, systemic administration of local anaesthetics by intravenous infusion may be considered. For systemic administration, long-acting local anaesthetics like bupivacaine are unsuitable as they are slower to dissociate from the cardiac sodium channels and are more likely to result in life-threatening cardiac arrhythmias. Lignocaine has a greater margin of safety (therapeutic window) and has been used as an infusion for post-operative analgesia.[10] A serum concentration of 1–3 µg/ml, maintained by infusion has been shown to be effective and reduced postoperative opioid requirements. However, very close cardiovascular monitoring and periodic neurological assessment is essential in view of potentially lethal side effects. This precludes it from being used routinely for acute pain management.

Lignocaine has also been used as an intravenous infusion for the management of various painful neuropathic illnesses.[11,12] The pathology of neuropathic pain is complex and more difficult to treat. In neuropathic pain, an exaggerated painful sensation may be perceived in the affected region due to structural changes or neuroplasticity changes in the nervous system. These changes may occur at any level, from the nerve endings to the sensory cortex in the brain. The condition may present as paraesthesia, dysaesthesia, hyperaesthesia, allodynia or hyperalgesia. Among other agents, antiarrhythmics and anticonvulsants have been shown to be effective in modifying the pain. The principle behind their action is probably a membrane stabilising effect on the nervous system by the blocking of sodium channels. Indeed, it has been seen that affected nerve cells demonstrate an increased density of sodium channels.[13] Lignocaine as an intravenous infusion, intranasal drops or topical patch has been shown to be effective in various studies, particularly in reducing the pain associated with diabetic neuropathy, post-herpetic neuralgia, post-amputation phantom limb pain or stump pain and thalamic pain syndrome.

Orally administered lignocaine is up to 70% metabolised by first-pass mechanism, leading to active metabolites, which can result in cardiac and central neurological side effects. The results can be very unpredictable and make it unsuitable for oral administration in chronic pain. However, as an intravenous infusion, it can be used as an assessment tool of the patient's response, in terms of lowering the pain scores. A reproducible reduction of pain scores compared to placebo control is taken as a positive response and the patient can be offered orally administered antiarrhythmics like mexiletine or tocainamide. These drugs also act on the sodium channels and have a membrane stabilising action. A response to an intravenous lignocaine infusion has been shown to predict the response to mexiletine.[14]

A trial of lignocaine infusion is done under close supervision with full resuscitation equipment available at hand. The theatre recovery area is used in most institutions, with the patient admitted in as a day case. The patient is monitored throughout the procedure with electrocardiograph (ECG), non-invasive blood pressure and pulse oximeter. A suitably qualified person stands by maintaining verbal communication and making periodic neurological assessments by looking for signs of confusion, slurring of speech and abnormal behaviour, which would necessitate immediate cessation of the procedure. The patient is asked to quantify the pain on a verbal analogue scale or a visual analogue scale (VAS) before the start of the procedure and thence every 5 min. It may be prudent to initiate the procedure with an infusion of normal saline for 15 min to identify a placebo response. The patient is kept blinded as to what is being administered in the infusion. If there is a positive response to saline infusion, it may not be considered necessary to proceed with the rest of the procedure. The trial is continued with an infusion of lignocaine 5 mg/kg patient's body weight, diluted in normal saline and infused over 30 min. The infusion is stopped immediately the observer notices any side effects, if the patient feels distressed, or else, cardiac rhythm abnormalities are noticed. It is not unusual for patients to report numbness of the tongue, facial paraesthesia and some slurring of speech. Convulsions may occur if early signs and symptoms are ignored.

Comparison of the patient's verbal analogue scale alongside a VAS recorded through the procedure would give an idea whether there is a significant response to the lignocaine infusion. Most positive responses have been noticed to occur at the dose of 5 mg/kg lignocaine infused over 30 min. Curiously enough, the plasma concentration reached at this infusion rate is not high enough to cause peripheral nerve conduction blockade. Such an infusion has not been shown to increase the pain threshold in normal individuals, but patients with neuropathic pain often show a relief of symptoms. This is possibly explained by abnormally sensitised nerve endings displaying an increased number of sodium channels that respond to a lignocaine infusion. Another postulate is that the circulating lignocaine acts selectively upon the spinal cord or the dorsal root ganglia.[15,16] Patients having displayed a positive response to lignocaine infusion may benefit from a trial of mexiletine.

Mexiletine

Pharmacology

Mexiletine, a class Ib antiarrhythmic agent, is rapidly and completely absorbed following oral administration with a bioavailability of about 90%. Peak plasma concentrations following oral administration occur within 1–4 hours and a linear relationship between dose and plasma concentration is observed in the dose range of 100 to 600 mg. Mexiletine is weakly bound to plasma proteins (70%). Its volume of distribution is large and varies from 5 to 9 l/kg in healthy individuals. Mexiletine is eliminated slowly in humans (with an elimination half-life of 10 h). It undergoes extensive metabolism in the liver to inactive metabolites.[17]

Mexiletine is structurally similar to lignocaine, but orally active. In patients with a normal cardiac conduction system, mexiletine has minimal effect on cardiac impulse generation and propagation. However, in symptomatic patients, mexiletine exhibits membrane-stabilising effects through its blocking action on sodium channels. It produces a significant reduction of ventricular arrhythmias.

Role in chronic pain

Mexiletine may be of benefit to patients with neuropathic pain, fibromyalgia and central pain conditions. The patients usually undergo a trial of lignocaine infusion first, under controlled conditions with close observation and monitoring. A positive response to a lignocaine infusion as indicated by a reduction of VAS pain scores increases the likelihood of them responding to oral mexiletine. The number needed to treat for mexiletine is of the order of 10. This is relatively high when compared to other agents used in the management of neuropathic pain.

It is usually started at 150 mg a day and titrated slowly to a maximum of 750 mg a day in divided doses. The usual stabilising dose is 450 to 675 mg/day to achieve a significant reduction of pain without intolerable side effects.

There is experimental evidence to suggest that there is an increased concentration of abnormal VGSCs in the nerves in patients with neuropathic pain.[18] These are in an excited state, resulting in spontaneous firing. Hence, a membrane stabilising drug may prove beneficial to patients with such painful conditions.

Toxicity

Clinically, mexiletine overdose is manifested by gastrointestinal disturbances, dizziness, diplopia, blurred vision, tremor, ataxia, slurring of speech and cardiac arrhythmias followed by convulsions.

KEY POINTS

- Local anaesthetics have a membrane stabilising action by blocking sodium channels in excitable tissues
- Local anaesthetics bind to the intracellular element of the VGSC molecule
- The duration of the block depends upon the drug characteristics, the rate of washout from the tissues concerned and additives added to the local anaesthetic solution
- Organic drug stays in equilibrium between two fractions, the ionised form and the non-ionised form. The former is the active form and the latter required for crossing membrane barriers
- The pH at which the two fractions are in equal proportions is called the pKa of the drug
- A drug with a low pKa will dissociate into a higher proportion of the non-ionised form compared to a drug with a high pKa
- Nerve fibres show varying susceptibility to blockade depending upon their cross-sectional diameter, presence of a myelin sheath and concentration of the local anaesthetic

- Central nervous system toxicity is likely to be seen before cardiovascular toxicity
- Regional block techniques are commonly used for acute pain management in the perioperative period. Their role in chronic conditions is more limited

References

1. Koller C. On the use of cocaine for producing anaesthesia on the eye. *Lancet* 1884; **2**: 990.
2. Corning JL. Spinal anaesthesia and local medication of the cord with cocaine. *NY Med J* 1885; **42**: 483.
3. Vanhoutte F, Vereecke J, Verbeke N et al. Stereoselective effects of the enantiomers of bupivacaine on the electrophysiological properties of the guinea-pig papillary muscle. *Br J Pharmacol* 1991; **103**(1): 1275–1281.
4. Marban E, Yamagishi T, Tomaselli GF. Structure and function of voltage-gated sodium channels. *J Physiol* 1998; **508(Pt 3)**: 647–657.
5. Ragsdale DS, McPhee JC, Scheuer T et al. Common molecular determinants of local anesthetic, antiarrhythmic, and anticonvulsant block of voltage-gated Na+ channels. *Proc Natl Acad Sci USA* 1996; **93**(17): 9270–9275.
6. Goldin AL, Barchi RL, Caldwell JH et al. Nomenclature of voltage-gated sodium channels. *Neuron* 2000; **28**(2): 365–368.
7. De Jong RH, Robles R, Corbin RW. Central actions of lidocaine – synaptic transmission. *Anesthesiology* 1969; **30**(1): 19–23.
8. Lund PC, Cwik JC. Propitocaine (citanest) and methemoglobinemia. *Anesthesiology* 1965; **26**: 569–571.
9. Richardson J, Lonnqvist PA. Thoracic paravertebral block. *Br J Anaesth* 1998; **81**(2): 230–238.
10. Bartlett EE, Hutserani O. Xylocaine for the relief of postoperative pain. *Anesth Analg* 1961; **40**: 296–304.
11. Kastrup J, Petersen P, Dejgard A et al. Treatment of chronic painful diabetic neuropathy with intravenous lidocaine infusion. *Br Med J (Clin Res Ed)* 1986; **292** (6514): 173.
12. Tanelian DL, Brose WG. Neuropathic pain can be relieved by drugs that are use-dependent sodium channel blockers: lidocaine, carbamazepine, and mexiletine. *Anesthesiology* 1991; **74**(5): 949–951.
13. Waxman SG, Dib-Hajj S, Cummins TR et al. Sodium channels and pain. *Proc Natl Acad Sci USA* 1999; **96**(14): 7635–7639.
14. Galer BS, Harle J, Rowbotham MC. Response to intravenous lidocaine infusion predicts subsequent response to oral mexiletine: a prospective study. *J Pain Symptom Manage* 1996; **12**(3): 161–167.
15. Woolf CJ, Wiesenfeld-Hallin Z. The systemic administration of local anaesthetics produces a selective depression of C-afferent fibre evoked activity in the spinal cord. *Pain* 1985; **23**(4): 361–374.
16. Devor M, Wall PD, Catalan N. Systemic lidocaine silences ectopic neuroma and DRG discharge without blocking nerve conduction. *Pain* 1992; **48**(2): 261–268.
17. Labbe L, Turgeon J. Clinical pharmacokinetics of mexiletine. *Clin Pharmacokinet* 1999; **37**(5): 361–384.
18. Gold MS. Sodium channels and pain therapy. *Curr Opin Anaesthesiol* 2000; **13**(5): 565–572.

Opioids

Introduction

Opioid drugs are widely used in medicine and are known to be extremely effective analgesics. As such, they are used to treat moderate or severe pain, rather than mild pain, which may respond to less potent analgesic drugs.

There are several terms used to describe this class of drug, and whilst they are generally used interchangeably, they all have slightly different meanings, as discussed below.

Definitions

- *Opioid* applies to all endogenous or synthetic compounds that produce morphine-like effects upon binding to a receptor. These substances are all related to the parent compound of *opium*, a naturally occurring drug that is an extract of *Papaver somniferum*, the poppy plant.
- *Opiate* is a term that is used less frequently, and refers to those naturally occurring drugs that are direct derivatives of opium (e.g. morphine and codeine).
- *Narcotic* is a term that has been widely used in the past, but is little used today. It is derived from the Greek word meaning 'stupor' and was originally used to describe a drug that precipitated sleep, but later became synonymous with the term opioid.

History

Opium and its derivatives have been used for thousands of years, and references to the drug can be seen in literature from as early as the 3rd century BC. This is the earliest reliable reference to opium and was reputedly used by

Arabian physicians. There are accounts of the usage of opium in ancient Roman, Greek and Egyptian literature.

In 1803 Friedrich Wilhelm Sertürner, was the first to isolate the active compound from opium and was named morphine, after Morpheus, the god of dreams.[1] E. Merck & Company was the first to commercially manufacture morphine in 1827. Isolation of further pure substances, such as codeine, followed shortly after this initial discovery. Since then a series of synthetic opiates (e.g. fentanyl, oxycodone) have been developed along with a variety of delivery systems (e.g. slow-release tablets, transdermal preparations, patient-controlled delivery systems).

Pharmacodynamics

Structure

The structure of opioid drugs varies depending on whether the drug is a derivative of morphine or is a synthetic drug.

Morphine is a phenanthrene derivative (Fig. 10.1).

Other drugs that are related to morphine in structure are known as morphine analogues, and include, among others, the full agonists diamorphine and codeine, the partial agonist nalorphine and the antagonist naloxone. These relatives of morphine are produced by exchanging either the nitrogen atom or a hydroxyl group for another atom or molecule.

Diamorphine (diacetylmorphine) is a direct derivative of morphine, produced by acetylation at the 3 and 6 positions and is thus semisynthetic. It is more lipid soluble than morphine (i.e. it more readily crosses membranes, such as the blood–brain barrier) and, therefore, higher concentrations are achieved in a shorter time, providing the 'hit' sought by addicts. It is metabolised to morphine, and produces almost identical effects to morphine. Because of the increased solubility, lower concentrations are needed to produce analgesia than with morphine.

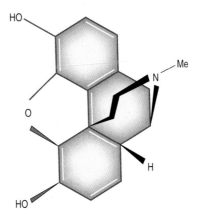

Fig. 10.1   Structure of morphine

Codeine is also a direct derivative of morphine. Its structure is methylmorphine, the methyl substitution is on the phenolic hydroxyl group.[2] Codeine is a pro-drug, like diamorphine it is metabolised to morphine. It is classed as a much less potent analgesic (approximately 75–85% less potent than morphine). This is because approximately 10% of the codeine dose is converted to morphine. It is available in the UK over the counter in doses of 8 mg or less combined with paracetamol (acetaminophen). Higher doses are used clinically, commonly 30–60 mg codeine. Codeine is, therefore, used to treat mild-to-moderate, rather than severe pain. It is also known to cause less addictive behaviour, and as such is available as a 'pharmacy' medicine, rather than a 'prescription only' medicine.

Adverse effects are common even at clinical doses. It is, therefore, important to discuss how the effects of these drugs can be reversed. Opioid antagonists exist (e.g. naloxone and naltrexone), and are extremely effective at reversing the effects of opioids, both the analgesic and side effects. The details of these drugs are discussed later.

Opioid drugs may also be synthetic derivatives, with structures dissimilar to morphine. These drugs include pethidine, fentanyl, methadone, dextropropoxyphene, pentazocine and buprenorphine (Table 10.1).

Endogenous opioids

Opioid drugs (e.g. morphine) are known to bring about their actions by mimicking the naturally occurring opioids within the body, known as endogenous opioids.

The endogenous opioid system is complex, with many known naturally occurring peptides and is only briefly discussed here.

TABLE 10.1 Table of some available opioids and their classification

Drug name	Classification	Half life (hours)
Morphine	Naturally occurring Pure agonist	2–3
Diamorphine	Semi-synthetic Pro-drug Pure agonist	0.5
Codeine	Semi-synthetic Pro-drug Pure agonist	2–3
Methadone	Synthetic Pure agonist	12–>150
Fentanyl	Synthetic Pure agonist	7–12
Alfentanil	Synthetic Pure agonist	1–2
Remifentanil	Synthetic Pure agonist	0.1
Buprenorphine	Semi-synthetic Partial agonist	2–3
Tramadol	Mixed action	7

There are three different families of endogenous opioid peptides, known as enkephalins, endorphins and dynorphins. Each family has an individual polypeptide precursor and these are: preproenkephalin, preproopiomelanocortin and preprodynorphin. Each of these precursors undergoes modification to produce the various endogenous opioid peptides. The commonly known peptides are leu-enkephalin, met-enkephalin, β-endorphin and dynorphin.[3] These endogenous peptides are found throughout the brain, however, within the spinal cord, there is slightly more distinction. The enkephalins are generally found in the descending pathways down to the dorsal horn and dynorphin is more commonly found in interneurones.[3]

It is via these endogenous peptides that the receptor system for opioids has been understood.

Mechanisms of action

Cellular level

The overall effect of opioids at a cellular level is inhibitory. This inhibitory effect occurs via the interaction of the opioid drug at an opioid receptor. These receptors are G-protein-coupled receptors, and inhibit adenylate cyclase (a membrane-bound enzyme). This inhibition of adenylate cyclase causes a decrease in the intracellular concentration of the second messenger, cyclic 3′,5′-adenosine monophosphate (cAMP), which in turn inhibits downstream processes, via the inhibition of protein kinase A (PKA).

The G-protein-coupled receptors are also directly coupled to specific ion channels. By binding to the opioid receptor, drugs cause potassium channels to open, whilst preventing the opening of voltage-gated calcium channels. The action on these membrane ion channels is to reduce the excitability of neurones (via hyperpolarisation caused by opening K^+ channels) and also reduces the release of transmitter (by inhibiting Ca^{2+} influx into the cell). Thus, the overall actions are inhibitory.

Effects on pain: The nociceptive pathway

Opioid receptors are found throughout the central nervous system (CNS), thus allowing opioid drugs to act at a relatively global level within the CNS. Areas of the brain known to be rich in opioid receptors include the periaqueductal grey matter, pontine reticular formation, median raphe, nucleus raphe magnus and the gigantocellular reticularis in the rostral ventromedial medulla and spinal cord. These areas project to many other parts of the brain and, by stimulating or inhibiting them, inhibit pain transmission. Also, the dorsal horn itself is known to be sensitive to opioids, as are the peripheral terminals of nociceptive afferent neurones.

At a central level, substantial analgesia is achieved by intrathecal injection of very low concentrations of opioid, thus proving their central action.

At a spinal level, opioids prevent the transmission of pain through the dorsal horn, again proving the presence of opioid receptors at a spinal level.

In the periphery, it is thought that opioid drugs act upon the peripheral terminals of afferent neurones, thus preventing ascending nociceptive transmission. This is demonstrated by a local injection of opiate, such as morphine, to a painful area of the body (e.g. a joint, providing analgesia).

Opioid receptors

There are generally thought to be three major classes of opioid receptor within the nervous system that are involved in analgesia. These receptors are named: mu (μ), kappa (κ) and delta (δ) and they mediate the pharmacological effects of opiates. These receptors are all G-protein-coupled receptors and thus inhibit adenylate cyclase. Each of the three major receptor classes can be further divided into subtypes.

μ Receptors

Most of the opioid drugs used for analgesia are thought to be relatively selective for μ receptors and so it is surmised that μ receptors are responsible for most of the analgesic effects of opioids and also the major adverse effects of these drugs.

μ receptors can be subdivided into:

- μ_1: thought to act supraspinally
- μ_2: thought to act at a spinal level.

In practice, when morphine is given systemically, it acts predominantly through the central μ_1 receptors.

κ Receptors

A few opioid analgesics are selective for κ receptors. The analgesia produced tends to be at a spinal or peripheral level rather than central, and drugs that selectively act at these receptors tend to produce few adverse effects and no dependence.

There are three receptor subtypes known for κ:

- κ_1: mostly present at a spinal level
- κ_2: little is known of these receptors
- κ_3: receptors are found supraspinally.

δ Receptors

δ receptors are found more in the periphery than in the central nervous system, and so the effects mediated by these receptors are spinal and peripheral. δ receptors are further divided into δ_1 and δ_2.

A fourth receptor type is known to mediate the effects of opioid drugs and this is the sigma (σ) receptor type. This receptor type is not a true opioid receptor, but opioids and other psychotomimetic drugs are known to act at these receptors.

It is important to remember that different opioid drugs have different affinities for each of the receptor types, and that there is also the genetic variability of individuals meaning that the density of each type of receptor will vary from person to person. This may explain why some patients respond to one opioid in a different way to another.

Pharmacokinetics

Absorption

Most opioid analgesics when administered via the intravenous, intramuscular, subcutaneous and transmucosal (such as inside the nose and mouth) routes have high bioavailability. By definition intravenous administration of any drug has 100% bioavailability. More recently, the transdermal route of administration has been used to administer opioid analgesics (e.g. fentanyl) as a patch worn on the skin.

Opioids may also be taken orally; however, many drugs in this class undergo significant hepatic first-pass metabolism. The compounds undergo glucuronidation in the liver, which decreases the bioavailability (i.e. only a proportion of the administered dose reaches the systemic circulation). This essentially means that a higher oral dose of the drug is required to produce a meaningful therapeutic effect. For approximate bioavailabilities of opioid drugs see Table 10.2.

Distribution

Opioid drugs bind to plasma proteins in the blood, and are carried to distant sites in the body. The drugs dissociate readily from the plasma proteins and tend to accumulate in areas of highest perfusion, such as the liver, lungs and kidneys. The brain tends to be an area in which there is less accumulation of opioid drugs. This is due to the blood–brain barrier, which prevents many opioid drugs accessing the brain. However, some opioids are able to traverse the blood–brain barrier, such as diamorphine (heroin) due to the lipophilic nature of the compound.

Accumulation also occurs in fatty tissue, and this is important to remember when administering particularly lipophilic drugs, such as fentanyl.

As these drugs are largely transported bound to plasma proteins, it is important to consider the protein-depleted patient. A lack of plasma protein will inevitably increase the free concentration of a drug, and this should not be forgotten when prescribing opioids in these patients.

TABLE 10.2 Bioavailabilities of some opioid drugs in common clinical use

Opioid drug	Percentage bioavailability (%)
Morphine	25
Codeine	50
Tramadol	75
Oxycodone	60
Methadone	80
Buprenorphine	30 (sub-lingual administration)
Pentazocine	47
Data from[4]	

Metabolism

The main route of inactivation of opioid drugs is via hepatic metabolism, usually in the form of conjugation with the compound glucuronide. Compounds that have free hydroxyl groups, usually at the 3- and 6- positions are readily conjugated with glucuronide (e.g. morphine). The metabolite of morphine, morphine 6-glucuronide is also a potent analgesic (Fig. 10.2).

It is important to note that some opioid drugs are metabolised to produce morphine. Examples are diamorphine and codeine, and once metabolised to morphine, undergo glucuronidation to produce the same active metabolites. It should be noted that codeine is metabolised by the P450 system in the liver. Approximately 10% is metabolised to morphine (hence its use for mild-to-moderate pain). In the Caucasian population, genetic variation of the enzyme system is such that 10% are unable to effectively metabolise codeine and thus it is ineffective in those patients.

It should also be remembered that many of the metabolites of opioids are pharmacologically active and may have longer half-lives than their parent compound (e.g. morphine and morphine-6-glucuronide).

Excretion

The majority of the opioid conjugates are excreted in the urine via the kidneys. A small proportion of the metabolites find their way to the gut via biliary excretion, and here they are hydrolysed back to morphine and reabsorbed via the enterohepatic circulation, to eventually find their way back to the liver for further metabolism.

It is important to understand that there is the potential for accumulation of active metabolites in renal insufficiency.

Pharmacological actions

Effects on the CNS

Analgesia

In humans, analgesia without loss of consciousness can be achieved with morphine and morphine-like drugs. Opioids are used mainly for the treatment of

Fig. 10.2 Metabolic products of morphine

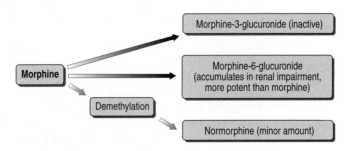

moderate or severe pain, which may be acute or chronic. These drugs are, therefore, useful in treating pain associated with cancer (tumour growth), inflammation, bone pain and soft-tissue injury. Opioids are also often used for the treatment of postoperative pain. It is generally believed that opioid drugs are better at treating dull pain that is continuous in nature rather than sharp pain that may be intermittent or sporadic. However, opioids are potent enough analgesics to treat the severe intermittent pain of biliary or renal colic.

The mechanism by which analgesia is achieved has been described previously, opioids work by acting upon the nociceptive pathway to inhibit the transmission of pain. Some opioids, e.g. morphine and diamorphine, are also thought to have some effect on the psychological impact of pain, at the level of the limbic system within the brain. However, this is not the case for all opioid drugs.

Respiratory depression

This is a significant adverse effect, particularly with the more potent drugs, such as morphine, and respiratory depression must be taken into consideration when prescribing or administering opioids for analgesic use. Although significant this is uncommonly seen, as pain stimulates respiration and if the dose and effect are properly monitored significant levels of respiratory depression are avoided.

Both analgesia and respiratory depression are mediated by the μ receptors, and so by increasing opioid concentration to achieve analgesia, the chance of producing respiratory depression increases.

Respiratory depression occurs due to a reduction in the sensitivity of the respiratory centre in the brain to the arterial partial pressure of carbon dioxide ($PaCO_2$) and as a result, the $PaCO_2$ increases. The increase in carbon dioxide in itself has a narcotic effect in the sense that is results in drowsiness and eventually loss of consciousness.

Unfortunately, respiratory depression occurs at therapeutic doses of opioids, and such is its significance, it is the commonest cause of death in acute opioid poisoning.

With careful controlled titration of dose this side effect can be avoided or minimised with little risk to the patient in both the acute and chronic setting. Greater care is required in the elderly and frail patients who may respond to lower doses of opioid due to their altered physiology. As a general rule starting with a low dose and titrating it slowly to effect will result in appropriate analgesia and minimal side effects.

Euphoria, sedation and confusion

Some patients, after administration of morphine, experience a pleasant feeling of freedom and contentment. This feeling of euphoria is mediated mainly via μ receptors, but is tempered by the dysphoria produced by activation of κ receptors. The euphoria produced by opioids is clinically important when attempting to alleviate pain, as it lessens the agitation associated with pain. These effects along with confusion and potentially hallucinations are more common in the elderly. Such effects are very frightening for the patient and dose modification or alteration to another opioid may be required.

Drowsiness is a frequently seen effect of opioid drugs. It is more commonly seen in the elderly or frail than younger patients, usually the patient is woken easily from sleep. Sedation is commonly seen with the phenanthrene derivatives such as morphine, but less often with synthetic drugs such as fentanyl.

Nausea and vomiting

This is a common adverse effect of opioid drugs, particularly morphine, occurring in approximately 35–45% of patients. It is dose-related, and if problematic, anti-emetics can be administered. The nausea usually resolves with repeated administrations of the opioid. Interestingly, some patients will tolerate one opioid better than another and this may be a reason to swap drugs. This is more commonly done in patients who are on opioids chronically.

The nausea and vomiting occur due to the central action of the drug in the chemoreceptor trigger zone (area postrema) in the medulla.

Immunosuppression

There is evidence that opioid drugs cause immunosuppression with long-term use. This leads to an increased susceptibility to infection and decreased tumour suppression. It is thought to occur by a complex process, whereby opioids have a direct effect on the cells of the immune system and an indirect effect via centrally mediated neuronal mechanisms.[5]

It is thought that acute immunosuppression may be mediated by the sympathetic nervous system, and that chronic immunosuppression involves the hypothalamic–pituitary–adrenal axis.

Papillary constriction

This is a normal and insignificant effect of opioids probably mediated in the same way as the gastrointestinal and urinary effects.

Peripheral effects

Effects on the gastrointestinal and urinary system

Constipation is a well-recognised side effect of opioid drug use. This is a dose-dependent effect and may not settle with continued use. In long-term use concomitant administration of drugs (e.g. gastric stimulants or stool softeners) to counteract this side effect should be considered.

Tone is generally increased throughout the gastrointestinal tract and motility reduced. This is brought about due to a high density of opioid receptors in the gastrointestinal system. Constipation occurs because there is a lack of propulsive or peristaltic action in the small and large intestines, delaying the passage of digested material. This results in more water reabsorption from the gastric contents resulting in constipation. However, in a patient with diarrhoea, the action of opioid drugs on the bowel is desirable (i.e. the increased absorption of water) and some opioids (e.g. loperamide) are licensed for the treatment of diarrhoea.

It is also important to remember that reduced motility and increased tone in the stomach cause a delay in gastric emptying. This has implications for patients taking other medications, which may not be absorbed as well due to this delay. This would include drugs not absorbed from the stomach or that are altered by the gastric contents.

The mechanism of action for this effect is thought to be mediated locally by the enteric nervous system and centrally via the CNS.

A similar effect on the muscle of the urinary tract results in sphincter contraction and the development of acute urinary retention.

Itch[5]

Itch is a common and sometimes significant side effect that necessitates the withdrawal of the opioid. It is thought to be a μ receptor mediated effect.[6] It is reversed with opioid antagonists and may be more apparent with one agent over another. Using an alternative opioid may reduce the severity of this side effect.

Other side effects

There are other side effects to consider, some of which will be of greater relevance in chronic use. These include weight gain or loss, reduced adrenal function and altered sexual function.

Opioid antagonists

To combat the adverse effects of opioid drugs (that may occur in overdose) opioid antagonists exist. The two most common antagonists are naloxone, which is relatively short acting and naltrexone, which is longer acting. These drugs can be administered to reverse the effects of morphine and other opioids if overdose is known, or even suspected. Naloxone and naltrexone are direct antagonists of morphine and other opioids. They act by binding to opioid receptors, preventing the occupancy of the receptors by the agonist drug. They work very rapidly, within minutes, and can be life-saving in overdose. However, naloxone, which is more commonly used than naltrexone, has a very short half-life as it is rapidly metabolised by the liver, and, therefore, repeated doses may be required.

The use of opioid antagonists needs to be done with close observation of the effects. The reversal of undesirable effects should be the objective. The analgesic effects will also be reversed, which will have a detrimental effect on the patient and may precipitate an acute withdrawal effect in patients who are taking opioids in the long term.

Common controversies with opioids[7]

Tolerance

A definition of tolerance of a drug is the need to increase the dose of the drug in order to maintain its pharmacological effects. Put another way, the same dose of drug will have diminishing effect. This is a pharmacological phenomenon.

Tolerance to morphine and other opioid drugs occurs rapidly, it has been demonstrated at 24 hours after administration, although generally it is thought to occur after approximately 2 weeks of continuous treatment.

Tolerance occurs with most of the pharmacological effects of opioids (pain relief, euphoria and respiratory depression) but there is little tolerance with respect to papillary constriction and constipation. For example, an addict who increases the dose of morphine or diamorphine to maintain a given level of euphoria will not experience further respiratory depression, but they will have increased constriction of the pupils and further reduction in bowel motility.

The mechanism by which tolerance to opioids is thought to occur involves the cellular pathway previously discussed. Opioids are known to inhibit the membrane-bound enzyme adenylate cyclase, which in turn inhibits the formation of the second messenger cAMP. Over time, even in the presence of the opioid drug, expression of adenylate cyclase increases in a bid to overcome the inhibition by the opioid and the levels of cAMP increase accordingly. Therefore, to continue to produce a pharmacological effect, the amount of opioid must be increased in order to re-inhibit adenylate cyclase.

In long-term clinical use for pain management the dose of opioid does not appear to increase after the initial titration to reach analgesia. Tolerance does not, therefore, seem to occur at steady therapeutic levels.

Withdrawal

This is a syndrome that manifests when a drug is stopped or the dose reduced in patients who have been habitual users (this may be clinical or recreational use). For opioids this may be psychological withdrawal with craving and agitation or physical withdrawal with diarrhoea and tachycardia. Giving the opioid antagonist naloxone may also induce a withdrawal response.

Withdrawal is again a pharmacological effect and is common with many medications that are in clinical use.

Dependence

Physiological and/or psychological dependence on any drug is demonstrated by an abstinence syndrome (i.e. a withdrawal response on stopping the drug); characteristic signs are seen that are directly attributable to the abstinence from drug use. This is to say that the continued use of the drug is required in order to prevent a physiological withdrawal response.

There is confusion over the difference between dependence and addiction both within the medical fraternity and the lay public. This causes confusion and reluctance in patients who refuse to take medication that causes dependence, misunderstanding this for addiction.

Abrupt withdrawal of morphine and morphine-related drugs, or administration of an opioid antagonist, results in a typical pattern; some of the first signs of withdrawal are sweating, yawning and rhinorrhea, seen at 12 hours post-withdrawal, and these are followed by restlessness, piloerection (cold-turkey), shaking, pupillary dilatation, insomnia and irritability. By day 3, abdominal cramp, muscle spasms, increases in heart rate and blood pressure, nausea and diarrhoea are seen.

These signs are usually accompanied by psychological signs of withdrawal, a strong craving for the drug, which may result in violent behaviour and erratic moods.

Withdrawal symptoms last approximately 10 days, with a peak on day 2 or 3 of abstinence. However, the psychological dependence may last much longer.

The abstinence syndrome from morphine and other strong opioids can be immediately relieved by administration of the opioid drug. The degree of withdrawal that a patient has to undergo can be minimised by slowly titrating the dose down over a period of weeks or months (depending on the drug concerned, the dose they are on and for how long they have been taking it).

Addiction[7,8]

This is a syndrome and pattern of substance misuse. There are several criteria and published classifications. Usually three of the following elements are required to occur at the same time within the previous 12 months:

- The drug and related stimuli become increasingly important. There is frequently a change in behaviour focused on drug seeking at any cost
- Loss of control in using the drug
- Tolerance having developed
- A withdrawal response being evident on stopping the drug
- Relapse to dependent use after a period of stopping the drug
- Modification of mood with positive effects or lifting of a negative mood state.

This is clearly different to dependence and requires a misuse of the agent responsible. In clinical practice addiction is uncommon, although dependence is seen. Patients using opioids for modifying their pain tend to find any alteration in their mood or feelings of loss of self control unpleasant and will stop taking the drug at an early stage. Clinical trials tend to be too short to be able to comment on dependence or addiction, but are able to identify the side effects of opioids.[9]

KEY POINTS

- There is an endogenous opioid system (enkephalins, endorphins and dynorphins) within the brain and spinal cord
- Opioids work via specific receptors (μ, κ and δ) resulting in a reduction in excitability of nociceptive neurones. Different opioids have differing affinities to each receptor
- Opioids are highly protein bound in the blood stream. Plasma protein levels will affect the free drug available. Dose reduction may be required under such circumstances
- Codeine is a prodrug with approximately 10% being converted to morphine
- Respiratory depression should not be a problem if the dose of opioid is titrated to effect with regard to pain
- Nausea is a common side effect but can be reduced when indicated by concomitant use of antiemetics
- Confusion and hallucinations may occur especially in the elderly. Careful dose titration to effect or rotating the opioid will minimise this problem
- Constipation is very common and appropriate drugs should be administered to counteract this. This is particularly true in long-term use
- A physical dependence and withdrawal syndrome does occur, but can be managed by slow withdrawal of drug. Addiction is uncommon when opioids are used for analgesia
- Opioids are potent analgesics for moderate-to-severe pain with good efficacy in acute and cancer pain settings. They have a role (but much more limited) in chronic pain and should only be used when appropriate patient supervision is available

References

1. Huxtable RJ, Schwarz SKW. The isolation of morphine – first principles in science and ethics. *Mol Interv* 2001; **1**(4): 189–191.
2. Gutstein HB, Akil H. *Opioid analgesics* in *Goodman and Gillman's the pharmacological basis of therapeutics*, 11th edn. In: Brunton L, Parker J, Lazo K (eds). New York: McGraw Hill Publishing; 2005.
3. Rang HP, Dale MM, Ritter JM et al. Analgesic drugs. In: *Pharmacology*, 5th edn. Edinburgh: Churchill Livingstone; 2003: 562–584.
4. Heffernan AM, Rowbotham DJ. Clinical pharmacology: opioids. In: Rowbotham DJ, Macintyre PE (eds) *Clinical pain management*. Arnold: London; 2003: 43–54.
5. Sharp B, Yaksh T. Pain killers of the immune system. *Nat Med* 1997; **3**(8): 831–832.
6. Ko MC, Song MS, Edwards T et al. The role of central mu opioid receptors in opioid-induced itch in primates. *J Pharmacol Exp Ther* 2004; **310**(1): 169–176.
7. The British Pain Society. *Pain and substance misuse: improving the patient experience. A consensus document for consultation*. London: The British Pain Society; 2006.
8. The Pain Society. *Recommendations for the appropriate use of opioids for persistent non-cancer pain. A consensus statement prepared on behalf of the Pain Society, the Royal College of Anaesthetists, the Royal College of General Practitioners and the Royal College of Psychiatrists*. London: The Pain Society; 2004.
9. Kalso E, Edwards J, Moore RA et al. Opioids in chronic non-cancer pain: systematic review of efficacy and safety. *Pain* 2004; **112**(3): 372–380.

Further reading

Suggested reading for developing an understanding for pharmacology and therapeutics:

Brunton L, Parker, J, Lazo K (eds) *Goodman and Gillman's The Pharmacological Basis of Therapeutics*, 11th edn. New York: McGraw Hill Publishing; 2005.

General references for understanding opioid use in clinical practice:

The British Pain Society. *Pain and substance misuse: improving the patient experience. A consensus document for consultation*. London: The British Pain Society; 2006.

The Pain Society. *Recommendations for the appropriate use of opioids for persistent non-cancer pain. A consensus statement prepared on behalf of the Pain Society, the Royal College of Anaesthetists, the Royal College of General Practitioners and the Royal College of Psychiatrists*. London: The Pain Society; 2004.

Websites

www.britishpainsociety.org/misuse_0806.pdf (accessed 20/11/06)

Adjuvant and miscellaneous drugs used in pain management

Introduction

Analgesic drugs are generally considered to be those compounds that reduce the perception of pain in either clinical or experimental models of nociception. In animal studies, this reduction in pain is assessed by means of the behavioural alterations seen following administration of the analgesic. In humans, subjective assessments of pain are generally used. In practice, particularly at a preclinical level, this generally means that robust experimental models of pain are developed that reliably produce pain. This experimentally generated pain is reduced by a relatively limited group of drugs, which have become standard and familiar agents in pain management. These drugs generally work well when dealing with straightforward acute pain in the clinical setting. However, where more complex acute pain presentations are encountered, or in the inescapably complex scenario of chronic pain, the limited scope of these familiar drugs becomes evident and alternative compounds need to be sought. Furthermore, potentially serious problems have been identified with the use of many classical analgesic agents and means of reducing these risks are also being sought.

Adjuvant drugs are those drugs used to enhance the efficacy of other drugs used in pain management and are used in combination with those drugs, typically the opioids. However, a number of these drugs have significant analgesic activity in circumstances where classical analgesics, such as opioids, are ineffective or poorly effective. In these circumstances, the drugs are used alone.

From a practical perspective, the majority of drugs described in this chapter possess little potential for addiction or misuse (with the notable exception of the cannabinoids); this is an important consideration when any medication is to be used in the long term.

It will be obvious that adjuvant agents will often be prescribed simultaneously with other analgesic medication. In addition, more than one adjuvant may be prescribed at the same time. However, this will increase the likelihood of both adverse events and drug interactions, some of which are described below. Where unusual or unfamiliar drugs are concurrently prescribed liaison with an experienced pharmacist is essential to avoid potentially hazardous interactions.

Antidepressant agents

Antidepressant drugs have been used in pain management for over 40 years. They have been used for the management of both pain as well as coexisting depressive symptoms that are common in patients suffering from chronic pain. They remain an effective and useful component of the analgesic pharmacopoeia.

The first antidepressant drugs available for clinical use were the monoamine oxidase inhibitors (MAOIs), developed in the 1950s and early 1960s.

Antidepressants and pain management[1,2]

Their use in pain management was first reported in the mid-1960s. As is often the case in clinical medicine, the application of a pharmacological solution to a clinical problem was more a case of serendipity than logic. Chronic pain presentations have always perplexed health professionals and frequently, patients with such presentations have been dismissed as presenting with primary psychiatric pathology. As is noted elsewhere in this book, whilst psychosocial factors do strongly modulate an individual's experience of pain, it is relatively infrequent to see individuals in whom pain is a presentation of pure psychopathology. Nevertheless, this viewpoint has always attracted a following and a particularly persistent paradigm has centred around the 'masked depression' hypothesis. This postulates that complaints of chronic pain are an expression of existential and emotional distress in individuals in whom direct expression of such feelings is either personally or culturally unacceptable. This paradigm was particularly popular in the 1960s and 1970s and, fortuitously, led to the newly developed antidepressant agents being prescribed to patients with chronic pain.

The beneficial effect of these drugs in certain groups of patients with chronic pain was seen as a vindication of the masked depression hypothesis, although by modern standards, the quality of the early research was very poor. Later studies, using randomised, double-blind designs, with appropriate analysis of confounding factors, yielded much more interesting information. Firstly, whilst benefit was seen across a variety of pain syndromes, the most significant benefit was seen in neuropathic pain syndromes, such as diabetic neuropathy, postherpetic neuralgia and demyelination. Secondly, whilst patients' mood did tend to improve, pain relief occurred irrespective of whether the patients initially presented with depressed mood; in other words, the analgesic and antidepressant effects appeared to be separate. Similarly, subsequent studies have also shown that even in situations where antidepressant agents do not appear to provide significant pain relief, depressed patients benefit in terms of improved mood.

A large number of antidepressant agents are available for clinical use. The research evidence indicates that those compounds likely to be useful in chronic pain management are rather fewer. As noted above, the first agents to be used were the MAOIs, such as phenelzine. This group of drugs causes irreversible inhibition of monoamine oxidase. They have potentially serious interactions with many pharmacological compounds and even some foods; hence they are generally not used outside specialist psychiatric practice. In more recent years, reversible MAOIs, such as moclobemide, have become available and there is some evidence of analgesic activity in clinical pain states, although currently other agents have a better evidence base.

Tricyclic antidepressants

For many years, tricyclic antidepressant drugs have been the benchmark compounds in terms of antidepressant analgesia. Randomised controlled trials support the use of imipramine, amitriptyline, nortriptyline, desipramine and doxepin in a variety of clinical pain states, although in reality, the analgesia is probably a class effect of these drugs and the choice of agent is more dependent on the tolerability of a specific agent in an individual patient. The dose required to produce useful analgesia is of the same order of magnitude as that required to produce benefit when used for the treatment of depression. For drugs such as amitriptyline or imipramine, this generally will require doses in excess of 100 mg daily. Lower doses are unlikely to be effective. Treatment duration is also an important consideration. Useful responses are rarely seen before 2 weeks and an appropriate treatment trial should be of at least 6–8 weeks' duration.

The use of more modern antidepressant drugs has yielded rather mixed results. The selective serotonin reuptake inhibitors (SSRIs) have been studied quite extensively and the conclusion here is fairly clear; they have little if any analgesic activity. On the other hand, drugs having a mixed monoaminergic profile, the so-called serotonin/noradrenaline (norepinephrine) reuptake inhibitors (SNRIs), do appear to have similar activity to the tricyclic drugs and a limited evidence base does support the use of the SNRI venlafaxine in neuropathic pain (Table 11.1).

TABLE 11.1 Antidepressant drugs used in pain management with some of the common side effects

Drug class	Examples	Side effects
Tricyclic antidepressants	Amitriptyline	Sedation
	Nortriptyline	Dry mouth
	Imipramine	Cognitive function
	Desipramine	Postural hypotension
	Doxepin	Weight change
Serotonin/noradrenaline reuptake inhibitors	Venlafaxine	Caution in heart disease
		Constipation
		Nausea
		Hypertension

Mode of action

The mode of action of the antidepressant agents in modulating pain is, essentially, unknown, although it is likely that a number of mechanisms are relevant.

It has been known for many years that descending pathways from the brain stem project to neurones in the superficial dorsal horn of the spinal cord. These projections appear to involve serotonergic and noradrenergic transmission onto neurons that, in turn, inhibit the transmission of pain signals within deeper layers of the spinal cord. It has been postulated that antidepressants enhance this activity and, hence, enhance the analgesic response. The problem with this model is that antidepressants appear to have no short- or long-term activity on somatic pain.

Over recent years, it has been discovered that serotonin in particular has very varied effects on pain transmission within the spinal cord with inhibitory effects at some sites but facilitatory effects at others.

Other models of antidepressant action in neuropathic pain have discarded the notion of neurotransmitter potentiation altogether and have suggested a mechanism by which antidepressant drugs enhance the plasticity of the nervous system, allowing the reversal of some of the pathological changes seen following nerve injury. Two important candidate mechanisms for this process are the activation of glial cells to release neurotrophins (nerve growth factors) and activation of neurological stem cells. Both of these are known to occur following antidepressant administration and are thought to represent a major part of the action of these drugs in the management of depression. Similar mechanisms may well be active following their use in pain management, although direct evidence is currently lacking.

Side effects

Side effects are fairly common with antidepressant administration and are generally similar across all classes. The most common are sedation, dry mouth and altered cognitive function, particularly with the tricyclic agents. Sexual dysfunction is also very common and appears to be dose related. Erectile impotence in men and loss of orgasmic function in both sexes is common and can cause great distress. It is rarely volunteered as a symptom by patients and direct questioning is often required.

A rare adverse event seen with the antidepressant agents is the serotonin syndrome, characterised by delirium and autonomic instability. This is a dose-related phenomenon and is rare when a single agent is used alone. However, it may occur when two agents are inadvertently co-prescribed and can be precipitated by the concurrent use of an antidepressant agent and tramadol as the latter has strong serotonergic activity.

Anticonvulsant drugs[3-6]

Anticonvulsant drugs have been used for many years in the management of certain chronic pain conditions. The first description of the use of anticonvulsants in pain management dates back to 1947 when phenytoin was described in the treatment of trigeminal neuralgia. Since that time, many new compounds have been developed and a number of these have found a role in pain management.

Anticonvulsants are used in the management of chronic neuropathic pain as well as migraine and some less common headache syndromes. In this respect, their role is probably more limited than the antidepressant drugs. Anticonvulsants have no effect on acute somatic pain and, indeed, some appear to show a slight enhancement of the pain response when used in acute somatic pain.

Mode of action

The mode of action of anticonvulsants is far more varied than, say, the antidepressant drugs. In many cases, the mode of action is poorly understood. However, in the broadest sense there are two main modes of action:

- Firstly, a drug may decrease the maximum firing rate of neurones by interfering with the activity of ion channels in the cell membrane.
- Secondly, a drug may either mimic, or potentiate the effect of an inhibitory neurotransmitter, such as gamma-aminobutyric acid (GABA).

Many clinically used drugs have effects on several different systems and some display effects both on ion channels and inhibitory neurotransmitters. For others, sodium valproate in particular, the mode of action remains unknown despite 30 years of clinical use. This heterogeneity of pharmacological activity means that if one particular drug proves ineffective, another drug from a different class can quite reasonably be tried and may still prove effective.

Unlike antidepressant drugs, anticonvulsants are active from the commencement of therapy and this may be attractive where a rapid drug titration is possible. This is often the case in inpatient settings. On the other hand, side effects are common and rapid titration, particularly in the outpatient setting, may yield an unacceptably high level of adverse effects, compromising compliance.

Side effects

Side effects with anticonvulsants are common. Some, such as sedation, ataxia, nausea and fatigue, are reported with virtually all compounds. They are usually self-limiting and improve with the maintenance of treatment. Other side effects are more persistent and may be potentially hazardous. Hepatic dysfunction has been reported with a number of anticonvulsants, carbamazepine and sodium valproate in particular, and whilst this is usually fully reversible on cessation of the drug, severe hepatotoxicity has been reported.

Skin rashes have also been reported and once again, whilst these usually resolve with drug cessation, severe skin damage, occasionally associated with the Stevens-Johnson syndrome, has been reported.

Many anticonvulsant agents have been shown to have adverse effects on the developing foetus and a specific foetal anticonvulsant syndrome has been reported. Around 6% of infants born to mothers taking anticonvulsants have malformations, including neural tube defects, and a further proportion show developmental delay in later childhood. The cause is unknown, although it may be due to altered folate metabolism. Clear associations have been found

TABLE 11.2 Anticonvulsants used for chronic pain and their side effects

Drug	Common side effects	Serious side effects
Phenytoin	Sedation	Hepatic dysfunction
Carbamazepine	Ataxia	Skin rashes
Sodium valproate	Nausea	Stevens-Johnson syndrome
Newer drugs appear to be better tolerated	Fatigue	(occasional)
Gabapentin		Blood dyscrasia
Pregabalin		

with phenytoin, carbamazepine and sodium valproate. Whether these considerations are relevant to other classes of anticonvulsant is unknown. However, whilst epilepsy is a potentially lethal illness, chronic pain is not and the use of anticonvulsants in pregnant women cannot be justified for the latter indication.

Many anticonvulsant agents are potent inducers or inhibitors of hepatic microsomal enzymes. This can lead to a variety of drug interactions similar to those described with antidepressant agents. Where multiple drug regimens are being used, great care must be taken to avoid potentially serious drug interactions, particularly where drugs such as methadone or buprenorphine (which are metabolised by microsomal enzymes) are being used (Table 11.2).

Ketamine[7–9]

Ketamine is an atypical anaesthetic agent that is similar to phencyclidine. Phencyclidine was also developed as an anaesthetic drug in the 1950s, but was abandoned due to severe psychotropic side effects. Nevertheless, it became a popular drug of abuse in the 1970s and attracted the name 'angel dust'.

Ketamine was known to possess powerful analgesic effects in subanaesthetic doses and its use became accepted into clinical practice, particularly in palliative care, during the 1990s. What was of particular interest was its ability to relieve pain in situations where other agents, particularly opioids, had failed. There also appeared to be useful activity in both acute and chronic neuropathic pain. Further experience has shown ketamine to have powerful analgesic activity in a variety of both acute and chronic pain states. Furthermore, there appears to be a strongly synergistic effect with other analgesic agents, particularly opioids.

Mode of action

Ketamine's major mode of action appears to be via its ability to block the activity of the N-methyl-D-aspartate (NMDA) receptor. This receptor is a complex ligand-gated ion channel that is primarily activated by glutamate, although a number of other cofactors are also required. Activation of the NMDA receptor is associated with long-term potentiation (LTP) within the central nervous system and is responsible for many effects, including the development of neural pathways, learning and memory. Within pain pathways, LTP has been shown to promote the development of central sensitisation to pain, resulting in an increased level of pain transmission for a particular level of stimulus.

It is noteworthy that whilst a number of compounds demonstrate NMDA receptor blockade, ketamine is the only one that has been found useful in human pain. The reason for this appears to be that ketamine only binds to *activated* NMDA receptors, such as would be found in chronic pain states. It has no effect on the unactivated receptor.

Ketamine is not a particularly easy drug to use. The only available formulations are designed for injectable use and even whilst these can be administered orally, the oral bioavailability tends to be low and variable due to extensive first-pass metabolism. However, the major metabolite, norketamine, is highly active and has a longer circulating half-life than ketamine itself. Thus, in practice, whilst dose adjustments are frequently required, adequate therapeutic effects can often be attained. The major problem with ketamine use relates to the relatively narrow therapeutic index. In particular, dysphoria, hallucinations and cognitive impairment all occur at blood levels close to those associated with analgesia. Some benefit has been seen when using the purified S-isomer of ketamine as opposed to the more usual racemic mixture.

Side effects

Dysphoria, hallucinations and cognitive impairment are common as explained above. Apart from these, ketamine actually appears to be a relatively safe drug when used at the low doses employed in pain management.

There does however, remain a concern with long-term use. The NMDA receptor is ubiquitous throughout the nervous system and plays a major role in many systems. This is well demonstrated by the fact that genetic 'knockout' of the NMDA receptor is lethal in mammalian lines due to severe developmental abnormalities in the CNS. Reduced or suppressed function of the NMDA receptor also appears to be deleterious in humans. In schizophrenia for example, cognitive decline appears to be related to NMDA receptor hypofunction. Overall, this suggests that until further research becomes available, the use of ketamine in pain management needs to be confined to the short term only.

Skeletal muscle relaxants

Chronic musculoskeletal pain, particularly spinal pain, is often associated with abnormal muscle activation and muscle spasm. Lesions of the CNS, in addition to causing neuropathic pain syndromes, may result in painful muscle spasticity, often of a severe, paroxysmal nature. Skeletal muscle relaxants will usually help spasticity, but this may be at the cost of decreased muscle tone elsewhere, which may lead to a decrease in the mobility of the patient and thus make matters worse.

In the severely disabled patient, it is axiomatic that the underlying cause of the spasticity and any aggravating factors, such as pressure sores or infections, should be treated.

Baclofen

The drug of first choice is probably baclofen, which works on interneurones within the CNS; particularly the spinal cord. Baclofen is a derivative of the inhibitory neurotransmitter GABA and appears to be an agonist at the $GABA_B$ receptor. It appears to be effective for the treatment of spasticity caused by multiple sclerosis or other diseases of the spinal cord, especially traumatic lesions. There are reports of its use in trigeminal neuralgia and a number of painful conditions, including postherpetic neuralgia. There is also evidence of benefit during acute exacerbations of spinal pain where associated muscle spasm is occurring.

α-Adrenergic agonists[10]

α-adrenergic agonists appear to act on adrenergic receptors located in lamina I of the spinal dorsal horn as well as at target areas in the brain stem. In addition to analgesia, activation of these sites tends to produce a degree of sedation, although at clinically relevant doses, respiratory depression does not occur, offering a significant advantage over opioids.

Clonidine, tizanidine and dexmedetomidine have all been shown to possess useful analgesic activity. Dexmedetomidine has also found a role as a sedative drug in intensive-care medicine.

Clonidine[11]

The α-adrenergic agonist clonidine has been shown to produce analgesia, and there is evidence that both morphine and clonidine produce a dose-dependent inhibition of spinal nociceptive transmission that is mediated through different receptors for each drug. This may explain why clonidine has been shown to work synergistically with morphine when given intrathecally or epidurally. Clonidine also appears to work when given by other routes or even topically, but may cause severe hypotension by any route.

Tizanidine

The $α_2$-adrenergic agonist tizanidine has potent muscle relaxant activity and is an alternative to baclofen. It may also have some direct analgesic effects. Clonidine has similar effects (Table 11.3).

TABLE 11.3 Other adjunct agents and their side effects

Drug	Mechanism of action	Common side effects	Serious side effects
Ketamine	NMDA antagonist	Dysphoria Hallucinations Cognitive impairment	Psychotic effects
Baclofen	$GABA_B$ agonist	Sedation Weakness Cognitive impairment	Cardiovascular depression Angioedema
Clonidine	α-adrenergic agonist	Hypotension Dry mouth Sedation	Hypersensitivity reactions Bone marrow depression

Botulinum toxin[12]

The bacterium, *Clostridium botulinum* produces a range of potent toxins that interfere directly with neuromuscular transmission. The mode of action is complex and involves permanent inactivation of key proteins associated with the release of acetylcholine at the motor end-plate. There are also inhibitory effects on cholinergic transmission in the autonomic nervous system. Contamination of tinned or potted foods of low acid content with *Clostridium botulinum* is responsible for the condition known as 'botulism' in which systemic absorption of these toxins occurs, frequently with fatal results due to generalised muscular paralysis and autonomic dysfunction.

Purified preparations of clostridial toxins (generally termed botulinum toxin) are available and the type A toxin has been used for many years in the treatment of spasticity. Spasticity is often accompanied by pain and botulinum toxin has been shown to relieve the pain of spasticity and related dystonic conditions very effectively.

Interestingly, botulinum toxin has also been shown to have an analgesic effect independent of its effects on muscle relaxation. This was first noted in migraine but has been found in a variety of both musculoskeletal and neuropathic pain syndromes. The mode of action is unknown, although it is noteworthy that in animal models, botulinum toxin injected into peripheral muscle can be detected in the dorsal horn of the spinal cord in 24–48 hours. Inhibition of excitatory neurotransmitter release seems a likely candidate mechanism for its analgesic actions.

Botulinum toxin has a long duration of action and relief of muscle spasticity may last up to 3 months. Analgesia generally lasts at least as long as the muscle relaxation effect and has often been reported as lasting longer. Where treatment is successful, further treatment can be repeated at 3–4-monthly intervals, although with continuing use, particularly in high doses, there is a significant risk of developing antibodies to the toxin. This occurs in around 10% of patients receiving type A botulinum toxin for periods in excess of 1 year. Antibody generation is associated with a loss of clinical effect together with an increased risk of local inflammatory responses and more generalised hypersensitivity reactions.

Despite the dramatic systemic effects seen in botulism, administration of therapeutic quantities of purified botulinum toxins is generally very well tolerated. Significant paralysis has only occurred due to inadvertent overdose. Some local muscle weakness may occur, although this recovers fully as the effect of the toxin declines. This may, however, take some weeks and the effect may be troublesome where postural muscles are affected or where spasticity maintains an effective gait pattern.

Corticosteroids

Corticosteroids have only a very limited role in pain management. They still have an important disease-modifying role in many conditions associated with autoimmune activity where pain may be prominent, although the aim of treatment is not, specifically, analgesia.

Cancer pain

They are occasionally useful in the management of pain associated with aggressive tumour invasion of adjacent tissues, particularly invasion of bone and nerve plexuses. Dexamethasone has a specific role in the management of headache associated with raised intracranial pressure as may be seen with primary or secondary intracranial tumours (but not in so-called 'benign' intracranial hypertension). In these aggressive pain syndromes, high doses of steroids are generally required with a variety of potentially serious adverse events. Prolonged treatment is generally not an option.

Musculoskeletal pain

The use of 'depot' steroids has become well established in certain musculoskeletal pain syndromes, particularly arthritis and related degenerative conditions, although the evidence of efficacy is modest and local complications such as infection, synovial degradation and adverse changes in adjacent bone have all been reported. Certainly, their use in many chronic conditions, or to speed recovery from injury, must be questioned as they are strongly catabolic hormones and can tend to impair healing.

Radicular back pain

One area in which the use of depot steroids does have reasonable evidence of efficacy is in the management of painful radiculopathy following intervertebral disc prolapse. Whilst the efficacy is modest, the technique of epidural steroid injection is supported by metaanalysis and remains widespread. It should, however, be recognised that the technique only helps *radicular pain* and no effect can be expected on associated back pain. This often proves a major disappointment to the patient whose main problem is mechanical back pain.

Epidural steroid injection is not without risk. The steroid itself may predispose to local infection or even epidural lipomatosis where repeat procedures are performed. However, a more significant risk is potentially associated not with the steroid, but with the associated preservative. In many cases this is polyethylene glycol, which can act as a significant irritant if applied to exposed nerve roots or the internal surface of the meninges. In practice, there is no evidence that skilled administration, outside the dura, results in neurotoxicity. However, the procedure is probably overused, frequently in inappropriate clinical environments and in such circumstances, adverse outcomes are inevitable.

Drugs used in the management of migraine[13]

Migraine is but one of many headache syndromes. However, it is the commonest human neurovascular disorder and is a debilitating problem for many patients. The management of migraine differs considerably from many other acute or chronic pain conditions and specific pharmacological interventions may result in a significant improvement in quality of life. It is appropriate to discuss specific antimigraine drugs in some detail (Table 11.4).

Migraine is a complex phenomenon associated with abnormal excitability of the cerebral cortex. This in turn leads to episodic activation of cortical structures with secondary activation of the trigeminovascular system. The latter appears to be the key event in the generation of disabling pain in the head and face.

Migraine is common. Around 6% of adult males and 15% of adult females suffer regular migraine headache. Most patients self-medicate with simple analgesics or non-steroidal anti-inflammatory drugs (NSAIDs) and allow the acute episode to pass. Around half of patients with regular migraine suffer severe, recurring symptoms that respond poorly to simple measures. In these patients, both prophylactic and acute treatments should be considered.

As with many chronic pain presentations, chronic intractable migraine is frequently associated with lifestyle and psychosocial issues that must be addressed concurrently. Obvious examples are the use of alcohol and tobacco products, which are strong promoters of migraine. Psychological stress is also a frequent trigger of migraine and appropriate psychological management may be safer, cheaper and more effective than complex medication regimens.

TABLE 11.4 Drugs used in migraine

Drug group	Example	Mechanism	Side effects
Prophylaxis			
β-blockers	Propranolol	Possibly β_1 antagonist	Gastrointestinal upset
		5-HT_1 and$_2$ antagonist	Bradycardia Hypotension
Anticonvulsants (more modern agents may be better tolerated)	Gabapentin Topiramate All commonly used agents have some activity	Ion channel activity	See Table 11.2
Tricyclic antidepressants	Amitriptyline Nortriptyline	See above	See Table 11.1
Antihistamine	Pizotifen	Antihistamine	Weight gain Drowsiness
Acute episodes			
Ergotamine		Cerebral vasoconstriction	Vasospasm Nausea Vomiting Myocardial ischemia
Triptans	Sumatriptan Naratriptan Zolmitriptan	Serotonin agonists 5-$HT_{1B \text{ and } 1D}$	Coronary vasoconstriction Dizziness Fatigue Nausea

Prophylactic agents

β-Blockers

β-blockers have been used for many years in the prophylaxis of migraine and remain a useful group of drugs where tolerated. It does appear that the effects are limited to those drugs that cross the blood–brain barrier and in practice, propranolol remains the drug of choice.

The mode of action is essentially unknown and seems unlikely to be entirely related to β-adrenoceptor blockade. Whilst there is evidence that β-blockers may exert some of their therapeutic effects in migraine through $β_1$ adrenoceptor antagonist actions in the thalamus, it should also be noted that propranolol is a potent antagonist at the 5-hydroxytryptamine 1 and 2 ($5HT_1$ and $5HT_2$) receptors.

Anticonvulsants

Anticonvulsants are probably underused in migraine prophylaxis. As noted above, they are effective prophylactic agents and, in fact, their efficacy in migraine appears superior to their efficacy in peripheral neuropathic pain syndromes where their use is well established. The use of anticonvulsants in migraine may be particularly pertinent in view of the increasing evidence that migraine is one of a group of ion 'channelopathies', conditions in which inherited abnormalities of neuronal ion channels result in abnormal patterns of excitability. These conditions account for many cases of 'idiopathic' epilepsy and consistent evidence for channelopathies has also been found in subjects with recurrent migraine.

The commonly used anticonvulsant agents have been found to have prophylactic activity against migraine, although the more modern agents, such as gabapentin or topiramate, may be better tolerated.

Tricyclic antidepressant

Tricyclic antidepressant agents also appear to offer reasonable prophylactic effects. Effective doses are generally similar to those used in the management of neuropathic pain or depression, although, once again, side effects may limit compliance.

Other prophylactic agents

Other prophylactic agents include the serotonin antagonist, methysergide, and the antihistamine drug, pizotifen.

Methysergide is a potentially toxic drug and given the alternatives, its use is now difficult to justify.

Pizotifen appears moderately effective, but weight gain and drowsiness are relatively common and for a similar side effect profile, anticonvulsants are more effective.

Treatment for acute attacks

The best prophylactic agents tend to reduce the frequency of migraine attacks by around 50%, which is a substantial improvement, but migraine attacks still occur. Management of acute attacks should begin with appropriate trials of simple analgesics and NSAIDs. Nausea associated with gastric stasis may make absorption of orally administered drugs unreliable, although the rectal route can be successfully employed. For a significant minority of patients, simple analgesic regimens will prove ineffective and other remedies should be considered.

Ergotamine

Ergotamine has been used for many years for the management of migraine. The rationale for use was based around the properties of this drug to induce cerebral vasoconstriction and they are undoubtedly effective, although nausea may worsen and generalised arteriolar vasoconstriction may occur, particularly with repeat dosing. Rebound headache may occur after prolonged, repeat dosing. Ergotamine is often coadministered with caffeine to assist with the cerebral vasoconstrictor effect. A dose of 2 mg ergotamine/100 mg caffeine administered up to twice during an acute attack is appropriate, either via the oral or rectal routes.

Triptans

Migraine management has changed considerably with the advent of a specific class of serotonin agonist drugs: the triptans. The first triptan drugs were developed in the 1980s and a variety of different compounds are now available, although all of them appear to show powerful agonist activity at 5-HT_{1B} and 5-HT_{1D} receptors. Their mode of action appears to involve a specific reversal of the cerebral vasodilation and neurogenic oedema seen in migraine. Sumatriptan is the prototypical agent, although newer agents, such as naratriptan and zolmitriptan, show better oral availability and penetration of the blood–brain barrier.

Triptans are administered early in the acute phase of a migraine attack and will usually terminate it or prevent its further development. They can still be administered later in an attack and remain effective, although gastric stasis may impede absorption, under these circumstances a parenteral or transmucosal route may be more effective.

Triptans may be potentially hazardous in ischaemic heart disease as they can cause coronary vasoconstriction. Their use in patients with elevated cardiac risk must, therefore, be approached with some caution. Coadministration with ergot alkaloids or overdosage may cause coronary vasospasm in patients without coronary artery disease and must obviously be avoided.

Cannabinoids[14]

Cannabinoid drugs have been used throughout most of recorded human history. They have been part of the traditional healing practices of a number of cultures, although their use has generally not found much favour in scientifically based medical practice. The most important naturally occurring cannabinoids are those derived from the common hemp plant (*Cannabis sativa*) and of these compounds, the most active is δ-9-tetrahydrocannabinol. Other, synthetic cannabinoids have been developed, although only one, nabilone, has been used to any major extent in the clinical arena.

Mode of action

Cannabinoids exert their actions via cannabinoid 1 and 2 (CB$_1$ and CB$_2$) receptors:

- CB$_1$ receptors are found predominantly in the central nervous system where they are the commonest G-protein-coupled receptor yet found. They have an inhibitory role across a huge range of cortical and subcortical structures with particularly high concentrations being found in the frontal cortex, the limbic system and the cerebellar vermis. They are also found in the dorsal horn of the spinal cord in association with the pain pathways.
- CB$_2$ receptors are more usually found peripherally where they appear to have a role in modulation of the inflammatory response.

Classic cannabinoid actions are mediated exclusively via the CB$_1$ receptor, where drugs such as δ-9-tetrahydrocannabinol and nabilone are potent agonists. The most prominent actions are psychotropic, including altered mood states (euphoria or dysphoria), altered perception of time, altered perception of sound and sedation. Acute memory impairment also tends to occur and both paranoia and psychosis can be precipitated.

Analgesic effects

Amongst this *melee* of actions, a degree of analgesia is also induced, although detecting this, particularly in animal experiments, is not an easy task. In fact, many of the earlier experiments purporting to demonstrate cannabinoid analgesia in animals relied on the observation of behavioural responses to pain. Such responses become profoundly suppressed because of the drug-induced stupor caused by cannabinoids and this resulted in a misinterpretation of the analgesic potential of these compounds.

The same psychotropic effects that cloud the interpretation of cannabinoid experiments in animals have, of course, found favour with recreational substance users and worldwide, cannabis is the third most widely abused of all the recreational substances after alcohol and tobacco. The use of cannabis, even in purified preparations, remains illegal in most countries. As a general rule, no exception is made for medical use, although some state legislatures in North America have taken a more liberal view. Synthetic cannabinoids are generally accessible to clinicians in most countries.

The restrictions on recreational cannabis use have resulted in well-organised campaigns by cannabis users to have the drug legalised for recreational use. Regrettably, such groups have hijacked the medical debate, and opponents of the legalisation of cannabis are frequently portrayed as taking some form of pleasure in making patients suffer.

Clinical effects

The key question that must be asked is whether these drugs are actually clinically useful. Overall, the answer appears to be that they are not. Meta-analysis of cannabinoid trials has failed to demonstrate any useful effect in acute or chronic pain. More recent trials using cannabis sprays have tended to show small, positive effects, although the drugs are difficult to blind in a randomised trial and the novel method of administration employed may well contribute to the effect, independent of the therapeutic response.

Cannabinoid drugs are poorly tolerated by non-recreational users and the adverse event profile is broad, in keeping with the wide distribution of relevant receptors. Unless some way can be found of reducing adverse events, it is unlikely that cannabinoid drugs will provide any clinically useful alternative to the other, better-established drugs described above.

Clinical use of adjuvant and miscellaneous drugs in pain management

As has been highlighted above, the very nature of this group of drugs suggests that they will generally be used as part of a combination of compounds for the management of a pain condition. The increased risk of adverse events has been discussed, but it is also important to consider how these compounds can be safely used.

A guiding principle of combination therapy is that medications should be added to the regimen individually, the effects assessed over a reasonable period of time (and this may require several weeks) and ineffective drugs withdrawn before new drugs are added. Where possible, monitoring of blood levels can offer very useful information with respect to patient compliance and individual variations in drug handling that can explain unusual effects.

As noted above, the involvement of other professional disciplines can improve patient safety and monitoring. The services of an experienced clinical pharmacist can prove invaluable in this regard.

KEY POINTS

- Adjuvant agents are often used in combination with traditional analgesic drugs
- Adjuvant drugs may have analgesic properties in their own right, often when traditional agents have little benefit
- Combinations of drugs do increase the risk of interactions and side effects
- The tricyclic antidepressants have a good evidence for use in chronic pain but they are limited by the side effects and interactions with other drugs
- Anticonvulsants are commonly used in chronic pain and have no role in acute pain management
- Ketamine has a role in acute and chronic neuropathic pain but is limited by its variable bioavailability and potential for cognitive changes in long-term use
- Migraine is a common painful condition with simple analgesics helping many. The advent of the triptans has significantly helped the management of acute episodes
- Cannabinoids have had a lot of publicity but have not proven to be clinically important due in part to adverse side effects

References

1. Saarto T, Wiffen PJ. Antidepressants for neuropathic pain. *Cochrane Database Syst Rev* 2005(3): CD005454.
2. Sindrup SH, Otto M, Finnerop NB et al. Antidepressants in the treatment of neuropathic pain. *Basic Clin Pharmacol Toxicol* 2005; **96**(6): 399–409.
3. Jensen TS. Anticonvulsants in neuropathic pain: rationale and clinical evidence. *Eur J Pain* 2002; **6 Suppl A**: 61–68.
4. Wiffen P, Collins S, McQuay H et al. Anticonvulsant drugs for acute and chronic pain. *Cochrane Database Syst Rev* 2005(3): CD001133.
5. Wiffen PJ, McQuay H, Edwards JE et al. Gabapentin for acute and chronic pain. *Cochrane Database Syst Rev* 2005(3): CD005452.
6. Wiffen PJ, McQuay HJ, Moore RA. Carbamazepine for acute and chronic pain. *Cochrane Database Syst Rev* 2005(3): CD005451.
7. Bell RF, Dahl JB, Moore RA et al. Perioperative ketamine for acute postoperative pain. *Cochrane Database Syst Rev* 2006(1): CD004603.
8. Bell RF, Eccleston C, Kalso E. Ketamine as adjuvant to opioids for cancer pain. A qualitative systematic review. *J Pain Symptom Manage* 2003; **26**(3): 867–875.
9. Subramaniam K, Subramaniam B, Steinbrook RA. Ketamine as adjuvant analgesic to opioids: a quantitative and qualitative systematic review. *Anesth Analg* 2004; **99**(2): 482–495.
10. Smith H, Elliott J. Alpha2 receptors and agonists in pain management. *Curr Opin Anaesthesiol* 2001; **14**(5): 513–518.
11. Tryba M, Gehling M. Clonidine – a potent analgesic adjuvant. *Curr Opin Anaesthesiol* 2002; **15**(5): 511–517.
12. Bhidayasiri R, Truong DD. Expanding use of botulinum toxin. *J Neurol Sci* 2005; **235**(1–2): 1–9.
13. Goadsby PJ. Recent advances in the diagnosis and management of migraine. *BMJ* 2006; **332**(7532): 25–29.
14. Campbell FA, Tramer MR, Carroll D et al. Are cannabinoids an effective and safe treatment option in the management of pain? A qualitative systematic review. *BMJ* 2001; **323**(7303): 13–16.

Further reading

Ballantyne JC, Mao J. Opioid therapy for chronic pain. *N Engl J Med* 2003; **349**(20): 1943–1953.

Mao J. Opioid-induced abnormal pain sensitivity: implications in clinical opioid therapy. *Pain* 2002; **100**(3): 213–217.

Donald Graham

Peripheral interventions

Introduction

'Few experiences in life are more universal than pain, which flows like lava beneath the crust of daily life.'

The Gift of Pain, Yancey & Brand.

The reader should expect a chapter to be informative and up to date, but also stimulating, systematic and memorable.

The aims of this chapter are to cover the following areas:

- provide an overview of peripheral interventions for pain management
- provide a systematic framework for understanding and remembering the key elements
- provide a plan for treatment and supportive evidence
- link the preceding chapters looking at the basic sciences with those that follow, which apply them to the clinical setting.

Pain is subjective, emotional and personal. Commonly it is the least-liked symptom described by patients. Acute pain is a signal for alarm, its presence is key for survival. The cause of the pain may be internal, such as angina or colic, or interaction with our environment. As healthcare professionals our view of patients' pain may be skewed by the frequency and variety of pain we experience through patient contact, however, it is important to remember:

'Pain is what the patient says it is'

Nursing management of the patient with pain (McCaffery 1972)

There are seven frameworks built into the body of this chapter. Framework 1 provides an overview of the chapter structure. This will allow you to open a discussion on peripheral interventions in pain management. Subsequently, frameworks 2–7 provide increasing detail through logical steps developing the themes. The frameworks are easy to follow and each layer provides a basis for the next layer of information. Each layer is numerated on the left-hand side of the frameworks and is designed to emphasise levels of progression to increasing depth of knowledge.

Frameworks 6 (physical interventions) and 7 (pharmacological interventions) are followed by text and a structured table containing details of the method of delivery, indications for treatment and contraindications and precautions.

Framework 1 Peripheral interventions (Fig. 12.1)

Any clinical intervention demands a series of events, which are synthesised into a solution; you could perhaps call this parallel thinking. To provide this there has to be knowledge (neuroanatomy), a patient history, an examination, treatment options and planning. Each event generates its own framework (Figs 12.2–12.7) with increasing levels of detail.

Framework 2 Somatic peripheral neuroanatomy (Fig. 12.2)

Direct contact with our environment (internal or external) provides information on temperature, touch and pain through receptors and connections. Sensory landmarks relate surface anatomy to dermatomal levels (e.g. stubbing your toe enters the spinal cord at L5). The possible outcomes from tissue injury can then be considered.

Framework 3 Patient history (Fig. 12.3)

A thorough history is essential to form the correct diagnosis and formulate a plan. Patients best describe their pain in their own words and often use their hands to describe the site of their pain. It is important to have a systematic structured interview and framework 3 includes key questions you should remember when taking a pain history.

Framework 4 Examination (Fig. 12.4)

Further evaluation must include a relevant examination related to the pain problem and will often involve musculo-skeletal and neurological assessment, though other systems may also need to be examined.

Framework 5 Treatment planning (Fig. 12.5)

There are key essential requirements prior to discussing a management plan. These include the preceding history and examination, professional impartial behaviour and clear explanations of all relevant findings through direct discussion with the patient, staff and carers, if present. In addition, it is important to

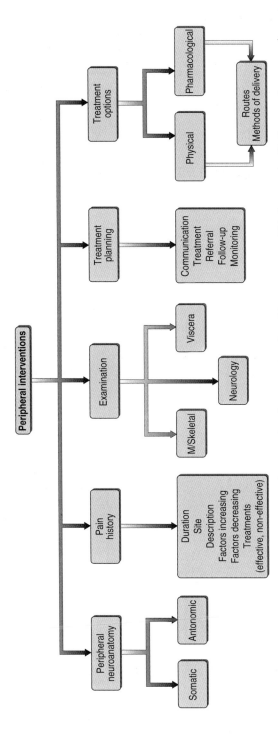

Fig. 12.1 Framework for understanding peripheral interventions in pain management. This framework will allow you to open a discussion on peripheral interventions in pain management. In essence this is a summary of the fundamental components for this chapter. For greater detail refer to each bold heading which will form a new heading in later pages in the chapter. Layers 1, 2, 3, etc., reflect increasingly greater depths of knowledge

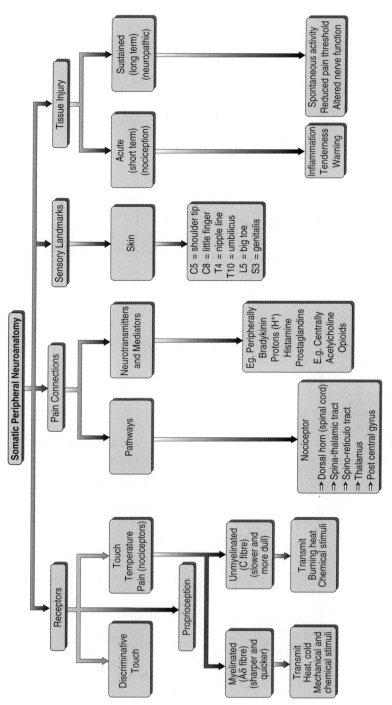

Fig. 12.2 Framework 2. See text for explanations

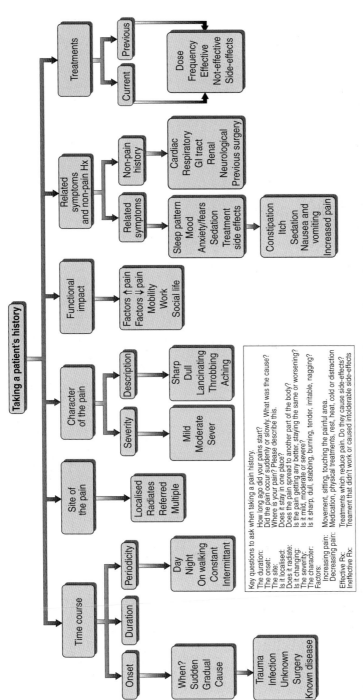

Key questions to ask when taking a pain history.
The duration: How long ago did your pains start?
The onset: Did the pain occur suddenly or slowly. What was the cause?
The site: Where is your pain? Please describe this.
Is it localised: Does it stay in one place?
Does it radiate: Does the pain spread to another part of the body?
Is it changing: Is the pain getting any better, staying the same or worsening?
The severity: Is it mild, moderate or severe?
The character: Is it sharp, dull, stabbing, burning, tender, irritable, nagging?
Factors:
  Increasing pain: Movement, sitting, touching the painful area.
  Decreasing pain: Medication, physical treatments, rest, heat, cold or distraction
Effective Rx: Treatments which reduce pain. Do they cause side-effects?
Ineffective Rx: Treament that didn't work or caused intolderable side-effects

Fig. 12.3   Framework 3. See text for explanations

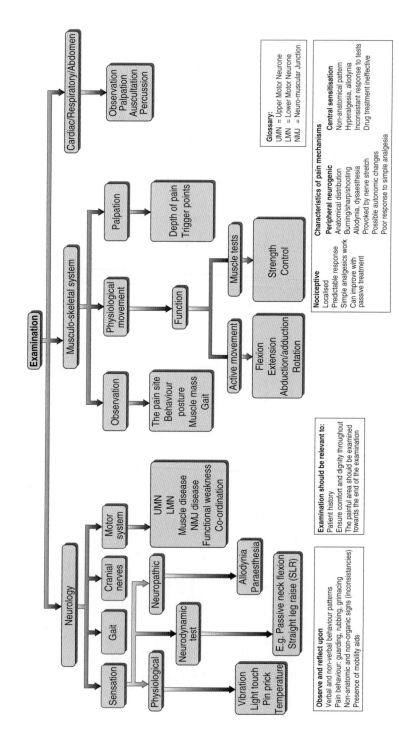

Fig. 12.4 Framework 4. See text for explanations

Cardiac/Respiratory/Abdomen

Observation
Palpation
Auscultation
Percussion

Glossary:
UMN = Upper Motor Neurone
LMN = Lower Motor Neurone
NMJ = Neuro-muscular Junction

Characteristics of pain mechanisms

Nociceptive
Localised
Predictable response
Simple analgesics work
Can improve with
passive treatment

Peripheral neurogenic
Anatomical distribution
Burning/sharp/shooting
Allodynia, dysaesthesia
Provoked by nerve stretch
Possible autonomic changes
Poor response to simple analgesia

Central sensitisation
Non-anatomical pattern
Hyperalgesia, allodynia
Inconsistant response to tests
Drug treatment ineffective

Examination

Musculo-skeletal system

Palpation
Depth of pain
Trigger points

Physiological movement
Function

Observation
The pain site
Behaviour
posture
Muscle mass
Gait

Muscle tests
Strength
Control

Active movement
Flexion
Extension
Abduction/adduction
Rotation

Examination should be relevant to:
Patient history
Ensure comfort and dignity throughout
The painful area should be examined
towards the end of the examination

Neurology

Motor system
UMN
LMN
Muscle disease
NMJ disease
Functional weakness
Co-ordination

Cranial nerves
Neuropathic
Allodynia
Paraesthesia

Gait
Neurodynamic test
E.g. Passive neck flexion
Straight leg raise (SLR)

Sensation
Physiological
Vibration
Light touch
Pin prick
Temperature

Observe and reflect upon
Verbal and non-verbal behaviour patterns
Pain behaviour: guarding, rubbing, grimacing
Non-anatomic and non-organic signs (inconsistancies)
Presence of mobility aids

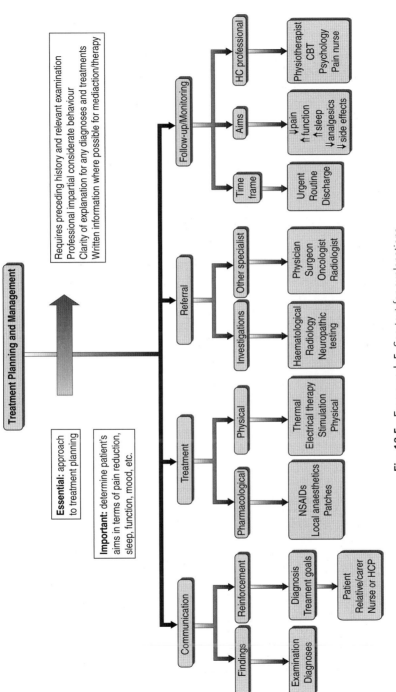

Fig. 12.5 Framework 5. See text for explanations

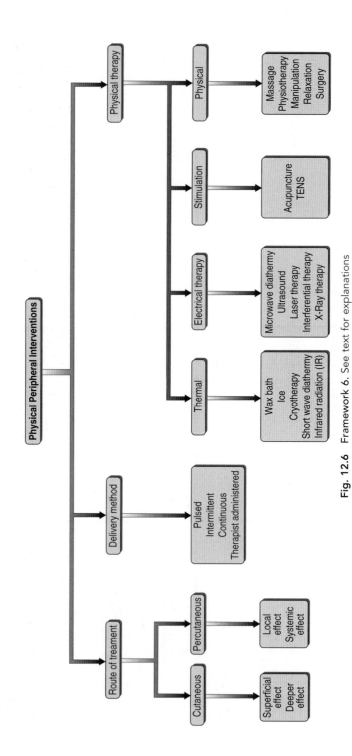

Fig. 12.6   Framework 6. See text for explanations

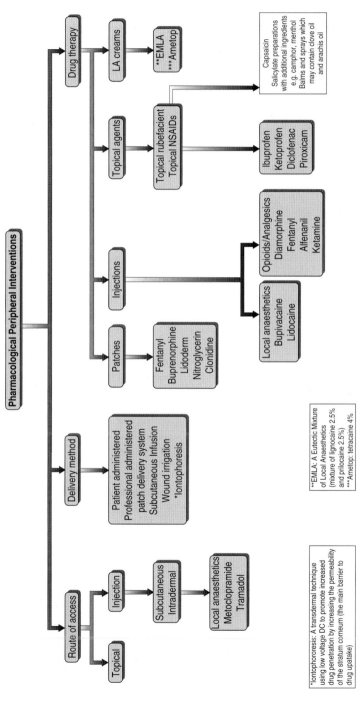

Fig. 12.7   Framework 7. See text for explanations

determine what the patient wants or expects to gain from any treatment. This may be pain relief, but at other times may be better mobility, sleep or improved mood. The process of planning involves communication of the findings and reinforcement of goals, treatment benefits and risks, appropriate referral and an agreed follow-up at an identified time and by whom. A thorough understanding of the basic science, psychology, therapeutics and anatomy is required before a considered discussion about management can be undertaken.

Frameworks 6 and 7 Physical and pharmacological treatments
(Figs 12.6 & 12.7)

Principally, these both involve the routes and method of delivery and in greater detail each of the treatments mentioned below.

Consider the immediate distress of a 'stubbed toe' or hitting one's 'funny bone'. The pain is sharp but usually short in duration. However, without this warning we would not protect or avoid further tissue damage to the affected area. On the contrary, a reduction in sensation or numbness increases the risk of tissue damage. This may occur due to diseases such as diabetes or leprosy, or may be iatrogenic following the use of local anaesthesia. Where nerve damage prevents the recognition of this symptom, severe damage can occur. The following anecdote is a true story taken from a personal account by Dr Paul Brand while in Papua New Guinea.

Nightmares of painlessness

'*A woman in a village near a leprosarium was roasting yams over a charcoal brazier. She pierced one yam with a sharp stick and held it over the fire, slowly twirling the stick between her fingers like a barbecue spit. The yam fell off the stick, however, and I watched as she tried unsuccessfully to spear it, each jab driving the yam farther underneath the hot red coals. Finally, she shrugged and looked over to an old man squatting a few feet away. At her gesture, obviously knowing what was expected of him, he shambled over to the fire, reached in, pushed aside the hot coals to retrieve the yam, and then returned to his seat. ... I immediately examined the old man's hands. He had no fingers left, only gnarled stubs covered with leaking blisters and scars of old wounds. Clearly, this was not the first time he had thrust his hands into a fire.*'

The Gift of Pain. Yancy and Brand

Fortunately, most of us exist constantly in a state of balance between no pain and various levels of pain severity, some of which require analgesia (Table 12.1).

TABLE 12.1 Examples of conditions leading to numbness and pain

Numbness	Sensory awareness	Pain
Protection	*Balance*	*Analgesia*
Examples		Examples
Local anaesthesia		Surgery
Diabetes		Trauma
Stroke		Neuralgia
Leprosy		

The sensation of pain is extremely variable not only between people but also within the same person. Pain remains a complex balance between physiology, behaviour and belief processes. Much of our pain experiences come from our interaction with the environment via our exterior tissues including the skin and subcutaneous tissues. They not only protect us from our environment but also provide an easily accessible route for pain management. Advantages include:

- avoidance of oral or more invasive routes of treatment
- improved patient compliance and satisfaction
- direct transdermal drug absorption of rubefacients and analgesics; drug action can occur locally or systemically as required
- ease of application of physical treatments (e.g. heat, ultrasound) and conduction to superficial or deeper tissues.

Peripheral interventions

A peripheral intervention is one that is delivered through: skin absorption (transdermal), the skin (percutaneous) or via conduction dependent upon the physical properties of the treatment.

Their action may be:

- superficial (e.g. a local anaesthetic cream acting on the sensory nerves in the skin)
- deep or more central (e.g. acupuncture or opioid patches acting on more proximal sensory structures or via the central nervous system).

Physical treatments

Heat treatments

Energy may be transferred to a patient with intent of increasing or decreasing heat and in turn increasing or decreasing blood flow to superficial or deeper tissues. Thermo therapy includes superficial and deep-heat treatments, cryotherapy and ultrasound.

Therapeutic heat

Therapeutic heat is one of the oldest physical modalities used to reduce and relieve pain. In general, heat modalities do not cure pain, but can be important additions to therapy.

Heat therapy can be classified by the depth of tissue penetration (superficial or deep) and how the energy transfer occurs. Heat energy may be transferred through the skin by conduction, convection, conversion or radiation.

The physiological effects of heat include:

1. Stimulation of thermoreceptors producing vasodilation by an axon reflex or by the release of nitric oxide.
2. Reduced sympathetic stimulation via sympathetic neurones.
3. Pain reduction through reduced muscle spasm and increased blood flow. This may help improve oxygen delivery and also wash out waste products or pain mediators.

Superficial treatments include hot packs, hot lamps, paraffin and whirlpool baths and fluidotherapy. The temperature can only be increased by a few degrees; the depth of effect is, therefore, a few centimetres only.

Deep heating treatments include ultrasound (U/S), short wave and microwave diathermy. These may be delivered by pulsed or by short-term continuous treatment.

Cryotherapy

Cryotherapy is the therapeutic use of cold. Mild cooling is used in rehabilitation to reduce pain and aid movement. It is thought that cooling decreases the intensity and duration of nerve conduction, thereby decreasing the perception of pain. Cold therapy also limits swelling by decreasing blood flow and leakiness of the capillaries, which in turn limits pain by decreasing painful stretch receptor transmission. All forms of cryotherapy in pain management are considered superficial cooling agents, but can reduce tissue temperature at a deeper level.

Cryotherapy treatments include cold packs, ice massage, cold water immersion and vapocoolant sprays (e.g. ethyl chloride). Vapocoolant sprays are used to determine sensory blockade during regional analgesia or aid in intravenous cannulation.

Thermotherapy

Thermotherapy (heat and cold) is commonly used for rheumatoid arthritis. Only paraffin wax baths have shown positive results for arthritic hands using a range of objective methods.[1]

Ultrasound

Ultrasound was first used during the First World War for SONAR (Sound Navigation and Ranging). This pulse-echo technology has been adapted for medical imaging and pain management. Therapeutic ultrasound consists of inaudible acoustic vibrations delivered at between 0.75 and 3.0 MHz (human hearing range is 0.16–0.2 MHz).

Ultrasound has a variety of physical effects classified as thermal and non-thermal. Thermal effects are due to tissue vibration, whereas non-thermal are due to acoustic streaming and cavitation. Passing a high-frequency alternating electrical current through a crystal that has piezoelectric properties produces these effects. This property enables the crystal to expand and contract at the frequency of the applied current. The change in crystal volume produces ultrasound waves. To be effective the ultrasound probe requires a good skin interface provided by acoustic conducting gel.

Pain reduction may occur due to stimulation of cutaneous thermal receptors, improved tissue extensibility due to increased tissue temperature, modulation of inflammation or to its non-thermal effects.

Several studies have examined the effects of ultrasound for a variety of musculoskeletal conditions, but there is little evidence to support its use.[2] Therapeutic ultrasound for the treatment of rheumatoid arthritis has been reviewed. Continuous treatment in water has improved hand grip (Table 12.2).[1]

TABLE 12.2 Heat treatments and ultrasound

	Method of delivery	Indications	Contraindications/ precautions
Superficial heat			
Hot packs Infra-red lamps Wax/paraffin baths (Temp. 110–120°F)	Direct contact or exposure Immersion Exposure time 20–30 minutes	Muscle spasm, myalgia, bursitis, contractures, stiff swollen joints	*Avoid*: Ischaemic tissues, acute injury, bleeding disorders, scar tissues, pregnancy and oedema *Risks*: Burns or skin damage
Fluidotherapy Occurs inside a cabinet using heated air convection	Heated air circulates particles that act like a fluid. Place body part in cabinet	Increase mobility in hands, wrists, ankles and feet (e.g. osteoarthritis)	As above
Deep heat			
Short wave diathermy (SWD) – Frequency 27MHz	A high frequency magnetic/electric field applied to the skin Continuous or pulsed therapy	Soft tissue injuries (e.g. ankle or neck) Deep or superficial wound healing	As for superficial heat therapy Eyes (wear goggles) *Avoid*: Exposure to implanted neural stimulators, cardiac pacemakers, pregnancy and testes
Microwave diathermy (MWD)	A higher frequency electromagnetic field Apply directly to affected area	Small tissue areas up too a depth of 5 cm	As above
Cryotherapy			
Cold packs, ice massage, cold-water immersion or vapocoolant sprays	Direct contact or immersion By pressurised spray	Reduce oedema or muscle spasm Sprays used for sensory assessment or cannulation	*Avoid*: Severe angina, arterial insufficiency Raynaud's phenomenon *Risks*: Mild peripheral vascular disease, insensitivity to the cold
Ultrasound			
High-frequency waveform Parameter variables: frequency, intensity and duration	Direct application of probe to skin in water or via air free gel on the pain site Can be continuous or pulsed	Soft tissue injuries, painful arthritic joints or reduced ROM	*Avoid*: Malignant tumours, pregnancy, joint cement, eyes and pacemakers *Risks*: Breast implants, fracture or acute inflammation

ROM: range of movement

Electrical therapy

The definition of what is meant by 'electrical therapy' varies from text to text. In this chapter electrical therapy includes interferential therapy and laser therapy.

Electrical therapy has been used for pain management as early as 46 AD using the electric discharge from a torpedo fish. The late 18th and early 19th centuries saw a revival, but it was Melzack and Wall's gate theory in the 1960s, which provided a scientific foundation for its use. Of course electrical stimulation is not only used for pain but internally for cardiac pacemakers or externally for DC shock.

Interferential

An interferential current is produced by the interference of two alternating current waveforms through electrodes applied to the skin. Treatment is based upon generating the required interference pattern to which tissues respond and focussing this pattern at the painful tissues. Electrical currents act physiologically by depolarising nerve membranes and producing an action potential (the nervous system does this anyway!). Stimulation may produce endogenous opioids (enkephalins and endorphins) and stimulate pain inhibitory pathways.

This technique involves a simultaneous AC generator using medium-frequency currents to produce a phasic waveform pattern. There is a continuous or pulsed delivery via skin electrodes. Variables include amplitude and pulse interval.

Indications include arthritic joint pains, muscular pains and recent soft tissue trauma.

The technique should be avoided in patients with demand pacemakers, thrombotic vessels, near the carotid sinus and in pregnant patients.

Laser therapy

The term *laser* is an acronym for light amplification by stimulated emission of radiation (LASER). Originally outlined by Albert Einstein laser light is monochromatic (one colour), coherent and directional. Therapeutic lasers for pain management are low-intensity 'cold' lasers, which use longer wavelengths and lower frequencies of light allowing deeper tissue penetration. Cold lasers may act by their cellular effects (increasing phosphate and nucleic acid production and cell stimulation), vasodilation and altered nerve conduction. A Cochrane Systematic Review has evaluated laser therapy for reduction of swelling and pain in hands and feet. Evidence suggests that treatment decreases pain and morning stiffness in the short term.[3]

Indications include arthritis,[3] low back and neck pain, chronic pain trigger points and wound healing.

This treatment should be avoided in haemorrhaging regions and for 4–6 months following radiotherapy. There is an increased risk in epilepsy, pregnancy and fever.

Stimulation therapy

Stimulation therapy acts upon the intact sensory nervous system by stimulating the large-diameter afferent fibres as occurs with TENS or through stimulation of peripheral sensory fibres leading to activation of endogenous opioids.

Transcutaneous electrical nerve stimulation

TENS is non-invasive, inexpensive, safe and easy to use. Since the 1970s technological advances have allowed smaller, cheaper, battery-operated units. The mode of action of TENS is complex and its physiological action is dependent upon which mode is used. TENS may stimulate Aβ fibres and spinal interneurones in addition to inducing endogenous opioid release. Clinically, TENS has a place in both acute and chronic pain states. Effective use of TENS depends upon a good practical knowledge of its capabilities and through patient education and literature. The clinical effectiveness of TENS for chronic pain[4] and knee osteoarthritis[5] has recently been reviewed. There is insufficient evidence to support the use of TENS in chronic pain; however, TENS is effective for pain control and knee stiffness in the short term.

Acupuncture

Acupuncture has been part of Chinese and Japanese traditional medicine for over 5000 years, but it wasn't until the 1970s following President Nixon's visit to China that its use in Western medicine grew in popularity. Acupuncture is administered via needle insertion through the skin into specific acupuncture points. Fundamental to classical acupuncture is the concept of *Qui* (Chi – the energy flow). The unobstructed circulation of Qui throughout the body is aided by placing needles at the acupuncture points found on the meridians below the skin. The meridians are characterised by *Yin* and *Yang*, which if out of balance can cause pain and disease. Classical acupuncture is the traditional practice according to the principles of Taoism, returning the body to harmony working with the body's energy and not against it (Box 12.1).

These acupuncture points can be stimulated by manual manipulation or by electrical current (electroacupuncture). Acupuncture points are closely related to the course of underlying peripheral nerves. Analgesia is thought to occur through stimulation of peripheral receptors and sensory fibres resulting in the activation of specific endogenous opioid systems. In addition, an intact sensory nervous system is necessary for success. In the UK needles should be single use and disposable. Acupuncture is more effective for chronic low back pain relief and improved function compared to no treatment,[6] and there is moderate evidence to support its use in the short term for chronic mechanical neck pain (Table 12.3).[7]

Manual therapy

This includes a vast array of treatments intended to promote motion and pain relief. The commonest methods include massage, joint mobilisation and manipulation and physiotherapy.

Massage

Massage is an ancient therapy and is used to mobilise soft tissue. Massage is thought to have a number of beneficial physiological effects, which may modulate pain but also relax, aid tissue repair, improve blood flow in superficial vessels and elevate mood. Pain reduction may occur through activation of segmental inhibitory pain pathways (via cutaneous mechanoreceptors) and by the production of endorphins. Massage for chronic low back pain has been

---

BOX 12.1 Tao of Pooh

Benjamin Hoff

Tao of Pooh

"You see Pooh," I said, "a lot of people don't seem to know what Taoism is..."

"Yes?" said Pooh blinking his eyes.

"So that's what this chapter is for – to explain things a bit."

"And the easiest way to do that would be for us to go to China for a moment"...

We see three men standing around a vat of vinegar. Each has dipped his finger into the vinegar and has tasted it. The expression of each man's face shows his individual reaction. The three masters are K'ung Fu-tse (Confucius), Buddha and Lao-tse, author of the oldest existing book on Taoism. The first has a sour look on his face, the second wears a bitter expression, but the third man is smiling... To Confucius the world was out of harmony with the Way of Heaven... To Buddha life on earth was bitter filled with attachments and desires that led to suffering... To Lao-tse the harmony that naturally existed between heaven and earth from the very beginning of time could be found by anyone at any time...it was only when men interfered with natural balance was struggle inevitable and life sour...

"But what does Taoism have to do with vinegar?" asked Pooh

Lao-tse is smiling because, although vinegar has an unpleasant taste by working in harmony with life's circumstances Taoists perceive the positive where others see the negative and life itself when understood and utilized for what it is, is sweet.

"Sweet? You mean like honey?" asked Pooh. "Well maybe not that sweet" I said

---

reviewed recently and trials show some relief from back pain over a period of weeks to months, especially if combined with exercise and education.[8] In addition, massage may be beneficial for cancer patients in the short term.[9]

Musculoskeletal physiotherapy

Musculoskeletal physiotherapy is a non-invasive intervention using therapeutic movement to overcome movement problems caused by pain.

This technique may suppress pain by activating neurophysiological mechanisms at either the spinal or supraspinal levels via peripheral mechanoreceptors.

Desensitisation techniques include passive and active movement involving changes of behaviour patterns and joint manipulation and mobilisation both of which may help reduce pain in chronic neck, low back and muscle tension headaches (Table 12.4).[10]

Non-pharmacological physical agents have widespread use in pain management. These approaches to pain management are particularly appropriate for superficial causes of pain in the peripheral musculoskeleton. Their actions are mediated by well-researched mechanisms of pain transmission including pain receptors, nerve conduction and spinal transmission. It is the manipulation of these mechanisms that can help generate analgesia (Fig. 12.8).

TABLE 12.3 TENS and acupuncture

	Methods of delivery	Indications	Contraindications/precautions
TENS Percutaneous electrical stimulation of the peripheral sensory nervous system	Via use of adhesive conductive patches directly over the painful area or dermatomally applied Use high- or low-frequency stimulation for continuous or intermittent periods	Labour pain Acute postoperative pain Angina Chronic pain	*Avoid:* Inflamed infected tissue, internal pacing devices, anterior neck, pregnancy, inability to use or understand equipment, topical patch drug-delivery systems and use while driving *Risk:* Skin damage through continuous use, cardiac disease
Acupuncture Ancient Chinese and Japanese needling technique often used in Asia with moxibustion (herbs being burnt) and dietary changes	Percutaneous needle placement at or near established points on acupuncture meridians Depth, frequency of treatment, needle numbers and duration vary	Most pain types Musculoskeletal neck and low back pain Angina Cancer Migraine Chronic headache Neuralgia Neuropathic pain	*Avoid:* Pregnancy, superficial or systemic infection, and acute migraine *Risk:* Severe cardiac disease, bleeding disorders, cardiac pacemaker

Future research on physical agents should concentrate on those physical approaches to pain management where prior studies, empirical evidence and anecdotal reports already exist. The application of physical therapies varies between countries and research may determine those who currently receive ineffective treatments and those who as yet do not benefit (see Framework 6).

Pharmacological interventions

Pharmacological peripheral interventions like other treatments may be organised initially into route of access, delivery method and drug therapy. It is important to recognise that some peripheral interventions predominantly act within the periphery (e.g. an intradermal injection of local anaesthetic for intravenous cannulation), whereas others (e.g. peripherally delivered opiates or opioids) predominantly act systemically on the brain or spinal cord through vascular absorption.

Here we will look at drugs that are peripherally administered either topically or by injection.

TABLE 12.4 Massage and musculoskeletal therapy

	Method of delivery	Indications	Contraindications/ precautions
Massage			
This technique is an art but research is accumulating of its advantage for well being, pain and relaxation	Manual technique using pressure via the hands or fingers to the affected area	Acute or chronic musculoskeletal pain associated with sports or disease states	*Avoid:* Local or systemic infection, bleeding disorders, local malignancy, fracture sites or recent deep vein thrombosis *Risk:* Cardiac disease skin disorders
Musculoskeletal physiotherapy			
This technique involves analytical assessment using theory and clinical history to develop a treatment plan It is a therapeutic process and requires careful monitoring of progress	Passive movement or active mobilisation by experienced professionals integrating theory and clinical history	Pain conditions associated with acute or chronic tissue injuries involving intra- and periarticular joint pains, and neuromuscular components	*Avoid:* No history of the injury, nerve root/peripheral nerve entrapment, fractures (immediate or pathological), severe unremitting night pain, significant trauma or obsessive personality *Risk:* Severity, irritability, stage of disease and patient behaviour influences relative risk

Fig. 12.8 Effect of peripheral interventions

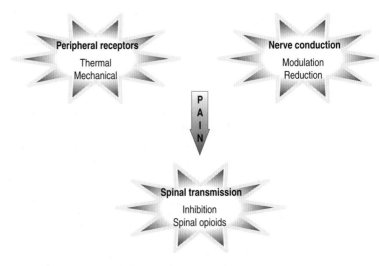

Peripheral receptors
Thermal
Mechanical

Nerve conduction
Modulation
Reduction

PAIN

Spinal transmission
Inhibition
Spinal opioids

Local anaesthetic creams

Local anaesthetic creams are simply and easily applied directly to the skin. In general, they are used to reduce the pain of needle insertion for children or where needle phobia may exist in adults (Box 12.2).

Considerations when using topical local anaesthetic creams:

- Commonly this is the dorsum of the hand for intravenous cannulation
- Skin must be clean and dry prior to application
- It is sensible to apply the cream to more than one site
- A thick layer should be applied to be effective
- Each application must be covered with an occlusive dressing.

There are two available preparations and both may cause redness, itching or swelling to the skin.

Ametop® (topical tetracaine 4% gel)

Amethocaine is a topical amide local anaesthetic agent. It is a white semi-transparent gel. It should be applied directly to the skin (without rubbing) for its anaesthetic action. It MUST be covered to be effective and left in situ for 30–45 min. Once removed the underlying area of skin is suitable for venepuncture or cannulation and will remain effective for between 4 and 6 h.

EMLA® (Eutectic Mixture of Local Anaesthetic: Lidocaine and Prilocaine)

EMLA is applied directly to the skin and can be applied 1–5 h prior to venepuncture, but its anaesthetic effect wears off rapidly (within 20–30 min) once removed.

Parents and professionals often ask which preparation is better at reducing children's pain with needle insertion? Although EMLA is effective in relieving children's pain, amethocaine is superior to EMLA for both intravenous drip insertion and for the duration of time it is applied.[11] EMLA has been used for analgesia during circumcision in newborn boys[12] and for venous leg ulcers,[13] and has been found to reduce pain in both Cochrane reviews (Table 12.5).

BOX 12.2 Needle phobia

Correct name is belonephobia – a fear of sharp objects such as pins or needles
The word phobia comes from the Greek and literally means 'fear' or 'suffering'
Suffering from a phobia generates an immense degree of fear and anxiety that is not in proportion to the actual danger
10% of the UK population has fear of the needle and it is increasingly recognised by doctors as a real problem
Causes of needle phobia may include a negative experience as a child at the dentist or hospital or through instruction from misinformed adults
The three main methods to manage such fear are to provide information, develop coping strategies or use topical anaesthetic preparations

TABLE 12.5 Topical local anaesthetics			
	Method of delivery	Indications	Contraindications/ precautions
Ametop			
This is an ester local anaesthetic Presented in a 1.5 g tube This product should be stored at 2–8°C	Can be applied for 30 min prior to venepuncture and 45 min prior to venous cannulation	It is used for taking a blood sample and for cannulation	*Avoid:* Allergy to local anaesthetics; open wounds; broken skin, lips, mouth or tongue, eyes and ears, anal or genital region and mucous membranes; premature infant or full-term child <1 month
EMLA			
This is an amide local anaesthetic 5% cream consisting of equal amounts of lidocaine (2.5%) and prilocaine (2.5%)	Must be applied for at least 60 min before a procedure Remove dressing immediately before use	Needle insertions, blood sampling, hair removal, superficial skin surgery (warts, genital warts and moles)	*Avoid:* As above including the anus and genitals of children, children <1 year *Risk:* Anaemia, pregnancy, methaemoglobinaemia and breastfeeding

Patches

Topical patches are a non-invasive peripheral intervention that can provide convenient drug delivery for therapeutic need. This delivery system is used for analgesia (e.g. transdermal fentanyl, buprenorphine, lignocaine, clonidine and nitroglycerin), but also commonly as an aid in smoking cessation (nicotine patches) or hormone replacement therapy (HRT).

The majority of these patch systems deliver the drug peripherally, it is absorbed and acts systemically, and these will be discussed briefly. The transdermal route provides a stable level of analgesia avoiding the peak serum concentrations with oral dosing and the associated side effects. In addition, with less 'tablets' to take compliance and satisfaction are improved. However, lignocaine (Lidoderm 5%) patches act locally with minimal systemic absorption and, therefore, act predominantly in the periphery.

Transdermal fentanyl

Fentanyl is a potent opioid which is highly lipid (fat) soluble making it suitable for transdermal administration. Fentanyl acts by binding to μ-receptors within the central nervous system producing analgesia. The patch is applied directly to the skin and is composed of four layers. There is an impermeable backing layer, a drug reservoir layer, a rate control membrane and an adhesive layer. Fentanyl diffuses through the rate control membrane in such a way to provide a 72-h drug-delivery system. A *'Fentanyl 25 patch'* will deliver the drug at 25 µg/h.

On applying a patch, changing dose or removal involves three phases:

1. A lag period after the first dose before therapeutic levels are reached.
2. A continual rise in blood concentration towards steady state by the second dose following initial treatment or where an increase in does occurs.
3. Once the patch is removed or dose reduced there is a delay in reduction of analgesia and side effects.[14]

Transdermal fentanyl is currently under investigation in a patient-controlled transdermal system design where fentanyl released into the skin is enhanced by iontophoresis after the patient pushes a button on the fentanyl patch (Box 12.3).[15]

Buprenorphine matrix-patch

Buprenorphine is a semi-synthetic opioid that is approximately 30 times as potent as morphine. Like fentanyl, buprenorphine is highly lipid soluble allowing transdermal penetration. Buprenorphine is characterised as a partial agonist at the µ-opioid receptor, this means it binds to a receptor but it can never produce 100% response no matter what dose is given. In addition, buprenorphine is an antagonist at the κ-opioid receptor and a weak agonist at the δ-receptor. Buprenorphine is incorporated into a polymer matrix, which allows continuous and reliable drug delivery through the skin into the systemic circulation.

Clinically, the patches are used for moderate-to-severe cancer and non-cancer pain and switching to these from weaker opioid analgesics is generally problem-free.

Local effects following patch application include transient erythema and pruritus, whereas the more common systemic side effects include nausea, dizziness and vomiting.[16]

Lidocaine patch (Lidoderm 5%®)

Lidocaine transdermal 5% patches are approved for pain secondary to postherpetic neuralgia, but have been used in other pain conditions. Lidocaine acts by blocking sodium channels on nerve membranes, inhibiting nerve conduction and thereby causing its analgesic effect. Interestingly, this formulation inhibits small dysfunctional pain fibres, but not large myelinated Aβ sensory fibres and, therefore, numbness does not occur at the site of application. Topical application of lidocaine avoids the potential toxic systemic effects and drug–drug interactions from other drug delivery routes. Older patients may benefit most from these advantages where sensitivity to adverse events increases risk and polypharmacy increases risk of unwanted drug potentiation or antagonism.

BOX 12.3 Transdermal opioids

Important message:
   All opioid patches contain a potent concentration of drug. They should be prescribed by experienced specialists and disposed of safely once removed.

Lidoderm patches are very well tolerated with minimal systemic delivery even when three patches are applied simultaneously. The amount of drug absorbed is directly proportional to the skin surface area covered and the duration of patch application. Patients can use the patches indefinitely without developing tolerance, physical dependence or addiction. The most common adverse event is erythema and irritation at the application site (28%).[17]

Clonidine patch (Cataprestts®)

Clonidine hydrochloride is a central α_2-agonist that may produce analgesia by activating central descending inhibitory pain pathways and inhibiting ascending pain pathways, but it may also act on peripheral pain receptors. The transdermal delivery system has been studied for postoperative pain control and reduction in opioid and anaesthesia requirements. However, the side-effect profile, including sedation, hypotension and bradycardia mediated by the central action, may limit its future use.[18]

Nitroglycerin patch (Nitroplast®, Minitran®)

Nitroglycerin is a nitric oxide generator. This may enhance the antinociception of opioids by helping activate inhibitory descending pathways, direct μ-receptor action or altering inflammation-induced vasoconstriction. Nitroglycerin patches have been used for both systemic and local pain relief; however, organic nitrates have limited anti-inflammatory and analgesic effects due to dose-limiting vascular dilatation causing hypotension and headaches (Table 12.6).[18]

Topical analgesics

This group of drugs includes rubefacients (topical capsaicin and salicylate preparations) and the non-steroidal anti-inflammatory drugs (NSAIDs). A miscellaneous group includes benzydamine, mucopolysaccharide polysulphate, salicylamide and cooling sprays.

A rubefacient is defined by the Royal Society of Medicine as 'a counter irritant'. The name is derived from the fact that these agents cause irritation of sensory nerve endings, which alter or mask pain in the underlying muscle or joint served by those same nerves. Reddening of the skin occurs due to dilation of blood vessels. Rubefacients are usually used as adjuvants to other therapies, such as oral analgesia, rest, and compression and may be of benefit where oral analgesics cause side effects. As the name suggests they are rubbed into the skin to alter or mask pain.

Topical analgesics are available as prescription-only medicine (PoM) and widely as non-prescription medicine. Consumers need to have the best information regarding risk and benefits.

Topical capsaicin

Capsaicin is the active compound present in chilli peppers, responsible for making them hot when eaten. In 1494 Columbus brought back chillies from his second voyage and so they entered into European cuisine.

Capsaicin was originally used in topical ointments for peripheral neuropathies (e.g. herpes zoster 'shingles'); it is highly fat soluble allowing skin

TABLE 12.6 Self-adhesive patch preparations

	Method of delivery	Indications	Contraindications/ precautions
Fentanyl			
Strengths available: 12.5, 25, 50, 75 and 100 µg patches (25 µg patch, oral morphine equivalent – approximately 100 mg/day for each day)	Apply patch to dry clean skin Leave in situ for 72 h Apply to different site for next patch DO NOT cut patch it will become ineffective May be administered by a patient-controlled transdermal system	Moderate-to-severe pain for cancer and non-cancer treatment where pain is opioid sensitive Stable pain, where the oral route is not available	*Avoid:* Opioid-naïve patients, acute postoperative pain, mild or intermittent pain, severe respiratory/airway risk or in children <2 years old *Risks:* Hypotension, asthma, renal or hepatic dysfunction and the elderly, fever or external heat may increase absorption, long duration of action the side effects need to be monitored on patch removal
Buprenorphine			
Strengths available: 35, 52.5 and 70 µg patches (35 µg patch oral morphine equivalent – approximately 30–60 mg/day for each day)	Apply patch to dry clean skin Leave in situ for 72 h Apply to different site for next patch Patch may be cut and shaped without loss of effect	Moderate-to-severe pain including degenerative musculoskeletal causes, neuropathic pain and cancer-related pain Stable background pain, where the oral route is not available Opioid dependence	*Avoid:* Opioid-naïve patients, mild or intermittent pain severe respiratory/airway risk patients <18 years old *Risks:* As for fentanyl patches
Lidocaine			
Each patch contains 700 mg of lidocaine in an adhesive compound with other ingredient Each patch measures 10 × 14 cm, but can be cut to size	Apply directly to affected area Keep patch(es) in place for 12 h then remove Do not reapply for 12 h	Postherpetic neuralgia, but also studied in lower back, neuropathic and osteoarthritic pain	*Avoid:* Allergy to amide local anaesthetics, open wounds, broken skin or mucosal membranes *Risk:* Hypotensive conditions or cardiac arrhythmias, self-limiting erythema may occur
Clonidine			
Catapres TTS patch 100 µg/ 24 h It is safe to cut the patch to size as needed	Apply to clean dry intact skin on the upper arm or chest	As an adjuvant to postoperative pain control and to reduce anaesthetic requirement	*Avoid:* Allergy to clonidine, in children aged <12 years or broken skin

(Continued)

TABLE 12.6 Self-adhesive patch preparations—cont'd

	Method of delivery	Indications	Contraindications/ precautions
	Change site for new patch		*Risk*: Hypotensive conditions or bradycardia
Nitroglycerin Patch strength used in studies is 5 mg	Apply to the chest wall on clean dry intact skin without hair May be worn continuously for 10–12 h	Nitroglycerin has been studied for its ability to augment analgesia and prolong time to first rescue analgesia postoperatively	*Avoid*: Allergy to nitrates, circulatory failure, severe hypotension, cardiogenic shock, children and closed-angle glaucoma *Risk*: Severe hepatic or renal impairment, hypothermia or head trauma

penetration and its use as a rubefacient. It binds to nociceptors (vanilloid receptor subtype 1 (VR1)) in the skin, causing initial excitation of the neurones and a period of enhanced sensitivity to noxious stimuli, usually perceived as itching or burning. This is followed by a refractory period with reduced sensitivity and persistent desensitisation from neurotransmitter release. It is this action that is exploited for therapeutic pain relief. Capsaicin is also used in a nasal spray form for headaches, sinus and allergy symptoms in addition to being the active ingredient in the chemical riot-control agent, pepper spray.

Topical capsaicin is available in two concentrations, 0.025% for musculoskeletal pain and 0.075% for neuropathic pain.

In systematic reviews for neuropathic conditions, topical capsaicin (0.075%) was better than placebo with numbers needed to treat (NNT) of 5.7 and for musculoskeletal conditions (0.025%) was better than placebo with an NNT of 8.1. Local adverse events occurred more frequently than with placebo, with a NNH of 2.5. More than 50% of patients have local symptoms and 13% withdrew from the studies due to adverse events.[19]

Topical salicylate

Topical salicylate is again a rubefacient and has been shown to be significantly better than placebo in acute conditions (NNT 2.1), but not in larger more valid studies for chronic conditions. Overall the evidence for its use in pain management is poor.[20]

Topical NSAIDs

Topical NSAIDs are used widely throughout the world both by prescription and as 'over-the-counter' preparations. For a topical NSAID to be effective it has to penetrate the skin, be absorbed, and be present in high enough concentrations to produce pain relief. Plasma concentrations of topical NSAIDs are generally less than 5% of those produced by the oral route. In contrast, meniscal cartilage and tendon levels are higher, with subcutaneous and muscle concentrations higher by a factor of a thousand. The low systemic concentrations probably account for the low occurrence of gastrointestinal side effects. Overall in acute conditions topical NSAIDs are shown to be effective. In acute pain studies effective analgesics have NNT values of 2.5 with ketoprofen proven to be highly effective. In chronic musculoskeletal pains, topical NSAIDs are better than placebo with a NNT of 4.6, but confidence is limited due to the short duration of the trials (Table 12.7) (see Framework 7).[21]

Wound irrigation

Wound irrigation is a peripheral intervention using local anaesthesia to improve postoperative pain management and thereby reduce the need for additional analgesia. A substantial amount of postoperative pain is associated with the site of incision. Studies have been performed using local anaesthesia (ropivacaine or bupivacaine) delivered either by subcutaneous catheter[22,23] or through post-surgical wound drains.[24] Effectiveness is determined by use of visual analogue scores (VAS) or reduction in postoperative analgesic requirements. Subcutaneous local anaesthesia would not be expected to have an effect

TABLE 12.7 Rubefacients and topical NSAIDs

	Method of delivery	Indications	Contraindications/precautions
Capsaicin 0.025% and 0.075% cream	Use sparingly Rub into skin of affected area only Apply 3–4 times per day	Neuropathic pains Diabetic neuropathy Postherpetic neuralgia Polyneuropathies Musculoskeletal pains: arthritic disorders Back pain or fibromyalgia	*Avoid:* Contact with eyes and inflamed or broken skin, use of excessive cream and hot bath/shower immediately before or after use *Risks:* Transient burning during initial treatment, wash hands immediately after use
Topical salicylate In general salicylate preparations occur in combination with other compounds	Apply with gentle massage 3–4 times per day	Musculoskeletal and neuropathic pains	*Avoid:* Contact with eyes, mucous membranes and broken skin; pregnancy or breastfeeding *Risk:* Overuse may cause hypersensitivity or worsen asthma or renal disease
Topical NSAIDs Gel, foam or compound topical applications Drugs include ketoprofen, piroxicam, feldene and ibuprofen	Apply with gentle massage 3–4 times per day	Sprains and strains and soft tissue injuries Chronic conditions including osteoarthritis and rheumatological disorders	*Avoid:* Contact with eyes and mucous membranes, pregnancy and breast-feeding; known NSAID allergy *Risk:* Known asthma or renal disease, photoallergic reactions may rarely occur

on visceral pain and with care dosing would not be expected to cause local anaesthetic toxicity. Such techniques require nursing and medical expertise and despite supportive evidence this technique is not yet used widely in the UK.

Intradermal anaesthesia

Intradermal injections provide almost instantaneous anaesthesia for percutaneous needling of the skin. A combination of the pharmacological drug action and physical tissue compression by the injectate produces the desired effect. Lidocaine is commonly used to site larger cannula or needles. Any concentration of lidocaine may be used intradermally before cannulation without affecting the degree of pain experienced,[25] but the addition of bicarbonate may further decrease pain.[26] Intradermal injection of metoclopramide (a commonly used anti-emetic agent) and tramadol (a centrally acting analgesic) may also produce this anaesthetic effect.[27] Metoclopramide has a similar structure to a local anaesthetics and tramadol (which is related to codeine) may act through a receptor-based mechanism.

KEY POINTS

- A thorough understanding of the basic science, psychology, therapeutics and anatomy is required before a considered discussion about management can be undertaken
- A peripheral intervention is one that is delivered through: skin absorption (transdermal), the skin (percutaneous) or via conduction dependent upon the physical properties of the treatment
- Local anaesthetic creams are commonly used prior to cannula insertion especially in children and needle-phobic adults (EMLA, Amatop)
- Transdermal opioids have gained favour in managing chronic pain and cancer pain, especially for those who cannot tolerate oral medication. The drugs used have to be highly lipid soluble
- Topical capsaicin has a role in managing neuropathic pain of limited area as part of a management programme
- Topical NSAIDs are of use in some chronic conditions where systemic use may put the patient at undue risk of side effects
- Wound irrigation has a role in the immediate postoperative period as has subcutaneous infiltration

---

References

1. Robinson VA, Brosseau L, Casimiro L et al. Thermotherapy for treating rheumatoid arthritis. *Cochrane Database Syst Rev* 2006; **2**: Reviews 2002.
2. van der Windt DA, van de Heijden GJ, van de Berg SG et al. Ultrasound therapy for musculoskeletal disorders: a systematic review. *Pain* 1999; **81**(3): 257–271.
3. Brosseau L, Robinson V, Wells G et al. Low level laser therapy (Classes, I, II and III) for treating rheumatoid arthritis. *Cochrane Database Syst Rev* 2005; **4**: Reviews 2005.
4. Carroll D, Moore RA, McQuay HJ et al. Transcutaneous electrical nerve stimulation (TENS) for chronic pain. *Cochrane Database Syst Rev* 2000; **4**: Reviews 2000.
5. Osiri M, Welch V, Brosseau L et al. Transcutaneous electrical nerve stimulation for knee osteoarthritis. *Cochrane Database Syst Rev* 2000; **4**: Reviews 2000.

6. Furlan AD, van Tulder MW, Chekin DC et al. Acupuncture and dry-needling for low back pain. *Cochrane Database Syst Rev* 2005; **1**: CD001351.
7. Trinh KV, Graham N, Gross AR et al. Acupuncture for neck disorders. *Cochrane Database Syst Rev* 2006; **3**: Reviews 2006.
8. Furlan AD, Brosseau L, Imamura M et al. Massage for low-back pain. *Cochrane Database Syst Rev* 2002; **2**: Reviews 2002.
9. Weinrich SP, Weinrich MC. The effect of massage on pain in cancer patients. *Appl Nurs Res* 1990; **3**(4): 140–145.
10. Zusman M. Mechanisms of musculoskeletal physiotherapy. *Phys Ther Rev* 2004; **9**: 39–49.
11. Lander JA, Weltman BJ, So SS. EMLA and Amethocaine for reduction of children's pain associated with needle insertion. *Cochrane Database Syst Rev* 2006; **3**: Reviews 2006.
12. Taddio A, Ohlsson K, Ohlsson A. Lidocaine-prilocaine cream for analgesia during circumcision in newborn boys. *Cochrane Database Syst Rev* 1999; **3**: Reviews 1999.
13. Briggs M, Nelson EA. Topical agents or dressings for pain in venous leg ulcers. *Cochrane Database Syst Rev* 2003; **1**: Reviews 2003.
14. Gourlay GK. Treatment of cancer pain with transdermal fentanyl. *Lancet Oncol* 2001; **2**(3): 165–172.
15. Chelly JE, Grass J, Houseman TW et al. The safety and efficacy of a fentanyl patient-controlled transdermal system for acute postoperative analgesia: a multicenter, placebo-controlled trial. *Anesth Analg* 2004; **98**(2): 427–433.
16. Griessinger N, Sittl R, Likar R. Transdermal buprenorphine in clinical practice – a post-marketing surveillance study in 13,179 patients. *Curr Med Res Opin* 2005; **21**(8): 1147–1156.
17. Gammaitoni AR, Alvarez NA, Galer BS. Safety and tolerability of the lidocaine patch 5%, a targeted peripheral analgesic: a review of the literature. *J Clin Pharmacol* 2003; **43**(2): 111–117.
18. Ball AM, Smith KM. Postoperative pain management: can transdermal patches help? *Orthopedics* 2006; **29**(3): 217–220.
19. Mason L, Moore RA, Derry S et al. Systematic review of topical capsaicin for the treatment of chronic pain. *BMJ* 2004; **328**(7446): 991.
20. Mason L, Moore RA, Edwards JE et al. Systematic review of efficacy of topical rubefacients containing salicylates for the treatment of acute and chronic pain. *BMJ* 2004; **328**(7446): 995.
21. *Topical analgesics: a review of reviews and a bit of perspective.* Bandolier Extra: Evidence-based health care. March 2005 [cited; Available from: *http://www.jr2.ox.ac.uk/bandolier/Extraforbando.*
22. Gottschalk A, Burmeister MA, Radtke P et al. Continuous wound infiltration with ropivacaine reduces pain and analgesic requirement after shoulder surgery. *Anesth Analg* 2003; **97**(4): 1086–1091.
23. Givens VA, Lipscomb GH, Meyer NL. A randomized trial of postoperative wound irrigation with local anesthetic for pain after cesarean delivery. *Am J Obstet Gynecol* 2002; **186**(6): 1188–1191.
24. Talbot H et al. Evaluation of a local anaesthesia regimen following mastectomy. *Anaesthesia* 2004; **59**(7): 664–667.
25. Criswell J, Gauntlett IS. Pain on intradermal injection with lignocaine. The effect of concentration. *Anaesthesia* 1991; **46**(8): 691–692.
26. Palmon SC, Lloyd AT, Kirsch JR. The effect of needle gauge and lidocaine pH on pain during intradermal injection. *Anesth Analg* 1998; **86**(2): 379–381.
27. Pang WW, Mok MS, Chang DP et al. Local anesthetic effect of tramadol, metoclopramide, and lidocaine following intradermal injection. *Reg Anesth Pain Med* 1998; **23**(6): 580–583.

Further reading

Cameron MH (ed.) Physical agents in rehabilitation. In: *Research to practice*, 2nd edn. London: Saunders; 2003.

Carroll D, Bowsher D (eds) *Pain: management and nursing care*. London: Butterworth-Heinmann Ltd; 1994.

Fuller G. *Neurological examination made easy*, 3rd edn. Edinburgh: Churchill Livingstone; 2004.

Linchitz RM, Sorell PJIII. Physical therapy techniques. In: Raj PP (ed.) *Pain medicine: a comprehensive review*. Philadelphia: Mosby; 2003: 327–333.

Petty NJ. *Neuromuscular examination and assessment*, 3rd edn. Edinburgh: Churchill Livingstone.

Wright A, Sluka KA. Nonpharmacological treatments for musculoskeletal pain. *Clin J Pain* 2001; **17**(1): 33–46.

Gwenda Cavill

Pain as a clinical entity

Introduction

The effective management of chronic pain is a challenge to the medical profession. It is a very common condition, but continues to be poorly understood by both suffers and their doctors. To manage chronic pain effectively, it is necessary for the clinician to understand the mechanisms of chronic pain, to be aware of treatments available for that pain and, perhaps most importantly of all, to understand the patient.

Acute vs. chronic pain

Acute pain and chronic pain are not the same entity. The differences are outlined in Table 13.1. In the Oxford English dictionary 'acute', when relating to a disease, is defined as *'coming sharply to a crisis; severe, not chronic'* while 'chronic' is defined as *'persisting for a long time'*. However, British colloquial use of 'chronic' means 'very bad; intense, severe'. This potential different understanding of the word chronic can cause communication difficulties between patients and healthcare professionals.

In the initial stages of chronic pain, the pain will be acute (i.e. of less than 3 months' duration). During this time, both patient and doctor are likely to deal with this as acute pain. The patient avoids activities that might exacerbate pain in the belief further damage is being avoided and the doctor possibly performs some investigations as to the cause of the pain. As the pain persists and the results of investigations are all normal, time passes and the pain becomes chronic. Strategies used to cope with the acute problem persist, but are now less appropriate and may contribute to the persistence of the pain.

Medical students are taught that pain is a symptom of disease, or effectively a signal that something is wrong. They are taught to investigate the symptom,

TABLE 13.1 Differences between acute and chronic pain	
Acute pain	Chronic pain
<3 months duration	>3 months duration
Protective, preventing further damage	Prevents normal functioning
Useful	Not useful
e.g. broken limb, appendicitis	e.g. post-herpetic neuralgia, chronic low back pain

pain, with the aim of making a diagnosis and then, ideally, providing a cure. This teaching is correct for acute pain, but when pain persists and the results of investigations are normal, both the patient and the doctor can become confused. The doctor reassures the patient that 'everything is normal' or 'there is nothing wrong'. However, this does not give the patient an explanation for the pain they are still experiencing. Investigations do not reassure patients there is nothing wrong with them, but confirm to them that their doctor is also concerned about the cause of their pain. If an investigation does not reveal the cause of the pain, it is not because the cause of their pain cannot be identified, but because the wrong investigation has been performed. Inability to identify a cause for chronic pain does not remind some healthcare professionals that medical science cannot yet explain all pain symptoms, but suggests to them that the patient's pain is in their head and is not physical. Eventually patients may also begin to wonder if they are not just imagining their pain and worry that they may be going mad. Family and friends of an individual with chronic pain may have the same thoughts.

Development from acute to chronic pain

For acute low back pain, the risk factors for developing chronic pain and long-term disability have been well researched and identified. These risk factors are called 'yellow flags' and are psychosocial barriers to recovery (see Table 13.2).[1] Essentially similar factors are associated with the development of chronicity for other pain conditions.[2] Psychosocial factors are more important than medical factors in the development of disability across cultures.[3]

Patients who believe the pain they are experiencing indicates tissue damage are more likely to rest and avoid any activity, including work. This is in the belief that any activity that precipitates their pain also indicates further damage. This lack of activity may result in muscle weakness, general loss of fitness and preoccupation with somatic symptoms.

Inappropriate expectations of treatment also predispose to chronicity. The expectations may be inappropriately high such as expecting complete relief of pain, or low where the patient does not believe active participation in treatment will affect the outcome.

A patient who is dissatisfied with their job may be less motivated to recover. If an employer is perceived to be unsympathetic, this may be an additional source of stress and promote further dissatisfaction with work. Well-meaning family and friends can reinforce the sick role in an individual taking time off

TABLE 13.2 Risk factors for developing chronic low back pain and long-term disability
Belief that pain and activity are harmful
Sickness behaviours such as extended rest
Social withdrawal
Emotional problems such as low or negative mood, depression, anxiety or stress
Problems and/or dissatisfaction at work
Problems with claims or compensation or time off work
Overprotective family; lack of support
Inappropriate expectations of treatment

work because of pain. They may advocate rest, discourage activities and to this end perform many little tasks with the intention of helping their family member or friend recover. This can promote the development of excessive pain behaviours. However, the converse is also true, as lack of support may also predispose to chronicity. This may take the form of inconsistent, critical or punitive responses from family or friends that make it more difficult for that individual to rehabilitate.

Lack of social contact is also associated with time off work. Working adults tend to make most of their daily social interactions at work. If someone feels they are not well enough to go to work, they may also feel they should not be doing light gardening, which may result in a chat with the neighbour over the fence, or going out in the evening for a quiet drink with friends, resulting in even less social contact. Social withdrawal may result. This is another predictor for chronic pain.

Premorbid problems with mood, depression, anxiety and stress also predispose to the development of chronicity. Chronic pain presents yet an additional problem to be dealt with by an individual with already compromised coping skills. Alternatively, these problems may develop as a consequence of chronic pain, when they will still predispose to chronicity. Substance abuse or dependence is also a risk factor. Again, this may be either a premorbid problem or develop as a consequence of chronic pain. Such individuals are likely to over-rely on medication and not comply with medical recommendations.

Dealing with insurance companies or making legal claims for compensation for injuries sustained in an accident is stressful enough at the best of times. However, during this process people with chronic pain may feel that the validity of their pain is being questioned, particularly if they do not have a diagnosis for their pain. There is little evidence that pain behaviours change significantly once a protracted claim has been settled, but problems settling such claims do predispose to chronicity of pain.

Duration of pain is also a factor. The longer pain persists, the more likely an individual is to have developed significant disability. A time period of 2 years is often considered the point by which many investigations and treatments have been performed and tried without success and a chronic pain syndrome has developed. For successful return to work the timescale is much shorter. Being off work with chronic pain for more than 6 months means the chance of someone returning to work is only 50%, while after 1 year off work it is only 10%.

Individuals who have a history of prolonged recovery from previous experiences of pain will tend to expect the same long convalescence will be required again and hence this is another risk factor for pain becoming chronic.

The correlation between a history of childhood psychological, physical or sexual abuse and the development of chronic pain is well accepted. Focusing on the pain may allow the sufferer to somatise their emotional trauma, but is likely to prevent resolution of pain. Hence, a history of abuse is also a psychosocial risk factor for the development of chronic pain.

Definitions of pain

There are many words and terms with precise meanings used by healthcare professionals to describe pain. These can enable efficient and effective communication between professionals, but can confuse patients if used during explanations of their pain. It is important that these words are used accurately in the clinical setting. Explanations of the meanings of these words to patients can reduce confusion and patient anxiety. For definitions see the Definitions section at the front of the book.

Some words that cause confusion include: allodynia, central pain, deafferentation pain, dysaesthesia and hyperalgesia. The following terms all have precise meanings but patients may consider them to be the same: neuralgia, neuritis, neuropathic or neurogenic pain, radicular pain or radiculalgia and radiculitis.

Understanding the mechanisms of chronic pain

An understanding of the mechanisms underlying the experience of chronic pain is essential to the effective management of such pain. This includes an understanding of both the sensory and the emotional components. It is important to remember that the physical and psychological factors described are not mutually exclusive, but combine in each individual to give a unique experience.

Sensory components of chronic pain

A traditional way of classifying the sensory component of chronic pain is by inferred mechanisms (see Table 13.3). This results in pain being described as either nociceptive or as non-nociceptive.[4]

Nociceptive pain

Nociceptive pain is presumed to be maintained by continual tissue injury and can be further subdivided into somatic and visceral pain.

TABLE 13.3 Classification of the sensory component of chronic pain			
Nociceptive		Non-nociceptive	
Visceral	Somatic	Neuropathic	Idiopathic

Somatic pain

Arises in tissues such as joints, bones and muscles and is well localised. An example is arthritic pain. It is often described as aching, stabbing or throbbing.

Visceral pain

Arises from viscera in the thorax, abdomen or pelvis. It tends to be rather diffuse and poorly defined and may be described as deep, dull or colicky. It is also referred to other locations. Chronic refractory angina is an example. Visceral pain is often associated with motor reflexes such as muscle spasm and with autonomic reflexes such as nausea and vomiting.

Non-nociceptive pain

Non-nociceptive pain can be subdivided into neuropathic and idiopathic pain.

Neuropathic pain

This is defined as being due to injury to the nociceptive pathway, either peripherally or centrally. Post-herpetic neuralgia is an example of peripheral nerve injury and post-stroke pain is an example of central injury. Clinical features include allodynia, hyperalgesia and hyperpathia. It is often described as burning or 'electric shock-like'.

Idiopathic pain

This refers to a wide spectrum of poorly understood pain states. Often there is no identifiable organic cause. Atypical facial pain is an example. The term 'psychogenic pain' has been used in the past, but this gives the impression that there is no physical cause for the pain, rather than admitting the underlying cause cannot be identified.

Emotional components of chronic pain

The International Association for the Study of Pain (IASP) states that pain is 'an unpleasant sensory and emotional experience associated with actual or potential tissue damage or described in terms of such damage'.[5] This definition clearly includes the emotional aspect of pain. This does not reflect different 'pain thresholds' between individuals, but does reflect the difference in the emotional components involved. There are many reports of soldiers on the battlefield sustaining serious injuries of which they remain unaware until after the fighting. Clearly, even the immediate reaction to tissue damage is dependent on factors other than the degree of tissue damage. In a different clinical scenario, asymtomatic individuals are often shown to have significant pathology on radiological imaging of their hip joints that might be expected to produce pain, while other individuals with minimal pathology report severe pain. The experience of pain is clearly not dependent purely on physical factors.

Individuals may report the worst pain they have ever experienced to be purely emotional, such as the death of their mother. Emotional states may influence both the reported severity of pain and the distress it causes. Anxiety and depression are commonly associated with chronic pain, as are frustration and anger. All these negative emotions may be aggravating factors.

The cognitive-behavioural approach to chronic pain essentially links thoughts, feelings and behaviours with the physical sensation of pain. It is based on the understanding that past experience leads to a pattern of beliefs and expectations about self, world, future and illness (Fig. 13.1).

This approach can be useful, as it aids understanding of the role of emotions and psychological involvement in chronic pain. Cognitive-behavioural therapies are designed to help people identify and correct distorted ideas and beliefs, with the aim of changing behaviours and are often used in the treatment of chronic pain. Patients are taught to recognise the connections between thoughts, feelings and actions. Spontaneous, negative thoughts are identified and the evidence for and against these often-distorted thoughts is examined. In order to substitute more realistic interpretations, the unhelpful beliefs that predispose to the negative thoughts are challenged and hopefully changed.

Thoughts

Illness beliefs

Feelings and behaviours are influenced by what an event means to an individual, rather than by the event itself. A patient presenting with chronic pain will have a variety of beliefs about their pain, which may be contributing to the perpetuation of that pain. It is important to establish an understanding of as many of these beliefs as possible. People naturally group their understanding of illness into the following categories:[6]

- Identity: the diagnosis and symptoms of the illness
- Cause: perceived cause, which may be biological or psychosocial
- Time-line: how long the illness will last
- Consequences: effects of the illness on the patient's life
- Cure/control: if the illness can be cured and to what extent the outcome can be controlled by self or others.

It is important that information to patients provided by healthcare professionals fits with patients' understanding of their pain, or overtly addresses any differences, in order for the information to be taken on board.

Identity. Approximately one-third of patients seen nationally in pain clinics do not have a diagnosis. Many patients understandably struggle to deal with the lack of a diagnosis and this can contribute to subsequent difficulties in understanding their condition. Often patients without a diagnosis seek multiple medical opinions and request investigations. This may be because they

Fig. 13.1 The hot cross bun of pain (or the cognitive-behavioural approach to pain)

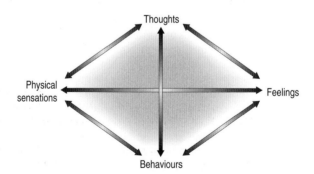

believe if a diagnosis could be found their doctor would be able to treat and cure them. It may also be because while they do not have a diagnosis, they feel there is doubt about the authenticity of their pain. When a diagnosis cannot be made, a clear explanation of the differences between acute and chronic pain, emphasising that the pain is due to damaged or abnormal functioning of pain or sensory nerves can be helpful.

Cause. It is important to ask patients what they believe is causing their pain. If pain is interpreted as ongoing tissue damage or potentially leading to severe disability, it will cause more distress than if it is interpreted as part of the healing process, which will eventually improve. Identifying the cause of a pain is sometimes easy, particularly when the pain had a sudden onset, for example following an obvious injury. It can be more difficult to explain to a patient that 5% of patients undergoing inguinal hernia repair experience chronic pain and that they are one of the unlucky 5%.

On occasion, the cause to which a patient attributes their pain can lead to more problems. A patient with back pain may attribute their pain to lifting a heavy object at work. However, if their pain did not begin until 3 weeks after they remember lifting the object, it is likely that their employer will not agree that this was the cause of their pain and, indeed, the employer is probably correct. This difference in opinion may become a 'yellow flag' as the patient attempts to obtain compensation from the employer for the perceived injury at work.

Time-line. Patients want to know what they can expect from their illness. From this, they plan their lives, particularly with respect to employment. Over-optimistic reassurance early on can be counter-productive. For example, if a casualty doctor reassures a patient that all their neck pain following a whiplash injury will be gone in 3 months, the patient may believe that if they just sit around and wait 3 months they will wake up one morning and be pain-free. However, with chronic pain it is often impossible to predict a time course, leaving the patient to face uncertainty.

Consequences. Chronic pain may have a huge impact on an individual's work, social life and physical and mental health. The perceived consequences of a diagnosis will depend on an individual's understanding of the impact of that condition on their life. If a relative was in a wheelchair due to 'arthritis', the diagnosis of arthritis may mean life in a wheelchair to the patient. The quality of life of patients living with chronic pain has been shown to be lower than that of patients on haemodialysis. In addition, patients with fibromyalgia syndrome have been shown to have a shorter life expectancy than matched controls.

Cure/control. If a patient is expecting or seeking a complete cure for their pain, they will almost certainly be disappointed. A treatment option that decreases their pain by 50% is unlikely to be considered effective by these patients, as they are only interested in a cure. Patients who have accepted there is no magical cure for their pain are much more likely to find a 50% decrease in their pain helpful and acceptable.

Individuals who believe their pain is a problem to be dealt with by health-care professionals, rather than something with which they must deal themselves, tend to expect passive treatments and are far less likely to actively participate in their treatment than individuals who believe their pain is their own problem to manage.

Self-efficacy

Effective coping depends on whether or not individuals believe they can cope with the pain. This is termed 'self-efficacy'. An individual's self-efficacy beliefs determine what activities that individual will begin, how much effort they will expend and for how long they will persist in that activity. If they don't believe they can perform graded exercises, they are unlikely to start such a programme of activity and very unlikely to complete it. Factors influencing self-efficacy include past performance at the task in hand or similar tasks, the performance of others perceived to be similar, verbal persuasion by others that one is capable and the patient's level of emotional and physiological arousal.[7] The mastery experience acquired through actual performance of a task is particularly important. Hence a graded exercise programme can be used both to improve levels of fitness and to improve self-efficacy. Perceived self-efficacy in chronic-pain patients predicts patient success at the conclusion of treatment.

Catastrophising

Catastrophisation, or the thinking of extremely negative thoughts, is now recognised as having a big influence on individuals with chronic pain and can predict reactions to pain and treatment. Catastrophisers report more pain than non-catastrophisers. It is easy to see that thoughts such as 'this pain is too much for me to cope with', 'I'm going to lose my job, my house and then my wife will leave me', induce feelings of distress and hopelessness, amongst others, that can result in more pain behaviours. Unsurprisingly, catastrophising is associated with lower self-efficacy.

Feelings

According to IASP, pain 'is unquestionably a sensation in a part or parts of the body, but is also always unpleasant and therefore also an emotional experience'. The emotions associated with pain are mostly negative and include fear, distress, anger, depression, guilt and hopelessness. Emotional disturbance in pain patients is more likely to be a consequence than a cause of chronic pain.[8]

There is no good evidence of severe emotional distress as a cause of pain, but complaints of pain may be exacerbated by emotional or social crises. Emotions such as anxiety, depression and anger cause a physiological response usually associated with noxious stimuli. This response includes increased sympathetic tone, endorphin production and muscle tension.

Emotional distress may occur in anticipation of pain. Many people dread the prospect of pain, so it is easy to see why many chronic pain patients try hard to avoid activities associated with pain or that they fear may exacerbate pain. Such anticipatory distress can be useful if it leads to problem-solving behaviour, but if excessive can produce serious debilitating effects. Emotional distress may also occur as a consequence of pain, as described in more detail below.

Pain problems may occur concurrently with emotional disturbances and also pain symptoms are relatively common in psychiatric patients. Making a physical diagnosis in the psychiatric population can be challenging, as these patients tend to use pain language rather indiscriminately.

Anxiety. An unexpected new pain generates fear. This fear is of the unknown, of the cause of the pain and its meaning and consequences. The amount of fear and what is feared will depend on the person and their experience. Fear produces anxiety about pain and this anxiety focuses attention on the pain. Anxiety may lead to muscle tension and consequently increase pain. Hence, there is a strong association between pain and anxiety. The anxiety may focus on the pain or be more generalised. There is a direct correlation between high anxiety levels and increased pain perception in people with recurrent low back pain.[9] The longer the pain persists and attempts at treatment fail the greater the anxiety.[10]

Depression. Depression and chronic pain are frequently associated, with 40–50% of chronic pain patients suffering from depression.[11] However, most people with chronic pain are not depressed.[12] While depression may predate the onset of chronic pain, it does appear that for most people with depression it is a reaction to their plight.[13] Whether pain predates the depression or *vice versa* remains under debate.[14]

Frustration and anger. There are many frustrations in living with chronic pain. These include the persistence of symptoms, lack of information about the causes of pain and repeated treatment failures. Higher levels of frustration than any other negative emotion are reported in pain patients.[15] Individuals may experience anger towards employers, insurers, benefit agencies, the health service, family members and themselves. Individuals with chronic pain often internalise their feelings of anger. Such bottled-up anger has been reported as being associated with pain intensity, pain behaviour and activity level.[16] Denial of anger by patients may lead the clinician to miss or underestimate this as a factor.

Control. Loss of control is also important in chronic pain. A person may perceive that things are under the control of external factors such as chance and luck rather than under their own control. As, despite their best efforts (seeking out more healthcare professionals, attempting to follow advice they have been given), individuals find themselves unable to find lasting relief from their pain and so feelings of hopelessness, helplessness and despair come to the fore. Patients with strong feelings of helplessness have higher levels of psychological distress.[17] Better coping is associated with a patient's higher level of perceived control.

Behaviours

It has been suggested that pain promotes behaviours aimed at healing, rather than behaviours aimed at reducing tissue damage.[18] However, with persistent pain, these recuperative behaviours can be unhelpful. Various behaviours associated with pain have been described,[19] including facial or audible expression (e.g. grimacing and groaning), distorted posture or movement (e.g. limping, protecting the painful area), negative affect (e.g. irritability, depression) or avoidance of activity (e.g. time off work, lying on sofa). These behaviours may be reinforced (see below). Emotions, such as anger, may be suppressed (see above). The lack of activity often resulting from pain behaviours can lead to deconditioning, no social contact and no distraction. These together can lead to a more developed sick role, which itself can increase pain perception.

By the time patients are seen in the pain clinic, they have often developed various pain behaviours that may be perpetuating the pain. The development of pain behaviours can be explained by psychological principles based in learning theory.[20]

Operant learning. Pain behaviour may be positively reinforced, hence encouraging the maintenance of the behaviour and also increasing the perception of pain. Reinforcement may take the form of attention (in response to limping) or permitted avoidance of undesirable activities (such as housework), i.e. secondary gains. The process does not require a conscious effort by the patient, but is learnt gradually. It is not malingering, as this requires the patient to consciously fake a symptom for some gain.

Respondent learning (classical conditioning). An association may develop between a response and a non-noxious stimulus. For example, a patient who has had a painful experience with a physiotherapist in the past may experience a negative emotional response to the presence of a physiotherapist, resulting in tense muscles and exacerbation of pain, thus reinforcing the association between a physiotherapist and pain.

Social learning (observational learning). A parent may have experienced health problems and behaved in a certain way (e.g. taking to bed when unwell). When faced with perceived ill health in the form of chronic pain, an individual exposed in earlier life to such behaviour may also take to their bed.

Overactivity/underactivity cycle. This is a pattern of behaviour that is strongly identified with the perpetuation of chronic pain. For reasons not fully understood, sufferers of chronic pain almost invariably describe their pain as varying from day to day. Sometimes the reasons for an exacerbation of pain are clear, such as overexertion the day before, but often no reason can be identified. On days when their pain is not quite so bad, or perhaps on days when the patient has no choice but to perform the activity, many patients perform unaccustomed activities, over and above their normal level of activity. Unsurprisingly this level of activity results in an exacerbation of pain on the following days with a consequent decrease in levels of activity on these days. Over time, this repeated pattern of behaviour results in decreasing levels of fitness and activity (see Fig. 13.2). To improve, a patient must first recognise their pattern of behaviour and its consequences, and then pace their activities so their level of activity gradually increases.

Stress

The term 'stress' means different things to different people, rather like the word 'chronic'. Laymen describe stress in terms of pressure, tension or an unpleasant emotional response. Psychologists define stressors as the external environment stress (e.g. financial problems), and the response to the stressor as stress or distress (e.g. the feeling of tension), i.e. stress is an interaction between an individual and the outside world. To psychologists, the concept of stress involves biochemical, physiological, behavioural and psychological changes.

Many life events, including chronic ill health, are considered to be stressful to various degrees. For example, 'death of a spouse' is considered a more stressful life event than 'a child leaving home' or 'going on holiday'. However, different individuals may consider different stressors as more or less stressful. A stress response is elicited if an individual appraises an event as

Fig. 13.2 The overactivity/ underactivity cycle

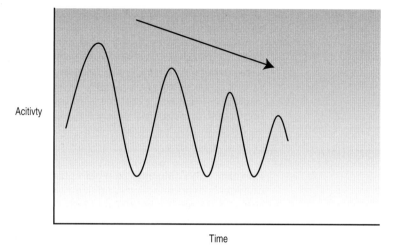

Acitivty

Time

stressful. Physiological responses may occur, including sympathetic nervous system arousal (affecting heart rate and blood pressure) and stress hormone release (catecholamines and corticosteroids). Psychological changes may also occur, including increases in fear, anxiety and anger and decreases in cognitive ability and sensitivity to others.

The stress response has often been described in terms of a 'fight or flight' response, with the physiological changes preparing the caveman to deal physically with potential threats. However, most of the stressors in modern life do not require a physical response so the hormones produced and the energy substrates released (glucose, fats) are not used. There is also no significant easing of the feelings associated with the stress response. Consequently, there may be long-term effects on physical health, such as atheromatous disease and diabetes, and also long-term effects on psychological wellbeing.

Actual or perceived control over the stressor may decrease the stress response. Positive self-efficacy may reduce the stress response in stressful situations. Successful coping and self-management decrease stress, while not coping and poor self-management result in the stress response. Stress-related illnesses are considered due to a prolonged failure of coping.

Coping. The way people cope with a stressful situation, such as chronic pain, depends on their view of the situation. This cognitive evaluation, or appraisal, is a dynamic process and changes according to an individual's perception of the consequences of an event, its importance to their wellbeing and the resources they believe they have available to deal with the threat.

There are a variety of coping styles, including the following:

- Problem-solving – forming a plan of action
- Problem avoidance – refusing to think about the problem
- Wishful thinking – dreaming about better times
- Emotional social support – talking to people about feelings
- Instrumental social support – asking people for advice
- Cognitive restructuring – redefining the problem
- Distraction – attentional diversion, drinking, taking drugs.

Most individuals use different techniques at various times, but depending on the situation, one or other technique may be preferable.

Coping styles may be overt behavioural coping strategies, such as rest, medication and use of relaxation, or covert coping strategies, such as distraction, reassurance the pain will improve, seeking information and problem-solving.[21] Active coping strategies (trying to function despite the pain) are associated with less pain and depression than passive coping strategies (depending on others to control the pain, restricting activities).

Personality

Personality also influences pain perception. Higher levels of the 'neurotic triad' of hysteria, hypochondriasis and depression are associated with an increase of chronic pain and can be related to less sleep, reduced social and work life, and feelings of exhaustion.[22] An increased preoccupation with pain may be associated with increased pain.

Management of chronic pain

To manage chronic pain effectively both the sensory and emotional components need to be addressed. While it is unrealistic to expect to be able to cure chronic pain, there are many treatments now available that may ease pain.

An understanding of the sensory mechanisms will guide choice of treatment. These include analgesics, adjunct analgesics, neurostimulation techniques, topical treatments, injections and neurolytic therapies.

An understanding of the patient and their psychosocial situation will guide decisions about other interventions that may be beneficial.

A clear explanation of chronic pain, addressing the patient's illness beliefs and any consequent anxieties or fears, will be required. Reassurance is possible, as there is evidence that chronic pain does not get worse with time. It would appear sensible to draw up a treatment plan with the patient, listing options that are appropriate for that patient with their pain. Unfortunately, not all patients are ready to engage in a treatment plan that does not promise a cure, or requires them to put in considerable effort themselves. Readiness for change is a topic in itself and is very relevant to chronic pain management.

Of great concern to the patient is the impact that chronic pain is having on his or her life and ways of improving and optimising that patient's level of functioning should be included in any treatment plan. Improving sleep, for example, can often make a big difference. Anxiety and depression may require specific treatment. Low levels of general fitness are often a problem and may be improved by a graded exercise programme. Addressing any over/under-activity cycling can be very important. Not all patients can comprehend the role that psychology plays in the maintenance of their pain and many are initially reluctant to consider any form of psychotherapy. Indeed, some patients refuse to ever consider this approach. However, by understanding the patient and providing appropriate information, other members of the multi-disciplinary team can help change how individuals view both their pain and themselves. Improvements in how a patient manages their chronic pain can be very rewarding for the healthcare professionals involved.

> **KEY POINTS**
>
> - The clinician has to understand the sensory and emotional components of chronic pain
> - The clinician has to be aware of treatments available for pain
> - Most importantly, the clinician has to understand the patient
> - Psychosocial factors are more important than medical factors in the development of disability
> - Being off work with chronic pain for more than 6 months means the chance of returning to work is only 50%, after 1 year off work it is only 10%
> - The emotional aspects must not be underestimated as there is wide variation in the reported severity of pain experienced by individuals in association with comparable noxious stimuli
> - Improvements in how a patient manages their chronic pain can be very rewarding for the healthcare professionals involved

References

1. van Tulder MW, Becker A, Bekkering T. *European guidelines for the management of acute nonspecific low back pain in primary care.* European Commission, Research Directorate General; 2004. Available at: *www.backpoaneurope.org*
2. Eimer BN, Freeman A. *Pain management psychotherapy: a practical guide.* New York: John Wiley and Sons; 1998.
3. Ormel J, Van Korff M, Ustan TB et al. Common mental disorders and disability across cultures. Results from the WHO Collaborative Study on Psychological Problems in General Health Care. *JAMA* 1994; **272**(22): 1741–1748.
4. Nagda J, Bajwa ZH. Definition and classification of pain. In: Warfield CA, Bajwa ZH (eds) *Principles and practice of pain medicine*, 2nd edn. New York: McGraw-Hill; 2004: 51–54.
5. Merskey H, Bogduk N (eds). *Classification of chronic pain.* 2nd edn. Seattle: IASP Press; 1994.
6. Leventhal H, Nerenz D. The assessment of illness cognition. In: Karoly P (ed.) *Measurement strategies in health psychology.* New York: John Wiley and Sons; 1985: 517–554.
7. Bandura A. Self-efficacy: toward a unifying theory of behavioral change. *Psychol Rev* 1977; **84**(2): 191–215.
8. Gamsa A. Is emotional disturbance a precipitator or a consequence of chronic pain? *Pain* 1990; **42**(2): 183–195.
9. Feuerstein M, Carter RL, Papciak AS. A prospective analysis of stress and fatigue in recurrent low back pain. *Pain* 1987; **31**(3): 333–344.
10. Fordyce WE, Steger JC. Chronic pain. In: Pomerleau OF, Brady J (eds) *Behavioural medicine: theory and practice.* Baltimore: Williams and Wilkins; 1979: 122–153.
11. Banks SM, Kerns RD. Explaining the high rates of depression in chronic pain: a diathesis-stress framework. *Psychological Bulletin* 1996; **119**: 95–110.
12. Magni G, Caudieron C, Rigatti-Luchini S et al. Chronic musculoskeletal pain and depressive symptoms in the general population. An analysis of the 1st National Health and Nutrition Examination Survey data. *Pain* 1990; **43**(3): 299–307.
13. Rudy TE, Kerns RD, Turk DC. Chronic pain and depression: toward a cognitive-behavioral mediation model. *Pain* 1988; **35**(2): 129–140.
14. Fishbain DA, Culter R, Rosomoff HL et al. Chronic pain-associated depression: antecedent or consequence of chronic pain? A review. *Clin J Pain* 1997; **13**(2): 116–137.

15. Wade JB, Price DD, Hamer RM et al. An emotional component analysis of chronic pain. *Pain* 1990; **40**(3): 303–310.
16. Kerns RD, Rosenberg R, Jacob MC. Anger expression and chronic pain. *J Behav Med* 1994; **17**(1): 57–67.
17. Keefe FJ, Crisson J, Urban BJ et al. Analyzing chronic low back pain: the relative contribution of pain coping strategies. *Pain* 1990; **40**(3): 293–301.
18. Wall PD. On the relation of injury to pain. The John J. Bonica lecture. *Pain* 1979; **6**(3): 253–264.
19. Turk DC, Wack JT, Kerns RD. An empirical examination of the 'pain-behavior' construct. *J Behav Med* 1985; **8**(2): 119–130.
20. Ogden J. *Health psychology a textbook.* Buckingham: Open University Press; 1996.
21. Jensen MP, Turner JA, Romano JM et al. Coping with chronic pain: a critical review of the literature. *Pain* 1991; **47**(3): 249–283.
22. Sternbach RA, Wolf SR, Murphy RW et al. Traits of pain patients: the low-back 'loser'. *Psychosomatics* 1973; **14**(4): 226–229.

Paul Wilkinson and Nilofer Sabrine

Epidemiology of pain

Introduction

Epidemiology is concerned with the study of populations or groups of people rather than individuals. It includes not only the study of illness and injury but also disability and mortality. The word epidemiology is derived from the Greek words *epi* meaning 'on or befall', *demos* which means 'people or population' and *logos* which can be translated as 'word or reason' with the suffix – ology meaning 'study of'. It is concerned with the distribution of health problems across different populations including age groups, social classes, occupational groups, geographical regions, gender, race and culture. It is also concerned with the determinants of disease; that is it helps us understand and explain the distribution of disease by identifying causal factors, which determine the presence or absence of disease. In addition, epidemiology helps us understand the impact of healthcare interventions within a population.

In relation to pain, epidemiology may help us answer the following questions:

- How many people get pain?
- Who gets pain?
- Why do people get pain?
- Can we prevent pain and its consequences?

The richness of the subject will be illustrated by considering carefully selected data focussing on back pain, which is common and where most information is available. Though there are considerable methodological difficulties, epidemiological studies into pain have provided searching, challenging and often tantalising insights into pain and its cause.

How many people get pain?

The frequency of pain can be considered in two ways:

- First, it can be classified by 'rates'; that is how fast pain is occurring. In this case, the term *incidence* is used to describe the number of new cases of pain that occur during a specified period of time in an at-risk population. An example would be the number of new cases of pain per million populations per annum. Essentially, incidence is a measure of risk.
- Second, the frequency of pain can be classified by 'proportions'; that is the fraction of the population having pain. *Prevalence* is defined as the number of affected persons present in the population divided by the number of people in the population at a specific time or during a period of time. *Point prevalence* refers to the prevalence of pain at a point in time while *period prevalence* refers to the people who have had pain over a period of time (frequently a year). Prevalence is most commonly used in pain studies.

Prevalence of pain

Estimates of the point prevalence of chronic pain in the community range from 2% to 45%. This is a great variation and reflects underlying methodological difficulties.

First, no tissue diagnosis or diagnostic test is available to diagnose pain unlike, for example, cancer and, therefore, it is difficult to clearly identify discrete groups of patients.

Second, when a descriptive diagnosis is used (e.g. chronic back pain), estimations of prevalence become vulnerable to the precise definitions used.

Finally, sampling from different populations may produce vastly different prevalences. Is the sample considering patients in the general population, patients who have attended a family practitioner or patients who attend a secondary care institution? Are the samples of adequate size and evenly matched across demographic factors such as age and gender to which prevalence is sensitive?

Here is a well-performed descriptive study:

A large random population of 5036 patients aged 25 and over in the Grampians of Scotland were sent questionnaires, 3605 responded. Self reported chronic pain (defined as 'pain or discomfort that persisted continuously or intermittently for longer than 3 months') occurred in around 50% with just under one-third reporting back pain and one-third reporting 'arthritis'. The authors standardised the sample for age and sex to arrive at a figure of estimated prevalence of pain in the population as a whole of 46.5% (44.8–48.2 95% confidence levels).[1]

This study clearly indicates that pain is common. The next question is how does the prevalence of pain vary by condition? In the UK, the 1-year prevalence of low back pain lasting 1 day or more in adults is around 40% and can be extracted from data in the population censuses.[2] In another UK study, lifetime prevalence of low back pain was 62%, annual prevalence was 48%, with a point prevalence of 16%.[3] In the USA, a number of large studies suggest life time incidence of chronic back pain as 45–65%, the point prevalence

TABLE 14.1 Prevalence of some common pain conditions	
Condition	Prevalence
Fibromyalgia/chronic widespread pain	Approx. 3–15% in the community
Amputation pain	Above 50% of amputees in most studies
Phantom limb pain	Around 50%
Phantom limb sensations	80–100% of amputees – mild pain
Stump pain	0–25% – moderate or severe pain
Pain after surgery	
Breast	10–20%
Thoracotomy	Overall, 5–50%. Pain at 1 year post surgery as high as 15–30% in some studies
Cholecystectomy	40% mild; typically 2–10% severe pain
Dental	Up to 15%
Central post-stroke pain	8% of people with stroke at 1 year
Orofacial pain	Up to 50% – mild pain; approximately 10% severe (point prevalence)
Migraine	7% male, 14% female (approximate average of trials)
Temperomandibular dysfunction	0.1–8% (point prevalence)
Shoulder pain	10–30% (point prevalence)
Knee pain	10–30% (point prevalence)
Neck pain	10–20% (point prevalence)

Data from Crombie IK et al. *Epidemiology of pain*. Seattle: IASP Press; 1999.

10–35% and 1-year period prevalence 25–35%.[4] The point, 1-year period and lifetime prevalence of back pain in some European countries may even reach, or exceed, 40%, 70% and 80%, respectively.[5]

Table 14.1 gives crude estimates of the prevalence of some other common pain problems. From this analysis, it can be safely concluded that pain is common and often severe. For more detailed analysis see the work of the IASP task force on epidemiology.[6]

Who is most likely to get pain?

Gender and pain

Females have a consistently higher prevalence of pain across a variety of conditions including joint pain, abdominal pain, temperomandibular pain and fibromyalgia, although pain from cluster headache and pancreatitis is commoner in men. The relative difference between sexes varies across the age span. For example, though back pain is commoner in women in most studies, the prevalence in men approaches or may even overtake the prevalence in women in middle age. The precise reasons for these gender differences are unknown.[7] Is this because females feel more pain or report more pain? Gender-based differences also occur in pain thresholds, analgesic requirements, attitudes toward pain management, coping styles and social roles.

Pain and increasing age

There is an increase in prevalence of joint pain, chronic widespread pain and fibromyalgia with age, but in contrast a decrease in abdominal pain and headache. Most studies indicate that the prevalence of pain rises with age and may be as high as 60–80% over 60 years of age. The prevalence would seem to plateau in many studies above 70 years but it is unclear if this is a genuine plateau or artefact due to reporting bias.

Pain and children

We know very little about the epidemiology of pain in childhood. In a Dutch study surveying 6636 children up to the age of 18 (5424 (82%) response rate), 54% had experienced pain within the previous 3 months. A quarter of the respondents reported chronic pain (recurrent or continuous pain for more than 3 months). The prevalence of chronic pain increased with age, and was significantly higher for girls ($p < 0.001$) with a marked increase in the reporting of chronic pain between 12 and 14 years of age.[8]

In existing studies, headache (either migranious or non-migranious) has a prevalence of 2–30%, abdominal pain 5–15% and musculoskeletal pains such as back 2.5–7.5% or knee 4–18%. Complex regional pain syndrome, juvenile arthritis, cancer pain and pain from sickle cell disease also contribute to the spectra of childhood pain problems.

It has been suggested that there is a strong association with psychological factors. For example, adolescents with chronic pain are more vulnerable in terms of neuroticism and negative fear of failure.[9]

Pain and socioeconomic class

Pain is usually commoner in lower socio-economic classes. For example, housing tenure, employment category and educational attainment were found to be independently associated with 'significant' pain; that is pain requiring professional help and treatment, and 'severe' or disabling pain.[10] In some studies differences may arise from confounding variables; for example, people from lower socioeconomic classes may undertake jobs that have more standing or heavy lifting, which may themselves increase the risk of back pain.[11] However, pain is not common just in lower social classes. In helicopter pilots the 1-year prevalence of back pain is high at nearly 80%.[12]

Pain and culture

Studying pain in different cultures may identify different coping strategies or social values to help us understand pain. There are many examples of cultural differences in prevalence. Let us briefly consider several findings selected in part from Dionne's analysis.[13] One-year prevalence of back pain was found to be almost twice as high in a British group compared to a Hong-Kong group. Is this because the Hong-Kong group has a different threshold for reporting symptoms or are there other risk factors to consider, such as stature or manual occupation? In a study of psychosocial and economic factors affecting the severity of disability from low back pain in the USA and New Zealand, the US group demonstrated consistently higher medication use, more mood disturbance and impairment of social, recreational and vocational function than the New Zealand group both before and after intervention. Thus, differences are evident even between advanced cultures. Finally, why does whiplash syndrome virtually not exist in some cultures? From this observation, it has been argued that expectation based on the witnessed suffering of others, hypervigilance and a compensation process that engenders anxiety, frustration and resentment amplify pain symptoms.[14]

It will be evident from these epidemiological studies that cultural differences raise interesting questions about the cause of pain even if the reasons for these differences are unclear.

Genetics and back pain

Though it is recognised that pain can be associated with genetic-linked conditions, such as sickle cell disease, recent advances also show that there may be a genetic effect on pain in other conditions. In one study, additive genetic effects explained approximately one-quarter of the liability to report back pain in men but none in women. The authors concluded that additive genetic effects are modest contributors to back pain in older men, but not in women.[15] It is anticipated that, in the future, findings, such as the association between lumbar disc disease and mutation of genes encoding subunits of collagen, will help our understanding of genetic differences.

In contrast, the prevalence of irritable bowel syndrome was 17% in monozygotic and 16% in dizygotic twins and genetic factors seem to be of little or no influence.[16]

Pain: the cost?

The cost of pain can be considered both as a cost to the individual and a cost to society. The individual cost can be measured as suffering, both the number of days spent suffering with pain and the level of severity. Pain can also have wider and more devastating consequences and the cost to the individual should consider psychological sequelae, disability and social consequences. For society as a whole, pain has a severe impact reflected in sick-leave, healthcare costs and welfare benefits. It is increasingly recognised that pain also has a cost burden due to poor performance at work.

Cost to the individual

During the course of 1 year, approximately 6% of people have longstanding chronic back pain and a similar percentage have associated difficulties with mobility or activities of daily living. The pool of patients is not static.[2] Based on simple questions to measure healthcare consumption from a sample of the general population around 50% suffered chronic pain, 15% reported the most severe grade of pain ('high disability, highly limiting') with an even higher percentage 30% having 'high expressed need'.[17] Despite this, the prognosis for a new episode of back pain is good, with around 65% requiring only one consultation, 60–70% are improved by 6 weeks, rising to 80–90% by 12 weeks.[4] This drops to only 50% beyond 12 weeks and historically the return to work after 2 years off work is quoted as close to zero. Recent evidence indicates that, with appropriate intervention, this is not the case.[18] With regard

Fig. 14.1 Illustrative pyramid of the severity of back pain based on a population sample of 100 000 and 1 year prevalence. Severe means severe chronic pain or significant disability. Data from Croft et al.[20]

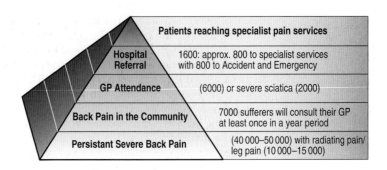

Patients reaching specialist pain services	
Hospital Referral	1600: approx. 800 to specialist services with 800 to Accident and Emergency
GP Attendance	(6000) or severe sciatica (2000)
Back Pain in the Community	7000 sufferers will consult their GP at least once in a year period
Persistant Severe Back Pain	(40 000–50 000) with radiating pain/ leg pain (10 000–15 000)

to back pain the prognosis for short-term recovery is lower if there is associated leg pain. Even so, classical studies show that 70% of patients with a diagnosis of sciatica of less than 14 days duration will be pain free one year later.[19] Croft et al[20] suggest a pyramidal structure of severity for back pain, which is developed in Figure 14.1 from available data.

Patients suffer from a high incidence of coexisting psychological morbidity in the form of anxiety, depression, frustration, stress and anger as well as disability. In a sample of patients attending a multidisciplinary pain unit 50% had clinically significant anxiety and 45% depression ($n = 102$) using a validated hospital anxiety and depression scale. Disability was also common, with around 10% virtually unable to walk and around 30–40% severely limited. From 30 to 40% of patients required some assistance for daily activities of bathing or making a meal. Over 80% of patients were not employed and 75% were receiving benefits (author's unpublished data). Patients have high expectations of cure; 100% ($n = 121$) agreed with the statement 'It is important to know the underlying cause of my pain in order to treat it effectively', a belief likely to lead to high levels of focus on medical care. Just under a half visited their family practitioners more than once every 4 weeks and over a half had visited at least two other specialists.

Life-time prevalence of psychiatric disorders in groups entering a pain rehabilitation programme suggest that around 50% met at least one criterion for a personality disorder and there was also a higher incidence of substance abuse than in the general population.[21] Social withdrawal, employment, family and relationship difficulties as well as sexual difficulties are also common.

Cost to employers

Work absenteeism is common amongst patients with pain. Nearly 5% of the working population is not at work due to back pain during any 4-week period. One-year period prevalence is estimated to be around 5–10%.[13] Back pain is commonly associated with work absence, but there are close associations with psychosocial factors and it is increasingly recognised that such factors are important in work abstinence in patients with pain problems.

Financial cost to society

As previously indicated, 7% of the population visit their general practitioner each year with back pain with around two-thirds being a new visit. Approximately half will receive a prescription.[4]

Grey and Mandiakis undertook a well-considered analysis of the impact of back pain and the socio-economic costs in the UK.[22] The authors estimated the direct healthcare cost of back pain in 1998 to be 1632 million pounds. With respect to the distribution of cost across different providers, 37% relates to care provided by physiotherapists and allied specialists, 31% is incurred in the hospital sector, 14% relates to primary care, 7% to medication, 6% to community care and 5% to radiology and imaging used for investigation purposes. Approximately 35% of this cost relates to services provided in the private sector. The authors concluded that these direct costs of back pain were insignificant compared to other costs of informal care and the production losses related to it, which total an astonishing 10 668 million pounds. The economic costs of back pain are enormous through high consultation rates, increased medication use and increased use of imaging and surgical resources. However, this is dwarfed by the socioeconomic costs.

Another important point is that costs are not equally distributed amongst patients with pain. In a study of the consequences of neck and back pain in a large Swedish survey of 3000 people ages 35–45 year it was noted that sufferers averaged 3.5 healthcare visits during the previous year, but notably the consumption of resources was highly skewed with about 6% of the sufferers accounting for over 50% of the costs.[23] This latter finding raises the issue of whether these individuals could be targeted specifically to improve the cost-effectiveness of care overall.

An epidemiological perspective on other issues

Why do people get pain?

We learn about pain as an alarm mechanism warning us that something is going wrong and linearity exists in the perceived relationship between tissue damage and pain severity. The question arises as to what are the determinants of chronic pain. Is chronic pain just acute pain for longer or with more injury?

Here we will use back pain as an illustration, but similar issues could be considered with other types of chronic pain.

Cross-sectional studies

Most pain studies relating to pain and causation are *cross-sectional* studies; that is information about pain, its impact and exposure status is collected at a point or period of time and usually compared against a control group without pain. Cross-sectional studies are relatively simple, inexpensive and can be conducted over a short time scale. However, associations do not mean causation and it can be difficult to separate true risk factors from the consequences of pain. For example, if a patient has pain and low mood, does the pain arise from the low mood or is it a consequence of it?

Longitudinal studies

One way of throwing light on this is to identify those factors that predispose to the chronicity of pain *before* the pain arises. This *longitudinal* approach is rare because of the time, cost involved and the difficulty in follow-up.

In an important study to examine the prevalence of pain in the community, data were collected on risk factors before the onset of pain that resulted in

TABLE 14.2 **Odds ratio is the estimated relative risk of developing back pain compared with non-exposed control**

Risk factor	Odds ratio (CI 95%)
Female	2.1 (1.1–4.1)
High levels of psychological distress	3.3 (1.5–7.2)
Poor self-rated health	3.6 (1.9–6.8)
Low levels of physical activity	2.8 (1.4–5.6)
Smoking	2.1 (1.0–4.3)
Dissatisfaction with employment	2.4 (1.3–4.5)
Factors related to the episode of low back pain	
Duration of symptoms, radiating to the leg	2.6 (1.3–5.1)
Widespread pain	6.4 (2.7–15)
Restriction in spinal mobility	3 (1.3–7.3)

Summarised from: Thomas E et al. Predicting who develops chronic low back pain in primary care: a prospective study. *BMJ* 1999; **318**(7199): 1662–1667.

consultation.[1] The authors then followed up these patients over time, allowing them to identify those factors that were likely to predict chronicity. These results are summarised in the form of odds ratios (Table 14.2). The most striking finding is that the components of the pain related to physical injury are relatively weak predictors of chronic back pain. There are other factors such as restriction in spinal mobility and psychological factors that collectively carry considerable weight. Interestingly, the greatest risk was attributed to those who had widespread pain. While one interpretation might be that this represents a group with overall worse physical disease for example degenerative arthritis that has not yet reached the back, this may not be the case. Increasingly, we are recognising that patients with widespread pain have pre-existing psychological distress and a poor outcome.

Other studies have confirmed the idea that pre-existing distress is important in chronicity. Increased risk of chronicity (persisting symptoms and/or disability) arose from psychological distress, depressive mood and, to a lesser extent, somatisation and catastrophising as a coping strategy.[24] In another study, prognosis was related to pain-related fear, catastrophisation (fearing the worst) and sexual or physical abuse.[25] Passive coping strategies have also been found to be important.[26]

Can we prevent chronic pain?

There are several possible levels of intervention to prevent pain.

Primary prevention

This involves halting the occurrence of pain before it happens. Primary prevention has mainly focussed on workplace interventions, such as training on handling, working techniques and body posturing. Though these approaches are widely believed to be valuable, where research has been undertaken results are usually modest. Many of the interventions inadequately consider important psychosocial factors.

Secondary prevention

This aims to provide interventions that halt the development of pain and disability early in its course and before chronicity occurs. Possible early interventions for back pain might be physical or manual therapy, surgery, psychological interventions, occupational intervention or some combination of these. In most cases, success has been poor. In manual therapy or exercise treatment, benefits were modest.[27] Surgery may be beneficial in many other situations but a large multicentre trial suggested that surgery was not cost-effective in chronic low back pain patients who have already failed standard non-operative care.[28] Psychological-based pain management interventions were disappointing in one study,[29] but questions arose about the competency of the intervention because of the difficulties of providing adequate training to those managing the conservative intervention. Occupational interventions have also had disappointing results.

Most success has occurred with clearly identified high-risk subgroups of the population and targeting them. Boersma and Linton[30] identified four risk groups in a population of patients in primary care in Sweden namely: fear-avoidant, distressed fear-avoidant, low risk and low risk-depressed mood. The distressed fear-avoidant group had an approximately 60% risk of developing long-term sickness compared to virtually none in the low-risk profiles. Furthermore, the group has shown that psychological interventions can reduce disability and sick leave.[31,32]

Tertiary prevention

Tertiary prevention refers to reducing disability once pain is chronic.

Tertiary prevention may involve improvements in:

- Triaging of those with chronic pain
- Earlier access to specialist services
- Care pathways
- Rehabilitation to work.

In the UK, waiting lists for scans and expert treatment have impeded care and resulted in patients presenting late to specialist pain services. Though rates of return to work after 2 years are low, successful intervention is possible. Eighty-six subjects in an occupationally orientated rehabilitation programme for long-term unemployed people with pain (mean duration of unemployment 38.9 months) were followed-up at 6 months to determine work status. Thirty-eight percent of subjects were employed and another 23% were in voluntary work or education/training.[18]

The question of preventing pain is of particular importance to government because of the huge economic burden and though results have been largely disappointing, there are some promising studies using interdisciplinary approaches.

Can epidemiology help us to organise and plan care in the pain clinic?

Pain may be a lifelong condition for many. Given its prevalence, if all patients were referred to a specialised chronic pain unit, units would be rapidly overwhelmed. Careful planning of resources is paramount. In a large study, clinics in the Northern Region of England, many with large waiting lists, had simple demographic data fed back to the practitioners. The function of clinics and the ability to manage waiting lists was closely linked to the number of reviews per new patient seen. In addition, it was recognised that there was a huge variation in the treatments undertaken prior to referral to specialist pain units;[33] a picture that changed over time.[34] If family practitioners provide more extensive pain services, it seems likely that the population as a whole will be better treated, accessibility to pain services will be improved and secondary care resources can be targeted more precisely to those in need. Initiatives such as intermediate clinics and educational initiatives are being undertaken in the UK to try to improve both access and quality of patient care.

Furthermore, epidemiological evidence provides support for comprehensive psychological care provision and physical therapy. The recognised impact of pain on an individual's life, such as sleep, sexual function or family, may allow appropriate intervention while epidemiological studies allow treatment outcomes to be measured from both the perspective of patients and society.

Is treatment cost-effective?

The treatment of pain is a basic human right, but in a health service of infinite demand and finite resources all treatments must be justified. Pain-management programmes are effective.[35,36] At long-term follow-up, patients treated in such a setting were functioning better than 75% of a sample that was either untreated or had conventional unimodal treatment approaches.[37] Treatment seems to be cost-effective in reducing healthcare and social consumption because the stakes are so very high. The savings in social costs for an individual returning to work after a programme of care can be as much as 60 times higher than the cost of care. This means that programmes are cost-effective even if the return to work rate is low. Given achievable rates of return to work,[18] the cost-effectiveness does not seem to be in doubt even if this one issue is considered in isolation. This analysis does not include other health and social improvements, such as reduced use of medicines and decreased consumption of healthcare resources.

Summary

Pain is common, often severe and disabling, and frequently has a wide variety of devastating consequences for individuals and society. Studies of chronic pain outwith progressive disease do not identify close links between physical damage and causality. Medical solutions to prevent and treat pain will not suffice; therefore, a broader multimodal approach has to be taken.

KEY POINTS

- Epidemiology is concerned with the study of populations or groups of people rather than individuals
- Estimates of the point prevalence of chronic pain in the community range from 2 to 45%
- No tissue diagnosis or diagnostic test is available to diagnose pain and, therefore, it is difficult to clearly identify discrete groups of patients

- In the UK, the 1-year prevalence of low back pain in adults lasting 1 day or more is around 40%
- Most studies indicate that the prevalence of pain rises with age and may be as high as 60–80% over 60 years of age
- It is increasingly recognised that patients with widespread pain have pre-existing psychological distress and a poor outcome
- Estimated direct healthcare costs for back pain in 1998 were 1632 million pounds. This is dwarfed by the cost to the community as a whole
- There is evidence for pain management being cost-effective, but that this needs to be multimodal

References

1. Thomas E, Silman AJ, Croft PR et al. Predicting who develops chronic low back pain in primary care: a prospective study. *BMJ* 1999; **318**(7199): 1662–1667.
2. Mason V. *The prevalence of back pain in Great Britain*. London: Office of Population Censuses and Surveys. Social Survey Division, HSMO; 1994.
3. McKinnon ME, Vickers MR, Ruddock VM et al. Community studies of the health service implications of low back pain. *Spine* 1997; **22**(18): 2161–2166.
4. Andersson GB. Epidemiological features of chronic low-back pain. *Lancet* 1999; **354**(9178): 581–585.
5. Raspe H. How epidemiology contributes to the management of spinal disorders. *Best Pract Res Clin Rheumatol* 2002; **16**(1): 9–21.
6. Crombie IK, Croft PR, Linton SJ et al. *Epidemiology of Pain*. Seattle: IASP Press; 1999.
7. LeResche L. Gender considerations in the epidemiology of chronic pain. In: Crombie IK et al. (eds) *Epidemiology of pain*. Seattle: IASP Press; 1999: 43–51.
8. Perquin CW, Hazebroek-Kampschreur AA, Hunfeld JA et al. Pain in children and adolescents: a common experience. *Pain* 2000; **87**(1): 51–58.
9. Merlijn VPBM, Hunfeld JA, van der Wouden JC et al. Psychosocial factors associated with chronic pain in adolescents. *Pain* 2003; **101**(1–2): 33–43.
10. Smith BH, Elliott AM, Chambers WA et al. The impact of chronic pain in the community. *Fam Pract* 2001; **18**(3): 292–299.
11. Bener A, El Rufaie OF, Siyam A et al. Epidemiology of low back pain in the United Arab Emirates. *APLAR Journal of Rheumatology* 2004; **7**(3): 189–195.
12. Bridger RS, Groom MR, Jones H et al. Task and postural factors are related to back pain in helicopter pilots. *Aviat Space Environ Med* 2002; **73**(8): 805–811.
13. Dionne ED. Low back pain. In: Crombie IK et al. (eds) *Epidemiology of pain*. Seattle: IASP Press; 1999: 289.
14. Ferrari R, Russell AS. Epidemiology of whiplash: an international dilemma. *Ann Rheum Dis* 1999; **58**(1): 1–5.
15. Hartvigsen J, Christensen K, Frederiksen H et al. Genetic and environmental contributions to back pain in old age: a study of 2,108 Danish twins aged 70 and older. *Spine* 2004; **29**(8): 897–901; discussion 902.
16. Mohammed I, Cherkas LF, Riley SA et al. Genetic influences in irritable bowel syndrome: a twin study. *Am J Gastroenterol* 2005; **100**(6): 1340–1344.
17. Elliott AM, Smith BH, Penny KI et al. The epidemiology of chronic pain in the community. *Lancet* 1999; **354**(9186): 1248–1252.
18. Watson PJ, Booker CK, Moores L et al. Returning the chronically unemployed with low back pain to employment. *Eur J Pain* 2004; **8**(4): 359–369.
19. Weber H. Lumbar disc herniation. A controlled, prospective study with ten years of observation. *Spine* 1983; **8**(2): 131–140.
20. Croft P, Papageorgious A, McNally R. Low back pain. In: Stevens A, Rafferty J (eds) *Health care needs assessment*. Radcliffe Medical Press Ltd; 1997: 145.

21. Polatin PB, Kinney RK, Gatchel RJ et al. Psychiatric illness and chronic low-back pain. The mind and the spine—which goes first? *Spine* 1993; **18**(1): 66–71.

22. Maniadakis N, Gray A. The economic burden of back pain in the UK. *Pain* 2000; **84**(1): 95–103.

23. Linton SJ, Ryberg M. Do epidemiological results replicate? The prevalence and health-economic consequences of neck and back pain in the general population. *Eur J Pain* 2000; **4**(4): 347–354.

24. Pincus T, Burton AK, Vogel S et al. A systematic review of psychological factors as predictors of chronicity/disability in prospective cohorts of low back pain. *Spine* 2002; **27**(5): E109–E120.

25. Linton SJ. A prospective study of the effects of sexual or physical abuse on back pain. *Pain* 2002; **96**(3): 347–351.

26. Mercado AC, Carroll LJ, Cassidy JD et al. Passive coping is a risk factor for disabling neck or low back pain. *Pain* 2005; **117**(1–2): 51–57.

27. Ernst E, Tillett R, Tveito TH et al. United Kingdom back pain exercise and manipulation (UK BEAM) trial: touch may have had non-specific effect, among other things. *BMJ* 2005; **330**(7492): 673–674.

28. Rivero-Arias O, Campbell H, Gray A et al. Surgical stabilisation of the spine compared with a programme of intensive rehabilitation for the management of patients with chronic low back pain: cost utility analysis based on a randomised controlled trial. *BMJ* 2005; **330**(7502): 1239.

29. Jellema P, van der Windt DA, van der Horst HE et al. Should treatment of (sub)acute low back pain be aimed at psychosocial prognostic factors? Cluster randomised clinical trial in general practice. *BMJ* 2005; **331**(7508): 84.

30. Boersma K, Linton SJ. Screening to identify patients at risk: profiles of psychological risk factors for early intervention. *Clin J Pain* 2005; **21**(1): 38–43; discussion 69–72.

31. Linton SJ, Andersson T. Can chronic disability be prevented? A randomized trial of a cognitive-behavior intervention and two forms of information for patients with spinal pain. *Spine* 2000; **25**(21): 2825–2831; discussion 2824.

32. Marhold C, Linton SJ, Melin L. A cognitive-behavioral return-to-work program: effects on pain patients with a history of long-term versus short-term sick leave. *Pain* 2001; **91**(1–2): 155–163.

33. Davies HTO, Crombie I. *Pain clinic – gaining commitment to change*. Occasional paper No39. The Scottish Office of Clinical Resources and Audit Symposium, 1993.

34. Anto J, Wilkinson PR. Utilisation of therapies for back-pain prior to referral to the pain clinic. *Proceedings of the Pain Society* 2004.

35. Guzman J, Esmail R, Karjalainen K et al. Multidisciplinary rehabilitation for chronic low back pain: systematic review. *BMJ* 2001; **322**(7301): 1511–1516.

36. Morley S, Eccleston C, Williams A. Systematic review and meta-analysis of randomized controlled trials of cognitive behaviour therapy and behaviour therapy for chronic pain in adults, excluding headache. *Pain* 1999; **80**(1–2): 1–13.

37. Flor H, Fydrich T, Turk DC. Efficacy of multidisciplinary pain treatment centers: a meta-analytic review. *Pain* 1992; **49**(2): 221–230.

38. Thomas E, Silman AJ, Croft PR et al. Predicting who develops chronic low back pain in primary care: a prospective study. *BMJ* 1999; **318**(7199): 1662–1667.

CHAPTER

15

Ashish Gulve

Pain assessment

Introduction

The American Pain Society has coined the phrase 'Pain: The 5th Vital Sign™' to increase awareness of pain treatment among healthcare professionals and recommended that patients' pain should be assessed every time pulse, blood pressure, temperature and respiration are checked.

The International Association for Study of Pain (IASP) defines pain as:

'an unpleasant sensory and emotional experience associated with actual or potential tissue damage, or described in terms of such damage.'[1]

According to this definition, pain is a complex, subjective, multidimensional symptom and often there is very little to find on physical examination and patients are usually treated symptomatically without ever having a definitive diagnosis. Hence, unlike many medical conditions, pain patients do not follow a clear path of history, examination, special investigations, diagnosis and appropriate therapy.

Pain assessment can be defined as a comprehensive clinical process of describing pain and its associated disability.

Pain measurement can be defined as a process to quantify pain and its dimensions. It is important to evaluate the response to therapy regularly.

Factors influencing pain perception

- Age
- Anxiety
- Culture
- Fear
- Gender

- Observational learning (family history of pain/patient's own previous pain experience)
- Personality: extroverts are associated with higher pain tolerance and introverts with greater sensitivity to pain. Introverts, however, may have fewer complaints about pain
- Psychological factors
- Religion
- Response of healthcare staff
- Sleep deprivation
- Society.

Barriers influencing pain assessment

Clinician influenced

- Insufficient knowledge
- Lack of pain training in medical school
- Lack of pain-assessment skills
- Rigidity or timidity in prescribing practices
- Over-estimation of risks involved in the therapy (e.g. opioids for non-cancer pain).

Patient influenced

- Reluctance to report pain (desire to be a 'good' non-complaining patient)
- Reluctance to take opioid drugs (social stigma, fear of addiction)
- Poor adherence to management plan (e.g. exercise regime, medication use).

Healthcare system influenced

- Low priority given to symptom control
- Unavailability or bureaucracy involved in opioid analgesic administration in some countries
- Inaccessibility of specialised care.

Objectives of pain assessment

- The aim is to make a working diagnosis and define the extent of injury or disease. Assessment helps to establish the underlying cause of pain, the associated biological effects and their magnitude. In contrast with the assessment of chronic pain, the need to establish the diagnosis is paramount to the management of acute pain.
- To determine the type of pain (e.g. neuropathic or nociceptive).
- To establish co-existing medical, emotional and psychological factors influencing the pain. Multiple factors shape the experience of pain, these include: fear, anxiety, sleep disturbances, illness, age, previous pain experience, the response of healthcare staff, drugs and analgesia, observational learning, level of information, personality and culture. The importance of psychological factors in determining the acute pain experience is well documented. Soldiers and sportsmen can sustain severe physical trauma without initially feeling pain.

- To determine a pain management strategy on the basis of information obtained as outlined above. This includes therapy for the underlying cause of pain as well as the appropriate analgesics for managing the pain itself. Acute pain could be initiated by: nociceptive, chemical, mechanical or thermal stimuli associated with surgery or trauma. Pain is often the presenting symptom of disturbances in biological function (e.g. myocardial infarction). The assessment process, therefore, must be adaptable and should take into account the clinical priorities and possible pressure on time. Treatment of the underlying disease process will often provide definitive pain relief.
- To evaluate the response to therapy. A lack of response to therapy indicates the need for reassessment and further investigations, an alternative diagnosis, reappraisal of the neurophysiology or mechanism of pain, the suitability of therapy for this mechanism, the mode of delivering analgesia or a more detailed understanding of an individual's pain, including non-physical dimensions.
- To compare and monitor progress of individual patients.
- To validate effectiveness of new treatments for clinical and research purposes.

Process of assessment

The underlying cause of pain may seem obvious in some patients, but to avoid mistakes and to assess clinical progress effectively it is essential to obtain:

- a detailed description of pain: including the history, current symptoms, pain measurement, past medical, surgical, family, personal, social, psychiatric and occupational history
- relevant physical examination to assess associated disability, i.e. functional impairment as well as general medical aspects
- appropriate investigations including special tests if indicated
- psychological, behavioural and emotional evaluation
- differential diagnosis.

Pain history

It is preferable to obtain a first-hand history from the patient. Patients feel this approach quite reassuring as they feel their pain is being taken seriously. As pain is a subjective experience, it is the patient's perception of pain and not that of the referring physician that should be documented. The history included in the referral letter may not exactly represent the patient's perspective of their pain. Along with a general medical history, a specific 'pain history' should also be taken. The interview and communication skills of the physician play an important role in determining the quality of evaluation. Important additional information may be obtained from relatives, medical records and other sources when appropriate.

Pain description

This aims to build a verbal picture of pain. The patient should be asked to describe the following characteristics of pain.

Primary or secondary complaint

The interview must establish the patient's chief complaint in their own words. Pain may not necessarily be the primary concern of the patient; it may be an associated symptom such as nausea or breathlessness, or it may be the anxiety or fear about an underlying cause or problem. This may suggest the need for a more detailed psychological assessment during the history when it is clinically appropriate.

Location and radiation

Location has a great diagnostic value and should be documented both in words and, ideally, on a body map. This should include any radiation or referral of pain and associated symptoms. Pain can be focal, multifocal, generalised, referred, superficial or deep. Focal pain is usually well circumscribed. Referred pain is experienced at a remote site from a presumed lesion. Referred pain can arise from injury in any deep tissues including viscera, muscle, bone and peripheral or central nervous tissue.

Specific site of pain

Ask if the patient can point to a specific site of pain or area involved. This can also be linked with the body map.

Mode of onset

The patient should be asked to describe the onset of pain, including its timing, precipitating events and associated factors (e.g. the type of injury may aid in diagnosis after trauma).

Intensity and severity

Pain intensity should be measured with simple and validated scales and be frequently reassessed. The intensity should be assessed at rest, with movement and with other relevant manoeuvres, such as breathing, coughing or moving the appropriate body region. The variation in intensity over time should be described. It should take into account current, least, worst and average pain intensity.

Character

Pain can be described as: aching, throbbing, sharp, shooting, lancinating, burning, numbing, gnawing, etc. Descriptors of pain quality can give clues to the underlying mechanism.

Neuropathic pain is usually described as burning, hot, shooting, electric-shock-like, tingling or lancinating, while somatic pain is often described as aching, throbbing or sometimes stabbing.

The quality of visceral pain varies according to the organ involved. Pain arising from a hollow viscous is often described as cramping or gnawing. Crushing chest pain is indicative of myocardial infraction.

A body map and a short McGill Pain Questionnaire[2] can be a useful adjunct in assessing the character of pain.

Temporal features

These include onset, duration, frequency and pattern of the pain. These features help to distinguish acute from chronic pain. While acute pain is well-defined, sudden onset and short-lived, chronic pain is waxing and waning. The presence of breakthrough pain should also be assessed. The time-course of the pain, including the duration and frequency of painful episodes, provide important diagnostic evidence (e.g. constant inflammatory pain and the colicky pain of an obstructed viscous).

Exacerbating and relieving factors

These are not only useful diagnostic pointers, but also a valuable guide to possible therapies for pain management. These can be classified as volitional or spontaneous; postural variation, activity, weight bearing, cutaneous stimulation, etc. Pain induced by light touch on normal-looking skin suggests a neuropathic component. Previous therapies and the response to these therapies should be inquired to help therapeutic decision-making. There may be variations with normal bodily functions (e.g. urination, bowel movements or with the menstrual cycle in women).

Associated symptoms

Open and then closed questions where necessary should be used to obtain evidence of other symptoms, such as nausea and vomiting, to support specific diagnosis, such as in abdominal pathology. Always ask about neurological symptoms, such as numbness, weakness and paraesthesia.

Somatic pain tends to be better localised, well defined, often sharp, painful in the area of injury or stimulus, and may follow the distribution of a nerve root or peripheral nerve.

Visceral pain tends to be poorly localised, more vague in definition, cramping, aching or colicky, and referred to a number of dermatomes, often in the midline.

How pain has changed since onset

A history of changes in the pain since it started, has it improved become worse or remained the same.

Treatments so far

An assessment of previous medical consultations, investigations, surgery, physiotherapy, occupational therapy, hydrotherapy, alternative therapies (e.g. acupuncture, chiropractor, osteopathy, herbal treatments and aromatherapy) is required. The outcome of these interventions should also be recorded along with any that the patient is still waiting for.

Medical aspects

The general medical history, including drug, occupational, marital, sexual, psychosocial and family history should be elicited when clinically appropriate.

Employment status, impact of pain on work and prospects of returning to work should be explored. If not in work then how does the patient occupy himself/herself?

Functional status

The assessment of disability associated with acute pain may focus on biological or organ dysfunction (e.g. the patient with an acute abdomen).

In other patients, such as those with musculo-skeletal pain, the assessment of acute pain and disability may include:

- The effect of pain on performing general activities, mobility and sleep
- The effect of pain on regional body movements and power
- The effect of medications and treatments on the pain.

Psychological assessment

- Hospital Anxiety and Depression Score (HAD)[3]
- Minnesota Multiphasic Personality Inventory (MMPI) used mostly in research and chronic pain practice.

  Refer to Chapter 16 for further details on the psychological components of pain.

Factors relevant to treatment

The following factors have a significant impact on what management to consider and patient's response to management:

- The patient's understanding about the cause of their pain (e.g. that they have cancer)
- Beliefs or concerns about the consequences of pain (e.g. the effect it has on their ability to work, or that the pain will inevitably increase with time)
- Benefits from having pain and disability (compensation, litigation, family or social benefits)
- Expectations from the healthcare system (e.g. to be cured or become pain free)
- Coping styles of the patient and family
- How family, friends or co-workers react to the person in pain
- Patient's, family's and employer's goals for treatment
- Treatment preferences when planning therapy
- The physical and mental ability to use particular therapies (e.g. patient-controlled analgesia [PCA], patient-controlled epidural analgesia [PCEA], transcutaneous electrical nerve stimulation [TENS], spinal cord stimulation [SCS]) are important in decision-making.

Physical examination

The physical examination follows the history, although in urgent clinical situations there may be some overlap to conserve time. Patients expect to be examined, but are likely to be anxious. It is essential to respect the need for privacy, confidentiality and modesty. The physical examination has multiple goals, such as identifying potential pain generators, neurological and functional impairments. It is an opportunity to gain the patient's trust, confidence and to further develop rapport. A verbal consent to examine should be obtained from the patient. This will also ascertain the patient's ability to tolerate examination.

The examination actually starts from the time of first meeting the patient. Patients will often give verbal and nonverbal clues as to the source and severity of pain, and urgency of the need for treatment. It is useful to observe how patients move, their gait, posture, facial expressions, general mood, anger and behaviour of the spouse or other attendants. The patient's appearance (general health, weight, muscle bulk, grooming), attitude and behaviour give lots of clues to the pain diagnosis.

After making preliminary observations, a regional examination is performed on the targeted body region as suggested by the history (e.g. low back pain/neck pain assessment). The structuring of a physical examination should be based on anatomical and physiological principles. Examination of the patient should be standardised and reproducible with regards to the observations and tests performed and the descriptive terminology used.

Pain elicited during examination should be described as concordant or non-concordant. Concordant pain is the pain in exactly the same location, nature or intensity with which the patient has presented while non-concordant pain is a pain different from the one with which the patient presented.

A directed pain examination would include the following.

Inspection

An inspection of the affected region is carried out, with particular attention to symmetry and cutaneous landmarks. Skin colour, rashes, scars, abnormal hair growth, pseudomotor dysfunction, oedema, muscular atrophy, hypertrophy or fasciculations, spinal curvatures and limb lengths should be noted.

Palpation

Palpation of the affected region gives insight into the abnormalities noted on inspection. Palpation performed in a systematic and comprehensive manner from the least painful to the most painful area will help to differentiate normal tissues from those in the painful region. This should elicit gross sensory changes, such as allodynia, dysaesthesia, paraesthesia, hyper/hypoalgesia, hyperpathia, hypoaesthesia and analgesia dolorosa (see Definitions list). Palpation also elicits painful muscle bands or nodules (tender/trigger points), neuromas in scars, peripheral pulsations and temperature.

Percussion

Pain on percussion over a sensory nerve can indicate nerve entrapment or presence of a neuroma (Tinel's sign). Pain on percussion of bony structures may indicate, fracture, dislocation, inflammation or infection.

Range of motion

This should be examined for articulated areas. Both active and passive range of motion should be examined. All the movements possible for that particular joint should be examined and described in degrees and its effect on pain should be assessed.

Motor examination

Functional motor examination can indicate the level of a lesion. Muscle bulk, tone, isolated muscle power and involuntary movements should be assessed and correlated with myotomal innervations.

Sensory examination

The sensory examination should include response to light touch, light pressure, pinprick or cold and vibration. Various sensory phenomena as described above and should be examined in addition to the proprioceptive evaluation. Matching any sensory changes to dermatomal and peripheral cutaneous nerve maps helps assess the anatomical significance of the changes.

Reflexes

A tendon reflex results from the stimulation of a stretch-sensitive afferent nerve from a neuromuscular spindle, which, via a single synapse, stimulates a motor nerve leading to a muscle contraction. Tendon reflexes are increased in upper motor neurone lesions and decreased in lower motor neurone lesions and muscular diseases. Superficial and deep tendon reflexes should be graded and described in the established manner.

Provocative tests

Certain manoeuvres would increase pain experienced in that region. The results of these would again be described as concordant vs. non-concordant pain. Some examples of these tests are Phalens' sign for the diagnosis of carpal tunnel syndrome, which involves tingling of the fingers by flexing the patient's wrist to a dorsal surface and holding it for 1 min indicating median nerve pathology; the Patrick/FABER (**F**lexion **AB**duction **E**xternal **R**otation) test for hip pathology; sciatic and femoral nerve stretching tests; straight leg raising test; Lasegue's test, which helps differentiate hamstring tightness and spondylolisthesis; crossed SLR – sensitive and specific; bowstring test and Valsalva manoeuvre.

Investigations

Additional investigations may be required to achieve all the objectives of pain assessment. Technological advances have provided methods of imaging body structures and function in great detail (e.g. radiological investigations such as plain X-rays, MRI, fMRI, CT, SPECT scan, etc.) and other tests like thermography, diagnostic nerve blocks, measurement of autonomic variables, Acti-watches, etc.

These investigations are sometimes helpful to rule out rather than diagnose the cause of pain. Chronic pain patients should be made aware of the role of these investigations, as they will invariably think we may find a completely curable condition.

Investigations may reveal abnormalities that are totally unrelated to the pain and patients get focused on these anomalies. A good clinical correlation of investigations and thorough explanation to the patient is essential. Frequently patients will have had multiple investigations prior to attending the chronic pain clinic and repeating them will have potentially negative effects on the patient's expectations of management and be an unnecessary expense.

Pain measurement

There is no 'ideal' measurement tool. Desirable characteristics of the ideal tool would be that it is: simple to administer, easy to understand, easily reproducible, clinically acceptable (appropriate for developmental, physical, emotional and cognitive status), valid, sensitive, reliable and suitable for experimental and clinical situations.

The multidimensional nature of pain offers many potential 'targets' for measurement. As pain is a subjective, personal experience, the logical and true assessments of a patient's pain must, therefore, be the patient's own report. The self-report is the gold standard of pain measurement.

Self-report measurement tools may be classified as unidimensional (e.g. categorical scales, numerical rating scales (NRS), visual analogue scales (VAS), picture scales or pain drawings) or multidimensional (e.g. McGill pain questionnaire).

Unidimensional tools

Unidimensional tools measure a single dimension or component of pain. The self-report of pain intensity is the most commonly used unidimensional measure of acute pain in the clinical environment.

Categorical scales/verbal rating scales

This is the oldest type of pain measurement tool. In its simplest form it could be a simple question, 'are you in pain?' – yes/no.

Commonly 4- or 5-point intensity scales are used with descriptors, such as none, mild, moderate, severe or excruciating. Pain relief can also be measured similarly: none, slightly, moderate, good or complete.

A numerical value (0, 1, 2, 3, 4) could be ascribed to each category for non-parametric analytical purposes.

Advantages
These tools are quick and simple to use. No special training is required as they are easy to learn and use. They are easier to complete than VAS or NRS. They are suitable for the elderly, older children and the visually impaired. They are also sensitive to gender and ethnic differences.

Disadvantages
Due to the limited number of descriptors there is a risk of oversimplifying the pain dimension, forcing the patient to choose a word that may not always be appropriate (e.g. an older patient may be in no pain, but have an excruciating ache). Patients generally tend to use a 'middle' option reducing the sensitivity of this scale. The simplicity of using the VRS may lead to haphazard use, with loss of validity.

They are subject to bias and being non-continuous can produce weaker data due to the use of non-parametric tests.

Numerical rating scales (Fig. 15.1)

This has a similar concept to the VAS. A line numbered from 0 to 10 with both ends having 'verbal anchors'. A variation of the NRS is verbal numerical scale (VNS).

Advantages
No special training is required and it is quick and easy to learn and use, and consistent and reproducible measurements are recorded, which correlate well with VAS.

The verbal form can be used in small children (e.g. poker chip tool in which chips represent 'pieces of hurt').

Fig. 15.1 Numerical rating scale

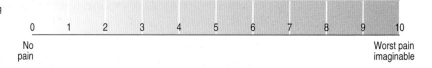

0   1   2   3   4   5   6   7   8   9   10

No
pain

Worst pain
imaginable

The NRS may be an appropriate tool for the retrospective assessment of pain. Statistical analysis is relatively easy and data can be compared between patients and within treatments.

Disadvantages

The scale is not necessarily linear. As pain intensity increases, a single point change in pain intensity from 7 to 8 may represent a greater subjective increase than a change from 1 to 2. On average, a reduction of 30% in the NRS for pain intensity represents a clinically important difference.

It is statistically weaker than the VAS as nonparametric tests are usually the most appropriate for analysing the data.

Visual analogue scales (Figs 15.2 & 15.3)

This is the most intensively studied pain measurement tool. It may be applied to measure pain intensity and pain relief, and can also be used to measure other aspects of pain experience (e.g. affective component).

The scale comprises a 10-cm straight line with 'verbal anchors' that define the boundaries. The score is obtained by measuring the distance in millimetres from left to right. The anchoring text can influence the scores depending on the patient's interpretation of the words used. This does present difficulties when these scales are used within research projects.

The line can be oriented vertically (thermometer scale) or horizontally without affecting the sensitivity of the VAS. The vertical alignment may be preferred in older patients. The VAS is more sensitive than the categorical VRS.

Advantages

It is quick and relatively simple to use for most patients. It avoids imprecise, descriptive terms, such as with the categorical scales, and allows a choice of many points or ratings. It is also suitable for use in children aged over 5 years.

Fig. 15.2 Visual analogue scale measuring pain intensity

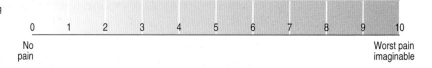

No
pain

Worst
imaginable
pain

Fig. 15.3 Visual analogue scale measuring degree of pain relief

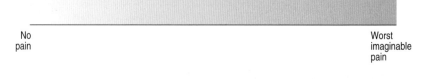

No
pain
relief

Complete
pain relief

Continuous data extraction can be used and parametric statistical tests with their greater statistical strength are appropriate.

Disadvantages

It is more demanding and requires greater cognitive skills (concentration, understanding and language skills) than the VRS and NRS. It may not be suitable for use at the extremes of ages, in the educationally subnormal, in those with impaired consciousness or those with deficient language skills. Up to 26% of patients find it confusing.

It may not be easy for patients to recall their initial or previous pain intensities when asked to repeat (or serial) measurements in either clinical practice or research studies. There may be problems with the minimum and maximum possible scores during repeat measurements, i.e. floor and ceiling effects (e.g. if the pain is reported as 100 mm, there is no way to increase the score at subsequent measurements if the pain intensity progresses).

The interpretation of pain relief can change over time, giving a different magnitude of pain relief for the same magnitude of pain intensity. Self-reports can be influenced by medication, sleep disturbance and affect.

Baseline or initial VAS measurements for pain intensity can vary widely between patients.

If a VAS is used to measure pain relief it has a more consistent baseline (e.g. no relief). Data from VAS to measure pain relief may, therefore, be more sensitive and easier to compare than data for pain intensity. This may be a more appropriate scale for use when interventions are used to relieve a patient's pain. In research projects it may be more appropriate to use both pain intensity and relief scales.

Picture scales

These are another form of unidimensional scale related to the categorical rating scales. These are advantageous for measuring pain and pain behaviour in children, the educationally subnormal and patients with poor language skills (e.g. faces pain scale). Several versions are available and have been validated in several patient groups (Fig. 15.4).

Both patients and observers can use picture scales, they are simple to use and are preferred by many patient groups.

Pain drawings

A sketch of the full human figure (both front and back) is printed and patients are asked to shade in areas corresponding to pain. Patients may be asked to use

Fig. 15.4 The faces pain scale (From: Benzon, Raja, Molloy et al. *The essentials of pain medicine and regional anaesthesia*, 2nd edn. Edinburgh: Churchill Livingstone; 2005)

various shades or patterns to mark different characteristics of pain (dull, sharp, stabbing, burning, etc.). This provides a high-impact record about the site and distribution of pain. Patients with more than one kind of pain are also able to describe their pain on a pain drawing.

These can be used as part of an initial assessment (common in the chronic pain clinic) and reused as the patient progresses through a period of pain management.

Multidimensional tools

Classically pain can be considered to have three dimensions:

- Sensory – discriminative
- Motivational – affective
- Cognitive – evaluative.

Patients use a characteristic language to describe these pain dimensions. As words are used as descriptors, which are often ranked as to their importance, it is necessary to assess what the words mean to the population under test. For example, elderly patients may not describe their pain as a pain, but as an ache, gripe or nuisance. It is, therefore, important to understand the use and meaning of language for the patient. This is true for validating these tools, but also in daily clinical practice in understanding patients. These concepts have led to the development of a vast number of multidimensional pain tools in many languages. Some of these tools are applicable to the general assessment of chronic pain, while others are designed for assessing specific types of pain. These tools for assessing pain have to be validated for the population they are used on. This becomes more complex when translating the tools to other languages.

Some examples of the multidimensional tools are the long and short forms of the McGill pain questionnaire, Minnesota multiphasic personality inventory, brief pain inventory.

Long form of McGill pain questionnaire[2]

This assesses the quality and character of pain by scaling pain in three dimensions: sensory, affective and evaluative. There are 20 sets of descriptors. The patient is instructed to select the sets relevant to their pain and then to identify (by circling with a pen) the individual words in each of these sets that are most appropriate. Three indices are produced from this information:

1. The pain rating index (PRI): each descriptor in each set has a rank value according to its implied intensity. The PRI is the subtotal of the ranked values of each chosen descriptor. There are separate scores for each of the three dimensions as well as a miscellaneous subclass. The PRI can be used to score acute and chronic pain conditions.
2. The number of words chosen (NWC).
3. The present pain intensity scale (PPIS): the patient is also asked to complete the categorical PPIS using descriptors from no pain through to excruciating.

The McGill questionnaires are at least as sensitive to changes in postoperative pain following oral analgesics as VRS and VAS. They have been validated in several settings, but due to the time taken to complete, remain principally for use as a research tool.

Short form of McGill pain questionnaire[4]

This is quicker to complete and suitable for multidimensional assessment of acute pain. It consists of three indices:

1. An index derived from 15 pain adjectives (11 sensory and four affective) that are ranked on a categorical scale of none, mild, moderate and severe.
2. A VAS.
3. A PPIS.

It correlates very highly with the PRI of the long form and is sensitive to changes brought about by various analgesic manoeuvres, including the types of analgesics used for postoperative pain. It is validated and is easier to use in the clinical setting (Fig. 15.5).

Brief pain inventory

The brief pain inventory asks the patients to rate the pain at its worst, least, average and current intensity. It is helpful to assess pain-related interference in seven areas: general activity, mood, walking ability, normal work, relationships with other people, enjoyment of life and sleep. This tool can be used both clinically and in research projects (Fig. 15.6).

Health-related quality of life measures

Several measures of health-related quality of life (HRQL) have been developed. These measures are multidimensional and include several domains, such as physical, psychological and social function, and various symptoms, which are prevalent in advanced medical illnesses. Pain is included as a single item or as a dimension in many of these measures. The European Organization for Research and Treatment of Cancer (EORTC) quality-of-life questionnaire is a type of tool that has been specifically designed for the use in oncology clinical trials. By using these tools a more comprehensive picture of the patient's total symptom burden and function might be obtained.

Hospital anxiety and depression scale[3]

The hospital anxiety and depression scale (HAD) is widely used as a measure of mood, emotional distress, anxiety, depression and emotional disorder in clinical populations with symptoms of physical disease. It attempts to measure anxiety and depression without confounding by somatic symptoms of physical disorder. The HAD only takes 2 to 5 min to complete, thus it is quick to use and easily acceptable to patients who may be quite unwell. With only 14 items each answered on a four-point verbal rating scale, it can be used to give measures of anxiety (seven items) and depression (seven items). The HAD achieves good internal consistency and test and retest reliabilities, is sensitive to change and gives valid assessments. It has been validated in a variety of settings over the years.

Other methods for measuring acute pain

None of these measures directly assesses pain but may help in the overall assessment of acute pain. Some are clearly research tools and none is a substitute for the patient's own reporting of pain. There are occasions when the patient is unable to be directly involved with pain scoring (e.g. unconscious).

Fig. 15.5 Short form of McGill pain questionnaire (From: Benzon, Raja, Molloy et al. *The essentials of pain medicine and regional anaesthesia*, 2nd edn. Edinburgh: Churchill Livingstone; 2005)

	None	Mild	Moderate	Severe
Throbbing	0) _____	1) _____	2) _____	3) _____
Shooting	0) _____	1) _____	2) _____	3) _____
Stabbing	0) _____	1) _____	2) _____	3) _____
Sharp	0) _____	1) _____	2) _____	3) _____
Cramping	0) _____	1) _____	2) _____	3) _____
Gnawing	0) _____	1) _____	2) _____	3) _____
Hot-burning	0) _____	1) _____	2) _____	3) _____
Aching	0) _____	1) _____	2) _____	3) _____
Heavy	0) _____	1) _____	2) _____	3) _____
Tender	0) _____	1) _____	2) _____	3) _____
Splitting	0) _____	1) _____	2) _____	3) _____
Tiring-exhausting	0) _____	1) _____	2) _____	3) _____
Sickening	0) _____	1) _____	2) _____	3) _____
Fearful	0) _____	1) _____	2) _____	3) _____
Punishing-cruel	0) _____	1) _____	2) _____	3) _____

Rate the intensity of your pain on the two scales below. Make a mark on the line to indicate where your pain falls between *No pain* and *Worst possible pain* and then circle the appropriate number on the second scale.

No
pain ├──┤ Worst
possible
pain

Circle the one of the following words that best describes your current pain:

0   No pain
1   Mild
2   Discomforting
3   Distressing
4   Excrutiating

Physiological and biochemical markers include heart rate, blood pressure, respiratory rate, arterial blood gas, catecholamine, cortisol and antidiuretic hormone estimation.

Neuropharmacological assessment of cerebrospinal fluid endorphin concentrations is used primarily as a research tool. Neurophysiological tests that may be appropriate include: EEG, evoked potentials, microneurography, EMG, nerve conduction and PET scanning.

Fig. 15.6 Brief pain inventory (From: Benzon, Raja, Molloy et al. *The essentials of pain medicine and regional anaesthesia*, 2nd edn. Edinburgh: Churchill Livingstone; 2005)

Please rate your pain by circling the one number that best describes your pain
DURING THE PAST WEEK:

Please rate your pain at its *worst* during the past week

| 0 | 1 | 2 | 3 | 4 | 5 | 6 | 7 | 8 | 9 | 10 |
No pain   Pain as bad as you can imagine

Please rate your pain at its *least* during the past week

| 0 | 1 | 2 | 3 | 4 | 5 | 6 | 7 | 8 | 9 | 10 |
No pain   Pain as bad as you can imagine

Please rate your pain on the *average* during the past week

| 0 | 1 | 2 | 3 | 4 | 5 | 6 | 7 | 8 | 9 | 10 |
No pain   Pain as bad as you can imagine

Please rate how much pain you have *right now*

| 0 | 1 | 2 | 3 | 4 | 5 | 6 | 7 | 8 | 9 | 10 |
No pain   Pain as bad as you can imagine

Circle the one number that best describes how, DURING THE PAST WEEK, pain has interfered with your:

General activity

| 0 | 1 | 2 | 3 | 4 | 5 | 6 | 7 | 8 | 9 | 10 |
Does not interfere   Completely interferes

Mood

| 0 | 1 | 2 | 3 | 4 | 5 | 6 | 7 | 8 | 9 | 10 |
Does not interfere   Completely interferes

Walking ability

| 0 | 1 | 2 | 3 | 4 | 5 | 6 | 7 | 8 | 9 | 10 |
Does not interfere   Completely interferes

Normal work (includes both work outside the home and housework)

| 0 | 1 | 2 | 3 | 4 | 5 | 6 | 7 | 8 | 9 | 10 |
Does not interfere   Completely interferes

Relations with other people

| 0 | 1 | 2 | 3 | 4 | 5 | 6 | 7 | 8 | 9 | 10 |
Does not interfere   Completely interferes

Sleep

| 0 | 1 | 2 | 3 | 4 | 5 | 6 | 7 | 8 | 9 | 10 |
Does not interfere   Completely interferes

Enjoyment of life

| 0 | 1 | 2 | 3 | 4 | 5 | 6 | 7 | 8 | 9 | 10 |
Does not interfere   Completely interferes

Assessment in special situations

Postoperative pain

The occurrence of acute pain is largely predictable and its intensity can be correlated with the operation site. The implementation of routine pain assessment after surgery is crucial and effective for improving the quality of pain management. A simple unidimensional tool to measure pain intensity is commonly used and pain measurement should be repeated regularly. The measurement must be a self-report where possible, as health professionals tend to underestimate patients' pain (this is true in the hospital and community setting).

Documented assessment of pain increases patient satisfaction and improves pain control, decreases anxiety and gives the patient greater control. It is the performance of assessment and not the measurement tool itself that is important. It provides an opportunity to educate and inform the patient about postoperative pain management.

Pain assessment should be used to assess the effect of therapeutic interventions on pain and function (e.g. pain intensity at rest, pain intensity during deep breathing and cough, and pain intensity during other manoeuvres, such as sitting up and getting out of bed). The intensity rating should always be documented together with the clinical intervention or response. This improves patient care, clinical accountability and aids clinical governance.

The possibility of an alternative diagnosis or complication should always be considered when a patient develops uncontrolled, unexpected or complex pain problems (e.g. wound dehiscence, compartment syndrome, peritonitis, neuropathic pain, etc.).

Assessment of pain in children

Children can experience pain soon after birth. Accurate assessment depends on the age and developmental abilities of the child. Improved assessment has greatly facilitated appropriate pain management.

Measures for pain assessment

Physiological
Assessment in this case involves heart rate, blood pressure, respiratory rate, palmar sweating, transcutaneous oxygen, serum catecholamine, glucagon and cortisol. It is not known to what extent they represent a general stress response rather than the appreciation of pain. They do, however, help guide management including pain.

Behavioural measures
This involves the assessment of crying, grimacing, irritability, etc. The neonatal facial action coding system is often used, where 10 facial actions are observed. It is not known to what extent certain behaviours represent pain rather than other forms of distress. In the preverbal child they can help in assessing weather pain is present or not.

Self-report measures
This is the preferred method of pain assessment in a child who can communicate verbally. Children of 18 months may be able to report the presence of pain and perhaps its location, but cannot give more information. Direct questioning is likely to yield better results than reliance on spontaneous reports. VAS can be used in children above 5 years of age and NRS in older children who understand numerical concepts. Categorical (faces scale: Fig. 15.4) are better in most but the very young, when the poker chip tool may be useful. Other scales that could be used are 'OUCHER' scale, the CHEOPS (Children's Hospital of Eastern Ontario Pain Scale) or the FLACC (Face, Legs, Activity, Cry, and Consolability) scale.

Assessment of pain in the elderly

The elderly will often be able to use the same tools as any adult. Dementia, cognitive deficit and confusion are more common in this age group. This is particularly true at the extreme of age and in those from care homes. A change in environment may precipitate confusion. Deafness or reduced hearing is also common as well as reduced speed of thought.

The elderly may not perceive or express pain in the same way as a younger age group. Their use of language may be different and it is important to ask specifically about pain and allow time for the patient to answer questions themselves.

The VAS vertically orientated may be easier for patient's to understand, verbal rating scores are also appropriate, but assessing the patient's meaning of the words used is important. There are also facial scales that can be used to assess pain in the older patient.

KEY POINTS

- Pain assessment is multidimensional including biological, psychological and social elements
- A thorough history is required along with what the pain means to the patient
- Patient expectations must be assessed before a management plan is produced
- Many scoring systems exist for scoring pain and are validated in a variety of clinical and research settings
- Patient self reports of pain and direct involvement in assessment is the gold standard. Observational reporting and proxy reporting are less reliable
- Pain should be considered as the 5th vital sign with documentation showing the intensity, action taken and response to intervention
- Many pain scales are (e.g. VAS, VRS, NRS) easy to use in the clinical setting

---

References

1. Merskey H, Bogduk N (eds) *Classification of chronic pain.* 2nd edn. Seattle: IASP Press; 1994.
2. Melzack R. The McGill Pain Questionnaire: major properties and scoring methods. *Pain* 1975; **1**(3): 277–299.
3. Zigmond AS, Snaith RP. The hospital anxiety and depression scale. *Acta Psychiatr Scand* 1983; **67**(6): 361–370.
4. Melzack R. The short-form McGill Pain Questionnaire. *Pain* 1987; **30**(2): 191–197.

Psychological impact of chronic pain

Introduction

'They can put a man on the moon but they cannot cure my pain.' In their quest to uncover solutions to unrelenting pain, patients often feel that a journey to the moon would be far less arduous.

It is indisputable that chronic pain is a complex and subjective experience that typically requires a multidisciplinary approach to assessment and management. The International Association for the Study of Pain defines pain as 'an unpleasant sensory and emotional experience associated with actual or potential tissue damage'.[1] The definition recognises the emotional component; irrespective of whether it pre-dates, is a consequence of or is a factor in the pain's development.

Recognising the emotional and sensory components of pain and giving them seemingly equal importance secures the integral place of clinical psychologists within pain management clinics. Of primary importance is the early introduction of psychology to the management of chronic pain. A preferable option would be for patients to be assessed by a multidisciplinary team, thus addressing the emotional, physical and social impact of pain head on. Such an approach would establish the ethos of the clinic from the outset. However, pressures on resources and ever-increasing pressure on waiting lists often prevent this from happening. The benefit of such an assessment would be to address misconceptions about the psychological input at an early stage. Moreover, this would lead to better management of emotional reactions and possibly prevent unnecessary chronicity. However, psychologists often find themselves being introduced to patients when options offered by the medical model are exhausted. Referral at this time can sometimes present a challenge for the psychologist and patient alike.

Seeing the psychologist

It is important to explore how patients perceive their referral to the psychologist. In some instances, the doctor may refer patients without a clear explanation as to why psychology is being recommended. Perhaps they suspect a psychological component to the pain and are unsure how to broach this with the patient in a sensitive manner. A sparse explanation regarding referral is often unhelpful for the patient and can sometimes result in an array of misconceptions, unnecessary anxiety and a refusal to attend.

If the patient does attend the appointment it has to be made explicit from the start that the psychologist believes their pain to be 'real'. Occasionally, patients may feel that a series of failed medical treatments are interpreted by doctors as implying *'psychogenic'* or *'psychological'* causes for their pain. Thus, referral to psychology reinforces the perception that the pain is perhaps 'imaginary' or that the patient is suffering from a mental illness. Without spending adequate time exploring these issues progressing with the assessment is fruitless, as information will undoubtedly be influenced by such views. It may be the first time that the patient has had contact with a psychologist, especially one in an acute healthcare setting and it is often worthwhile explaining the nature of their role and the difference between a psychologist and a psychiatrist as this may help minimise anxiety.

Pain journey

Usually offering appointment slots of 50 minutes or so, psychologists are able to provide the patient with an opportunity, without significant restraints of time, to tell their story. This may be the first opportunity that a patient has had to give a detailed account of their history to a single health professional and this in itself may prove very cathartic for them. Assessment should include enquiry into the patient's 'pain journey', that is, their interactions with often numerous health specialists, any suggested diagnoses and treatment outcomes. It is important to confirm the accuracy of the information that has been made available and identify any discordance between the patient's perception of these encounters and those of the professionals involved. Patients may be seeking the reassurance of a diagnosis particularly if several have been offered. Differing diagnoses often lead to confusion and distress, which can result in patients not being prepared for the possibility that a diagnosis may never be established. This leads to requests for further medical investigations and doctor–patient communication is vital at such times. Terms such as 'degenerative', 'crumbling' and 'wear and tear' may have been offered without clarification and patients may feel that they are being 'fobbed off'. Indeed, they may feel that if an accurate diagnosis has not been determined, something more sinister may be lurking. Patients may believe that if a definitive diagnosis were established they would receive the appropriate treatment, which would successfully reduce their pain.

Models of pain

The model of pain that the majority of patients are familiar with is the acute one. Until the commencement of their chronic pain, the medical model may have successfully treated any acute ailments they may have had. Despite explanations of the nature of their condition, chronic pain patients' expectations of a successful treatment often, and understandably, remain high. It is worth exploring patients' expectations of a clinic that specialises in what they often perceive as *'curing'* rather than *'managing'* chronic pain. Indeed, referral by health specialists may have been couched in terms of pain relief. Some treatments may have provided temporary relief from the pain thus reinforcing their belief that a cure may be possible. Patients' hopes will have been raised, however carefully they may have been counselled prior to the treatment.

Failed treatment is demoralising, depressing and reinforces a sense of helplessness and hopelessness. Being told that one's pain is unlikely to go away, that there is no diagnosis and that results of scans are not helpful can be very distressing for the patient.[2] In sheer desperation a patient will sometimes admit that they would prefer their scan to come back with a sinister diagnosis rather than no diagnosis. Occasionally, the continuous seeking for cures is driven by family members who themselves are working on the acute model of pain. Often, frustrated at being unable to help, family members sometimes reinforce the patient's need for a second medical opinion and their search for the elusive cure. Some may become very protective of the patient and prevent them from doing anything that might worsen the condition. Patients describe 'being wrapped up in cotton wool' and most find this frustrating and unhelpful.

Quality of life and loss

The problem with chronic pain is that it interferes with daily life and often prevents patients from engaging in activities that give them a sense of pleasure and purpose. Consequently, patients often report experiencing a number of emotional responses that often result in further unfavourable changes in behaviour. So when asked about quality of life the response from many patients is 'what quality of life?'. For some patients socialising is no longer a pleasure and this can result in a decline in self-confidence and social reinforcements. Financial restrictions may also force patients to limit social activities and interests, as employment may no longer be possible. Furthermore, some patients may not want to be seen socialising, as they fear judgement from others, e.g. 'she can't be in that much pain if she is out' or 'he looks happy enough, his back can't be too much of a problem'. Morley et al[3] discuss the interesting point that patients often fear that they will become socially isolated yet some deliberately avoid or withdraw from engaging in social activities in an attempt to reduce the burden on others and to maintain their self-esteem.

It is not surprising that patients often report experiencing numerous losses as a result of chronic pain. These may include the obvious physical, social and often financial losses that people mention but there are also losses related to identity and sense of self. Often patients who have endured chronic pain for a number of years will describe themselves as 'having changed' as a person and losing their identity. The assumptions they once held about themselves may have changed; for example, they may now perceive themselves as mentally weak and incapable of making decisions or feeling almost 'invisible' after losing their career. Furthermore, patients refer to the lost part of themselves, 'the person they were before'. For some they perceive that person as having gone forever, whereas others envisage their return when they are pain free. Furthermore, Hellstrom[4] purports that chronic pain disrupts the patient's expected development over time and there is the sense that patients have been propelled forward and are now functioning at a level where they feel 'old before their years'. This sentiment is often expressed by patients and causes a great deal of emotional distress and resentment towards the pain.

Sleep

The issue of sleep, or more accurately 'lack of it', actually follows on from the subject of loss and perceived identity. Patients often feel that their body does not have enough sleep and they wish they could return to the sleep pattern they had when they were younger. At this point it is often useful to educate patients that normal sleep for middle aged and older adults usually has more frequent periods of wakefulness.[5] Undoubtedly patients may experience disturbed periods of sleep but occasionally they will insist they have not slept in a number of days. Of course this is not technically true, because if deprived of sleep for a number of days people suffer significant mental deterioration. During assessment it is important to clarify why patients are unable to sleep. Is sleep disturbed because pain wakes them and they are unable to get back to sleep, or do they have difficulty going to sleep or are worrying thoughts preventing them from relaxing and 'switching off'.

Intervention will depend on the identified source of sleep disturbance, but it is always worthwhile encouraging patients to establish a sleep plan that consists of a standard wake-up time and bedtime. Furthermore, daytime napping should be discouraged, along with the intake of stimulants such as tea and coffee.

Mood

Assessment should include an account of the patient's premorbid psychological functioning and whether they have received any mental health input and in what form. The task is to determine whether the patient's feelings and symptoms relate to their pain history and to question whether these reactions are understandable. Perhaps the best way to gain the patient's confidence is to simply outline the normal consequences of chronic pain.[6] It is often a good idea to introduce the relationship between mind and body in simple terms and discuss how pain and emotions may impact upon each other.

In the majority of chronic pain patients it can be said that they may experience emotions such as anxiety, depression or anger. It is important to address some misconceptions and state that, whilst a number of patients experience emotional reactions, the majority of these people do not have a personality disorder, psychiatric illness nor are they malingerers. Indeed, patients usually react to the experience of chronic pain in ways that are largely understandable. Patients' distress can often be understood as a result of their symptoms or disability and it is of great value to clarify the meaning that such symptoms hold to them. Patients' emotions may have a number of sources, e.g. their interactions with health professionals, their perceived role within their family and so on.

Psychometric tests are used to support information gained from the psychologist's assessment. If the psychometric measures used have not been specifically standardised for use with chronic pain patients, the results should be interpreted with caution. The hospital anxiety and depression scale[7] is frequently used in hospitals and pain clinics in the UK, as it is easy to administer and score, it is familiar to various health professionals and it provides a score for anxiety and depression. However, caution must be used as it is not specifically designed for use with chronic pain patients. Numerous psychometric measures are available to measure specific psychological reactions (for a comprehensive list of measures see Gatchell).[8]

Anxiety

A degree of anxiety is fairly common amongst patients with chronic pain, particularly when they have not received a clear explanation or diagnosis. The prognosis may be uncertain and successful treatment options are not guaranteed ingredients in a recipe for an anxious patient. Feelings of being worried, nervous or tense may dominate alongside physical symptoms of increased heart rate, sweating, dry mouth and chest tightness, etc. Patients may report poor coping skills, reduced personal competence and a general feeling that they are reliant on others and large doses of medication to get them through the day. Eccleston et al[9] state that chronic pain patients report that they worry more about pain and their health than any other topic, and that they experience these worries as highly intrusive, unpleasant and difficult to diminish. Indeed, some patients have a preoccupation with bodily symptoms, sensations and changes, monitoring every twinge and ache. They may exercise selective attention and misinterpret sensations as evidence of further physical disease. From a diagnostic point of view it is important to gain a careful clinical history of the development of anxiety, which will help aid management. Cognitive approaches, such as cognitive restructuring, are commonly employed to treat anxiety disorders.

Depression

Over the course of time and a number of failed treatments patients may feel despondent and dejected. A fluctuating pattern of 'highs', e.g. that next treatment will work, followed by 'lows', e.g. another failed treatment can become an all too familiar picture. Such yo-yoing of emotions usually results in depression. Defined by a sense of hopelessness and pessimism, depression can be all consuming for patients faced with irrecoverable losses. However, diagnosis is not always straightforward and it is important to note that symptoms such as weight change, sleep disturbance and fatigue may also be a function of the chronic pain state.

The relationship between chronic pain and depression is complex and debate centres on the question of whether depression is a factor in the development of chronic pain or a consequence of it. For the most part depression is thought to be a consequence of pain[10] and may be understood in terms of the stress diathesis model in which loss of roles and personal competencies is central. Furthermore, it must be considered that some patients are reluctant to disclose low mood as they fear a diagnosis of depression could possibly prejudice further medical consultations and treatment.

Anger and frustration

The presence of anger is often self-evident from the manner and content of the patient's communications. The patient may be angry for a number of reasons and this may vary in intensity. Patients may be angry and frustrated with the medical profession, with repeated treatment failures, with the injustice of their situation, with not being able to work, with financial hardship, the medico-legal process, the pain and so on.

Once identified the task is for the therapist to move the patient forward and help them to develop strategies for managing their anger.

Beliefs and fear avoidance

It is important to examine the patient's belief system and identify possible cognitive distortions that may result in them experiencing accentuated emotional reactions (e.g. anger, depression and anxiety). Some patients may possess an array of unhelpful beliefs. Some of the common ones include thoughts that their pain is due to irreversible damage, perhaps due to serious disease that may have been overlooked or that the pain will lead to increased disability and greater dependency on others. Perhaps the most common underlying belief that patients' hold is where hurt is synonymous with harm. Such a belief is understandable as this is true for most acute conditions and this model is one which patients are often familiar with. The consequences of such beliefs are continued seeking of medical consultations, investigations and adopting 'ill' behaviour such as increased bed rest.[11]

Fear avoidance

Chronic pain patients often equate increases in pain with further physical damage. They follow the acute model rule that hurt equals harm and 'if it hurts, stop'. Consequently, patients try to avoid what could potentially lead to a further exacerbation in pain and increased disability.

Lethem et al[12] introduced the fear avoidance model. With respect to acute conditions such avoidance behaviour is an adaptive reaction as it serves to limit further damage. In the case of chronic conditions it can be a barrier to rehabilitation. When confronted with an activity that the patient believes will lead to increased pain it will be avoided. Therefore, no increase in pain is experienced and the patient learns that avoiding the situation is beneficial and they continue to behave in this way. However, if patients apply this rule to all experiences of pain they may actually be causing themselves greater harm. For example, the patient who believes muscle pain results in physical damage will learn to associate pain with activity, become reluctant to exercise and probably drop out of physical rehabilitation. This could potentially result in physical de-conditioning or the 'disuse syndrome'.[13] This is a detrimental condition in which performance of physical activities leads more easily to pain and physical discomfort, which in turn makes avoidance more likely. It has been reported that fear avoidance beliefs are more closely related to uncertainty of diagnosis than either severity or duration of pain. Some measures used to assess fear avoidance are the fear avoidance beliefs questionnaire[14] and the back beliefs questionnaire.[11]

Occasionally patients talk about 'discs slipping' and 'bones crumbling'; despite never encountering such consequences these beliefs have a powerful influence on behaviour. These beliefs may have been reinforced by medical consultations where such words are used in explanation with the patient taking a different message away than the one meant. There is a sub-group of chronic pain patients who express an intense fear of movement (kinesophobia) and a tendency to catastrophise the outcome. An example would be the patient who truly believes their back would snap after bending past a certain point. The therapist's task is to try to help the patient challenge this fear and focus on exercises that would specifically involve bending.[15] The Tampa scale for kinesophobia was developed by Miller et al in 1991, but unpublished. The scale was later published with permission by Vlaeyen[15] and can be used to assess fear of movement and re-injury; this is a valuable tool to enhance clinical assessment.

Interventions

Given that pain is a multidimensional construct, a number of psychotherapeutic and adjunctive techniques can be employed to help patients struggling with the impact of chronic pain. Therapy may be on a one-to-one basis, group or couple based. In pain management the preferred treatment paradigm is cognitive therapy, but it is important to tailor intervention to the individual and not the other way around.

Cognitive therapy

Cognitive therapy focuses on evaluating the patient's belief system and identifying dysfunctional thoughts that adversely impact upon mood, behaviour and pain. Time is often spent educating patients on the relationship between mind and body. A good way of demonstrating this link in a simple but effective way is to ask the patient to visualise a lemon, to describe it in as much detail as possible then ask the patient to imagine slicing it in half and taking a big bite. Usually they will grimace, thereby demonstrating the link between mind and body. However, this is not always successful and occasionally you come across a patient who loves eating lemons!

Patients are encouraged to identify dysfunctional thoughts, often referred to as 'cognitive errors', and identify the role they may serve in their current behaviour or emotional state. A common list of dysfunctional thoughts has been produced;[16] one that frequently occurs in chronic pain patients is that of 'catastrophising', whereby patients react be imagining the worst possible outcome. For example, 'if my pain continues I will end up in a wheelchair'. Providing the patient with this list can be a helpful tool in therapy as they can often identify with a number of thoughts. Once patients identify the unhelpful thoughts, the challenge is to generate less-threatening alternatives, a technique referred to as 'cognitive restructuring'. The aim is to alter unproductive behaviour, reduce emotional distress and develop effective coping strategies. Whilst reducing pain is not usually the aim of therapy, patients sometimes report an improvement in pain levels. This may be due to a number of reasons; for example, they may be engaging in more exercise as their previously dysfunctional thoughts regarding exercise have to be altered.

Therapy is structured with clear agendas set by the patient and psychologist focusing on specific areas of concern. Cognitive behavioural therapy incorporates behavioural techniques, some of which are outlined below.

A combination of cognitive and behavioural techniques, whether delivered individually or in group sessions, has been shown to be effective in helping patients with chronic pain.[17]

Behavioural techniques

Encouraging patients to set behavioural goals for themselves is a valuable technique in pain management. Some patients may stop some activities or interests due to increased pain but on closer examination it may be that they are able to reengage in that activity by adopting a different approach. For example, a patient may tell you that they were once a keen gardener, but after a day mowing the lawn they experienced an exacerbation in pain and thereby concluded that gardening makes their pain worse and no longer engage in the activity. This may result in the patient feeling depressed as the pain has prevented them from doing an activity they enjoy, they may have to depend on someone else to cut the grass and this may have financial implications which cause greater concern and so on. The task is to go back to the initial episode of increased pain and ask whether the gardening could be approached in a different way. It may be that the patient mows half of the lawn one day and the rest another, thus employing the strategy of pacing. The key is for patients to undertake the activity but to stop before they experience an increase in pain, have a rest and then go back to the task. The activity is, therefore, paced and, whilst it may take longer to achieve, the final result should be the same or similar and the patient will experience a sense of achievement rather than feeling despondent that the pain has taken control again. It must be noted, however, that patients sometimes struggle with pacing activities, often due to frustration, but if it is important that they complete the task themselves then increased time should not outweigh the sense of achievement.

Another behavioural technique is aimed at helping the patient diminish inappropriate verbal behaviours such as excessive 'pain talk'. With some patients, pain dominates their conversation and whilst this is often the requirement of a medical consultation, therapy aims to move people away from this and encourage them to focus on something productive rather than counterproductive. It is often helpful to encourage patients to think about how their 'pain talk' is viewed by others.

Relaxation

Relaxation has been demonstrated to be a valuable technique in pain management. It equips patients with a skill that in many cases can quickly lead to significant benefits, such as reducing anxiety, which sometimes leads to reports of decreased pain levels. Furthermore, it can empower patients as many feel helpless to impact upon their pain and finding a technique that they can control is very powerful. The impact of relaxation should not be underestimated and this must be evident in the way in which it is presented to patients. If professionals perceive it as, 'well, you might as well give it a try', then this will undoubtedly influence the patient's perception and commitment to the relaxation. It must be emphasised that relaxation is a skill that requires practice and discipline.

Psychologists should, however, be aware that for some acutely anxious or distressed patients, concentrating and focusing on relaxation techniques might be problematic. It is also important to consider patients who have strong religious beliefs, who may fear that relaxation invokes practices contrary to their spiritual experiences or cognitive styles.

Diaphragmatic breathing

Diaphragmatic breathing is at the very heart of relaxation and is often used in conjunction with the techniques mentioned below. Patients may think that this technique is simple as 'we breathe all the time', but it appears that most adults, unless professional singers, do not breathe from their diaphragm but their chest. When observing patients undertaking an exercise programme physiotherapists note that a number of patients hold their breath and guard against the prospect of increased pain. Such behaviour is not helpful as it leads to increased tension in the body, which makes the experience of pain more likely. Patients are instructed to breathe from their diaphragm rather than their chest as an aid to a deepened relaxation state.

Progressive muscle relaxation

With progressive muscle relaxation the patient is instructed to tense the muscles in a region of the body or a limb and then subsequently relax those muscles. For example, clenching a fist then releasing it. The tension and subsequent relaxation of muscle groups is conducted in a logical and sequential manner, generally from head to foot or the reverse. During the exercise patients are encouraged to focus their attention on the difference between a relaxed state and a tense state and to focus on any other sensations that occur. It is emphasised to patients that the tensing of muscles should not cause an increase in pain as this counteracts the purpose of the relaxation. If this is the case then they should miss out that particular part of the body or try reducing the tension slightly.

Autogenic training

This technique requires the patient to focus on sequential and progressive relaxation of parts of the body, but the step of tensing muscles is not required. Instead the patient is instructed to focus on sensations of warmth and heaviness extending throughout the body. They are also encouraged to develop their own phrases, e.g. my arms are heavy and relaxed. Some versions of autogenic training ask patients to focus on sensations in the extremities with the understanding that this facilitates increased blood flow to these parts and promotes peripheral warming and a reduction in sympathetic nervous arousal.

Visualisation/imagery

Visualisation involves talking the patient through vivid images that are particularly comforting or relaxing to them. Visualising somewhere where they feel completely comfortable, e.g. lying on a warm sandy beach, will hopefully encourage an emotional state that is inconsistent with anxiety or tension. The patient is then guided to vividly recapture as much of the imagined place as possible, the sights, sounds, smells, tastes, physical sensations and feelings, thus making it as real as possible. The aim is that the patient goes on to develop their own visualisations, but initially they may need to be guided by the psychologist. In this instance it is useful to check that the image is not distressing to the patient before the session begins; for example, if planning to talk them through a walk near the sea it would be a good idea to check that they are not frightened of the water.

Biofeedback

Biofeedback refers to a procedure whereby a patient's physiological processes, such as heart rate and muscle tension, are monitored, usually by electrical sensors linked to a hand-held machine, and then reported back to the patient. The biofeedback machine indicates any changes in physiological activity by means of audible or visual signals. For example, an increased beeping sound may signal an increase in tension and the patient is encouraged to develop strategies to reduce this. Such strategies may include diaphragmatic breathing or visualising a pleasant image. Biofeedback machines can be useful when working with patients who deny they are tense. Sometimes it is useful to ask patients to use the machine when they are watching television and to monitor whether tension is influenced by imagery or thoughts. Ultimately it is hoped that the patient will be able to invoke those strategies to reduce tension without the use of the biofeedback machine.

Pain management programmes

Pain management programmes are group-based approaches designed to help patients manage their pain. The aim is symptom management and improving quality of life rather than curing pain. The cognitive and behavioural foundations of pain management programmes were essentially established in 1976 by Fordyce[18] and Turk in 1983.[19] The nature of the programme is usually multidisciplinary involving input from psychology, physiotherapy, nursing/medical and occupational therapy. The first programme in the UK was developed at the Walton Hospital in Liverpool and Hope Hospital in Salford in 1983. An inpatient programme was developed in St. Thomas' in London in 1988, but the majority of programmes in the UK are run on an outpatient basis.

Selection criteria for entry onto programmes vary, but prior to referral clinics usually state that it is imperative that the patient has completed all medical investigations and treatment options. If this is not the case there could be the risk that they will not fully engage in the programme as they may be thinking about treatments that they have not yet tried. The emphasis is on managing pain as opposed to treating it. This should be made explicit from the start to prevent misunderstanding and unrealistic expectations. Patients should be at the point where they are not actively seeking a cure for their pain and their thinking is centred on self-management and improving quality of life using cognitive behavioural strategies, activity pacing, exercising, relaxation and so on.

Group work of this kind can be invaluable as patients often learn skills from each other and where some patients may be fearful of exercise, observing others engaging in it, is an opportunity for them to confront their beliefs. Due to the complexity of chronic pain and its impact on physical, cognitive, behavioural and social functioning a multidisciplinary intervention is often the best way forward for patients who are thinking in terms of management rather than curative approaches.

Summary

So, what of the man on the moon? As a psychologist the purpose is not to help patients discover the man on the moon and the ever-elusive cure; rather it is to help make sense of their journey, to manage their emotions and hopefully enable them to improve the quality of their life despite the presence of pain. However, I am not foolish enough to believe that patients ever lose sight of the moon (i.e. a cure), but perhaps a more achievable goal is to reposition it slightly, thereby preventing it from governing their lives. Understandably the task is potentially difficult, but encouragingly it is one that many patients achieve. Who knows, perhaps the future of medicine will one day make the moon far more accessible to those who live with chronic pain.

KEY POINTS

- Emotion, whether it predates, is a consequence of, or a factor in pain development needs to be addressed
- Exploring patients' expectations of a clinic that specialises in what they often perceive as '*curing*' rather than '*managing*' pain is vital
- Chronic pain interferes with daily life, having a direct impact on personal functioning and overall quality
- Alterations in sleep, and mood states such as anxiety and depression, are common in chronic pain patients
- Patients' beliefs about their pain may limit how they respond to its management
- Psychotherapeutic interventions can be employed to address some of the issues within the multidimensional construct of pain
- Pain management programmes offer a combination of interventions designed to help patients manage chronic pain

---

References

1. Merskey H, Bogduk N (eds). *Classification of chronic pain.* 2nd edn. Seattle: IASP Press; 1994.
2. van Tulder MW, Assendelft WJ, Koes BW. Spinal radiographic findings and nonspecific low back pain. A systematic review of observational studies. *Spine* 1997; **22**(4): 427–434.
3. Morley S, Doyle K, Beese A. Talking to others about pain: suffering in silence. In: Devor M, Rowbotham MC, Wiesenfeld–Hallin Z (eds). *Proceedings of the 9th World Congress on Pain.* Seattle: IASP Press; 2000: 1123–1129.
4. Hellstrom C. Temporal dimensions of the self-concept: entrapped and possible selves in chronic pain. *Psychol Health* 2001; **16**(1): 111–124.
5. Horne J. *Why we sleep: the functions of sleep in humans and other mammals.* Oxford: Oxford University Press; 1988.
6. Gatchell RJ. Psychological disorders and chronic pain: cause-and-effect relationships. In: Gatchell RJ, Turk DC (eds). *Psychological approaches to pain management: a practitioner's handbook.* New York: Guilford Press; 1996: 33–52.
7. Zigmond AS, Snaith RP. The hospital anxiety and depression scale. *Acta Psychiatr Scand* 1983; **67**(6): 361–370.

8. Gatchell RJ. *Clinical essentials of pain management.* DC Washington: American Psychological Association; 2005: 32.

9. Eccleston C et al. Worry and chronic pain patients: a description and analysis of individual differences. *Eur J Pain* 2001; **5**(3): 309–318.

10. Banks SM, Kerns RD. Explaining high rates of depression in chronic pain, a diathesis–stress framework. *Psychol Bull* 1996; **119**: 95–110.

11. Symonds TL et al. Do attitudes and beliefs influence work loss due to low back trouble? *Occup Med (Lond)* 1996; **46**(1): 25–32.

12. Lethem J et al. Outline of a fear-avoidance model of exaggerated pain perception—I. *Behav Res Ther* 1983; **21**(4): 401–408.

13. Bortz WM 2nd. The disuse syndrome. *West J Med* 1984; **141**(5): 691–694.

14. Waddell G et al. A fear-avoidance beliefs questionnaire (FABQ) and the role of fear-avoidance beliefs in chronic low back pain and disability. *Pain* 1993; **52**(2): 157–168.

15. Vlaeyen JWS et al. The role of fear of movement/(re)injury in pain disability. *J Occup Rehabil* 1995; **V5**(4): 235–252.

16. Beck AT et al. *Cognitive therapy of depression.* New York: Guilford Press; 1979: 261.

17. Morley S, Eccleston C, Williams A. Systematic review and meta-analysis of randomized controlled trials of cognitive behaviour therapy and behaviour therapy for chronic pain in adults, excluding headache. *Pain* 1999; **80**(1–2): 1–13.

18. Fordyce WE. *Behavioural methods for chronic pain and illness.* St Louis: C V Mosby; 1976.

19. Turk DC, Meichenbaum D, Genest M. *Pain and behavioural medicine: a cognitive behavioural perspective.* New York: Guilford Press; 1983: 452.

Sam Eldabe and Sivakumar Raghavan

Interventions in pain management

Introduction

Pain is the commonest symptom for which an individual seeks medical help. In recent years, advances in neurobiology have increased our understanding of mechanisms by which pain is produced and means by which it can be treated. Despite improved knowledge, however, pain largely remains undertreated.[1] The multidimensional nature of pain, subjective variation in response to pain and its treatment, difficulties in measuring and quantifying pain, and physicians' misconceptions regarding therapeutic interventions have all contributed towards pain being managed less effectively. Advances in technology have played a significant part in improving pain treatment and patient satisfaction. Patient-controlled analgesia devices, implantable intrathecal drug-delivery systems and spinal-cord stimulators are examples of sophisticated technology employed in the management of pain. Neuronal blockade with local anaesthetic agents or neurolytic agents is increasingly used in pain treatment and has diagnostic, prognostic, prophylactic and therapeutic applications. Psychological interventions and pain-management programmes have been developed to target the psychosocial components of pain. Some of the therapeutic interventions may in addition to pain relief, bring about favourable metabolic and endocrine responses. A holistic approach to pain management will address not only pain relief, but also the systemic, emotional, psychological and social factors that may have contributed to or have occurred as a result of pain. A multimodal pain recipe may include analgesics, neuronal blockade, physiotherapy and psychology sessions. In this chapter, we present an overview of various therapeutic interventions and their roles in pain management.

Acute vs. chronic pain

Acute pain can simply be defined as pain that occurs immediately after an acute injury or a disease process. Chronic pain on the other hand persists beyond the duration of injury or disease.

Clinical literature suggests that acute pain can progress into a chronic pain state. The human nervous system is adaptable and capable of substantial plasticity.[2] A huge nociceptive input can, through toxic effects of excitatory amino acids, permanently change spinal-cord function and, therefore, lead to chronic pain after an acute injury.[3] Acute pain should, therefore, be viewed as the initiation phase of an extensive, persistent nociceptive and behavioural cascade triggered by tissue injury.[1] This cascade subsides within weeks; but if pain is not suppressed, even a minor injury can sometimes progress to chronic pain.

Inadequate treatment of postoperative pain has been shown to decrease patients' quality of recovery in the immediate postoperative period.[4] Patients with chronic pain experience depression, fatigue, sleep disturbance, and decreased physical and mental function. Interventions in acute pain situations are, therefore, employed to minimise the risk of developing chronic pain (e.g. sciatic nerve block prior to leg amputation).

Chronic pain on the other hand is multidimensional in nature and interventions are used as part of a wider management strategy aimed at rehabilitation rather than complete cure.

Multidisciplinary pain clinics came into existence in order to address the multiple components of chronic pain. A typical pain clinic comprises of a pain management physician, psychologist, nurse specialist, physiotherapist, vocational counsellor and pharmacist.[5] Co-ordination, effective communication and teamwork amongst team members are vital in order to achieve high-quality care.

Systemic response to pain and treatment of pain[6,7]

The systemic response to injury, trauma or surgery involves endocrine and metabolic changes, which are referred to commonly as the 'stress response'. The endocrine response involves increased secretion of pituitary hormones like adrenocorticotropic hormone (ACTH), growth hormone and arginine-vasopressin; adrenocortical hormones such as cortisol and aldosterone; and glucagon from the pancreas. Secretion of insulin and thyroid hormone is reduced. The overall effect is an increase in catabolism that leads to increased breakdown of hepatic glycogen, skeletal muscle protein and fat stores. This can result in hyperglycaemia, muscle wasting and ketosis. Hypothalamic activation of the sympathetic nervous system results in increased catecholamine release from the adrenal medulla and increased norepinephrine release from presynaptic nerve terminals. This produces cardiovascular effects, such as tachycardia and hypertension, and modifies the function of pancreas, liver and kidneys. Increased secretion of aldosterone and arginine-vasopressin leads to increased sodium and water retention. Contrary to popular belief, similar endocrine and metabolic changes are observed in neonates in response to pain.[8]

Some of the interventions in pain management can favourably modify these responses. Opioids suppress hypothalamic and pituitary hormone secretion. Morphine, fentanyl and alfentanil have been shown to reduce cortisol and catecholamine levels in various studies. Thoracic epidural analgesia attenuates the sympatho-adrenal response to surgery. This may be beneficial to patients with ischaemic heart disease. Epidurals reduce thrombotic events by decreasing the hypercoagulability of blood in the perioperative period. Epidurals improve postoperative pulmonary function after upper abdominal and thoracic surgery. They also decrease paralytic ileus following abdominal procedures and thereby allow early use of enteral nutrition, which is important in reducing the risk of infectious complications. A multimodal approach of postoperative epidural analgesia and early mobilisation reduces pain scores, reduces hormonal and metabolic stress, and improves mobility and convalescence following surgery.[9]

Therapeutic interventions in pain management

An outline of interventions that are employed in the treatment of pain is depicted in Figure 17.1. Although there are similarities in the management of acute and chronic pain, some of the interventions are reserved almost exclusively for chronic pain. Examples of these include the use of antidepressants, anticonvulsants, neurolytic blocks and surgery to block nerve transmission. An extensive coverage of all interventions is beyond the scope of this book and the reader is referred to advanced textbooks of pain for further details.

Pharmacological interventions

A good history, examination and assessment of the severity of pain are important in determining the type of medication and route of administration for a particular patient. While analgesics are the mainstay in the treatment of acute pain, chronic pain often requires the addition of adjuvant drugs in addition to conventional analgesics.

Conventional analgesics

The commonly used analgesics include paracetamol, nonsteroidal anti-inflammatory drugs (NSAIDs) and opioids. These analgesics differ in their potencies and durations of action. There are differences in the intensity of various types of pain and patients' response to treatment. Hence, the choice of analgesics and dose should be tailored to the requirement of each patient.

Analgesics can be chosen in a stepwise fashion with low-potency drugs at the bottom and drugs with higher potency at the top. The World Health Organization (WHO) analgesic ladder (Fig. 17.2) described for the treatment of cancer pain is a classic example.[10] One can go up the ladder if pain worsens and come down as pain improves. A similar approach can be adapted for the management of acute and chronic nonmalignant pain. While considerable overlap exists between the treatment of acute and chronic pain, there are significant differences too.

The intravenous administration of drugs is popular in acute pain where a rapid onset of action is desirable and in the critical-care setting where oral administration may not be possible in sedated patients, and subcutaneous and intramuscular routes of administration may lead to unreliable absorption of drugs because of poor peripheral perfusion (Table 17.1). The side effect profiles of these drugs also influence their selection for a particular patient (Table 17.2). NSAIDs, for example, have serious complications with long-term use and may not be appropriate for chronic pain.

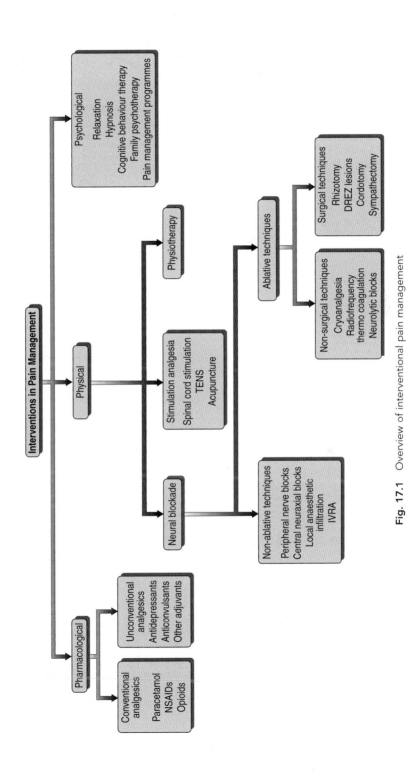

Fig. 17.1 Overview of interventional pain management

Fig. 17.2 The WHO analgesic ladder

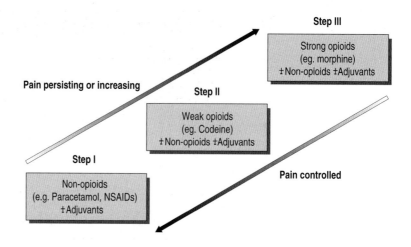

Pain persisting or increasing

Step III

Strong opioids
(eg. morphine)
±Non-opioids ±Adjuvants

Step II

Weak opioids
(eg. Codeine)
±Non-opioids ±Adjuvants

Pain controlled

Step I

Non-opioids
(e.g. Paracetamol, NSAIDs)
±Adjuvants

TABLE 17.1 Routes of administration of analgesics[35]	
Route	Comments
Oral	Ideal for chronic use
	Dependent on patients' ability to swallow, gastric emptying, food and pH
	Opioids have low oral bioavailability
Intramuscular	Pain and tissue irritation on injection
	Unreliable plasma concentration especially in low perfusion states
	Unsuitable for long-term use
Intravenous	Rapid action, can be titrated to effect
	High bioavailability, not dependent on patient characteristics
	Unsuitable for long-term use
Subcutaneous	Absorption is variable and dependent on tissue perfusion
	Used for long-term opioid administration especially in malignancy-related pain
Transmucosal	Sublingual, buccal and gingival modes of administration
	Offers rapid onset and patient comfort, oral transmucosal fentanyl citrate is useful for breakthrough cancer pain[36]
Rectal	Unreliable absorption and mucosal irritation
Transdermal	Improved patient compliance, long duration of action and steady plasma concentrations
	Slow onset makes it less useful for acute pain
	Fentanyl and buprenorphine patches are popular in chronic pain management
Topical	Topical NSAIDs are effective in acute pain[18]
Intra-articular	Not popular, intra-articular morphine provides good analgesia following arthroscopies;[18] steroid injections are used in treating arthritis
Inhalational	Limited use, inhaled entonox (50% nitrous oxide + 50% oxygen) is used for labour analgesia and change of dressings in burns

TABLE 17.2 Side effects of conventional analgesics	
Class	Complications
NSAIDs	Gastrointestinal ulceration/bleeding, impaired platelet function, fluid retention, reduction in renal blood flow, bronchospasm, Reye's syndrome and anaphylaxis
Opioids	Respiratory depression, nausea and vomiting, constipation, euphoria/dysphoria

Opioids and addiction

Addiction is often a concern that doctors have while prescribing opioids for pain relief, especially on a long-term basis. Oral morphine is frequently used for chronic pain management, especially cancer pain, and doses up to 500 mg may be needed in a day. Psychological addiction is rarely seen in clinical practice and an increase in demand for opioids usually reflects the development of tolerance or progression of the disease. Respiratory depression is also rare if the dose is titrated to the patient's analgesic requirements.[11]

Patient-controlled analgesia

Patient-controlled analgesia (PCA) is a method of pain relief that uses sophisticated electronic devices that allow self-administration of drugs by the patients. The intravenous route is commonly used, though epidural, subcutaneous and intranasal routes have been described. Commonly used drugs for intravenous PCA are opioids. PCA is extremely popular in the management of postoperative pain where its safety and efficacy are well established.[12] PCA devices allow patients to titrate doses of analgesics according to their needs. They also result in steady plasma level of drug being achieved. On-demand boluses with or without a background infusion can be programmed in the PCA. The size of bolus doses and the minimum time interval between doses (lockout) can be set, thereby minimising the risk of overdose. Nevertheless, respiratory rate and sedation scores need to be monitored and special care has to be taken in obese patients and those with obstructive sleep apnoea. Despite similar reduction in pain scores, there is higher patient satisfaction with PCA when compared to conventional analgesia.[13]

Unconventional analgesics

These drugs have limited use in the management of acute pain, but are extensively used on their own or in addition to conventional analgesics in chronic pain management. The pharmacology of these agents is discussed in more detail in Chapter 14.

Antidepressants

Though reported to be useful in many pain syndromes, antidepressants have proven efficacy in neuropathic pain, especially due to diabetic neuropathy and postherpetic neuralgia.[14] The mechanism by which analgesia is produced is unclear. However, analgesic properties are seen earlier and at much lower doses than that used for antidepressant effects.[15] The commonly used antidepressants include amitriptyline, nortriptyline, dosulepin, venlafaxine and fluoxetine.

Anticonvulsants

Anticonvulsants have proven benefits in neuropathic pain, especially trigeminal neuralgia and diabetic neuropathy.[16] A membrane stabilising action on neurones has been the traditional explanation for its action, but current thinking is that they interfere with the NMDA (*N*-methyl-D-aspartate) mechanism. The analgesic dose is similar to the anticonvulsant dose range, hence the similarity of adverse effects seen with anticonvulsants. Commonly used anticonvulsants are carbamazepine, sodium valproate, gabapentin, lamotrigine and pregabalin.

Adjuvants

These medications often find use in the management of chronic pain. Some of the commonly used adjuvants and their uses are shown in Table 17.3.

Physical interventions

Physical interventions can be broadly divided into:

- Nonablative methods of neuronal blockade
- Ablative (destructive) methods of neuronal blockade
- Stimulation analgesia
- Physiotherapy.

Nonablative neuronal blockade

Peripheral nerve blocks[17]

Peripheral nerve blocks are more commonly used in the management of acute pain especially in the perioperative setting. The advantages include high-quality and long-lasting analgesia, a reduction in opioid requirements and, thereby, a decrease in side effects including nausea, vomiting and respiratory depression. A multimodel approach works better in the treatment of acute pain and would include a combination of nerve block, paracetamol, NSAID and opioid.

TABLE 17.3 Adjuvants used in pain management

Medication	Indication
α_2-agonists (clonidine, dexmedetomidine)	Neuropathic pain
Baclofen	Spasm of cerebral palsy, multiple sclerosis, hemiplegia and spinal cord injury
NMDA receptor antagonists (ketamine, dextromethorphan)	Neuropathic pain
Anxiolytics (fluphenazine, haloperidol, diazepam)	Affective component of pain
Steroids (dexamethasone)	Cancer pain, nerve compression pain
Bisphosphonates (pamidronate, clodronate)	Pain from metastatic bone disease
Membrane stabilizers (lidocaine, mexiletine, flecainide)	Neuropathic pain

The role of temporary peripheral nerve blocks in chronic pain is understandably limited because pain will return when the block wears off. A series of local anaesthetic injections or nerve blocks, however, are thought to break the cycle of pain, aid mobilisation and physiotherapy, thereby assisting in overall functional improvement.[18] Due to unknown mechanisms, the duration of pain relief sometimes outlasts the duration of action of local anaesthetics and, hence, may have a role in chronic pain management.[18] Peripheral nerve blocks can also be used diagnostically to identify the nerves carrying nociceptive signals and thereby assess the value of blocking the nerve permanently for the treatment of chronic pain.

The administration of nerve blocks should be done under aseptic precautions. Standard monitoring as for any other operation should be used and full resuscitation equipment readily available. Local anaesthetic drugs are used to achieve blockade of nerve transmission. Adjuvants like opioids, clonidine and ketamine are sometimes added to potentiate nerve blocks. The role of steroids is controversial. Care should be taken not to exceed maximal safe doses of local anaesthetics (Table 17.4).

A precise knowledge of anatomy is vital in order to attain an effective block and to avoid complications like intravascular injections and block of neighbouring nerves. Peripheral nerve stimulators are increasingly used to locate nerves with precision and thereby obtain more effective blocks. Nerve blocks using ultrasound guidance are also gaining popularity.

Contraindications for nerve blocks include patient refusal, allergy to local anaesthetics, coagulation abnormalities and infection at the site of administration of the block.

Some of the commonly performed peripheral nerve blocks are summarised in Table 17.5. Detailed descriptions of peripheral nerve blocks can be found in standard textbooks of regional anaesthesia. The axillary brachial plexus block is described as an example to highlight the importance of knowledge of anatomy and complications associated with nerve blocks.

Brachial plexus block (axillary approach). The axillary plexus block is the most commonly performed block for surgical procedures of the upper limb and is safer than other approaches to the brachial plexus. The axillary artery is a continuation of the subclavian artery in the axilla where the median, ulnar and radial nerves (the three major nerves of the upper limb) are related laterally, medially and posteriorly to the artery respectively. With the patient

TABLE 17.4 Maximal safe doses of local anaesthetics	
Agent	Maximum safe dose (mg kg^{-1})
Lidocaine (lignocaine) without adrenaline (epinephrine)	3
Lidocaine (lignocaine) with adrenaline (epinephrine)	7
Bupivacaine	2
Levobupivacaine	2
Ropivacaine	3.5
Tetracaine (amethocaine)	1.5
Cocaine	3
Prilocaine	5

TABLE 17.5 Common peripheral nerve blocks

Nerve blocks	Description
Upper extremity blocks	
Brachial plexus block[23]	Interscalene, supraclavicular, infraclavicular and axillary approaches
	Useful for upper limb surgery, diagnosis and treatment of complex regional pain syndrome type 1 and painful peripheral vascular disorders
	Continuous blockade through a catheter is helpful in prolonging the duration of the block
Wrist block	The ulnar, median and radial nerves can be blocked at the wrist
	Useful for hand surgery
Digital nerve blocks	Block done on the ulnar and radial sides of a digit to block nerve branches entering the digit
	Nerve injury is the main complication
Suprascapular nerve block	Pain relief in rheumatoid arthritis, rotator cuff lesions of the shoulder and arthroscopic shoulder surgery
Lower extremity blocks	
Femoral nerve block	Blockade of the femoral nerve, which lies just lateral to the femoral artery and below the inguinal ligament
	Offers good pain relief in femoral fractures and knee surgery. Combined with sciatic nerve block to provide anaesthesia of entire lower limb
Sciatic nerve block	Approached anteriorly or posteriorly in the thigh to provide anaesthesia of the posterior aspect of thigh and entire leg
Ankle block	Block of 5 nerves (saphenous nerve, deep peroneal nerve, superficial peroneal nerve, tibial nerve and sural nerve)
	Useful in foot surgery
Head and neck blocks	
Gasserian ganglion block	Radiographic guidance is necessary
	Used in treating trigeminal neuralgia and facial cancer pain
Facial nerve block	Relieves spasm of facial muscles following herpes zoster of the facial nerve
Glossopharyngeal nerve block	Useful for pain from malignancies at the base of tongue, epiglottis and palatine tonsils
Superficial cervical plexus block	Useful for pain relief during and after carotid endarterectomies and shoulder surgery
Deep cervical plexus block	Used in cancer pain originating from cervical spine or shoulder
Blocks of the trunk	
Intercostal nerve blocks	Provides analgesia following thoracic and upper abdominal surgery, rib fractures, herpes zoster and cancer
Inguinal nerve block	Ilioinguinal and iliohypogastric nerves are blocked to provide postoperative pain relief after inguinal herniorrhaphy/orchiopexy

supine, the shoulder is abducted and elbow flexed at 90° so that the wrist lies near the patient's head. The axillary artery is palpated as high as possible in the axilla. After proper skin preparation with an antiseptic solution, a local anaesthetic wheal is raised on the skin in front of the artery. A 22-gauge needle is inserted to a position just above the artery. A distinct click is felt when the needle pierces the neurovascular sheath. Paraesthesia is sometimes elicited. A nerve stimulator may be used to locate specific nerves around the artery and response of appropriate muscles looked for. A catheter can be placed through the needle to provide continuous analgesia. Complications of this procedure include nerve damage, intravascular injections and haematoma formation (Fig. 17.3).

Central neuraxial blocks

Central neuraxial blocks include spinal (intrathecal) and epidural blocks. These blocks are used in the perioperative period either alone or in combination with general anaesthesia. They are very popular in obstetric anaesthesia and continuous analgesia, where implanted catheters are employed in chronic pain. A thorough knowledge of spinal anatomy and technical expertise is vital to achieve a successful block and avoid potential complications. Central neural blocks may not be appropriate for all patients. Some of the main contraindications are given in Table 17.6. Besides producing reliable analgesia and motor block for surgery, these blocks have other physiological effects, some of them beneficial (DVT prophylaxis, reduction in stress response) and some detrimental (hypotension). The common physiological alterations noted with central neuraxial blocks are as follows:

1. Cardiovascular system
   Blockade of sympathetic nerves causes hypotension. A high block can involve cardiac accelerator fibres (T1–T4) and cause bradycardia and even cardiac arrest. Patient monitoring and administration of intravenous fluids and vasoconstrictors (e.g. ephedrine, metaraminol and phenylephrine) may be necessary to maintain adequate perfusion to vital organs. A degree of hypotension, however, reduces surgical bleeding. Central neural blocks also reduce the incidence of thromboembolic events following surgery.
2. Respiratory system
   Motor block of abdominal and intercostal muscles can impair the ability to cough. Patients with obstructive airways disease may be dependent on accessory muscles of respiration to exhale actively. These patients may develop respiratory distress due to motor block of these muscles. High

Fig. 17.3 The axillary brachial plexus block. The line marks the position of the axillary artery pulsations

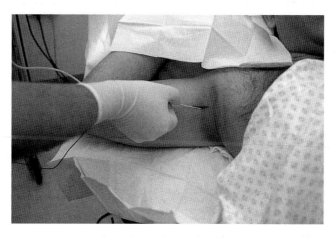

TABLE 17.6 Contraindications to central neuraxial blocks

Absolute	Relative
Patient refusal	Uncooperative patients
Local infections	Psychiatric patients
Septicaemia	Neurological abnormalities
Raised intracranial pressure	Fixed cardiac output lesions (e.g. aortic stenosis, mitral stenosis)
Therapeutic anti-coagulation	Heparin, aspirin and other antiplatelet drugs
Coagulopathy	Prolonged surgery
Hypovolaemic shock	

central blocks can cause apnoea by blockade of the phrenic nerve (C3–C5), but more often apnoea is seen due to brain stem ischaemia secondary to hypotension.

3. Metabolic/endocrine effects

Central neural blocks reduce catecholamine release from the adrenal medulla (in pelvic and lower limb surgery) in response to surgical stimuli and hence reduce complications like hypertension, myocardial ischaemia/infarction and hyperglycaemia.

4. Urinary system

Blockade of the sacral nerve roots (S2–S4) can impair bladder emptying and result in urinary retention.

5. Splanchnic perfusion

Splanchnic blood flow is reduced as a result of reduction in mean arterial pressure, however, this is not often a practical problem due to autoregulation in individual organs.

Spinal (intrathecal/subarachnoid) blocks. As the name indicates, these blocks involve administration of local anaesthetics into the subarachnoid space surrounding the spinal cord. Cerebrospinal fluid (CSF) circulates in this space. Local anaesthetics injected into the CSF act on the spinal nerve roots and prevent neurotransmission. The level of spinal segments blocked will depend on the extent of spread of the drug up the intrathecal space. The spread of local anaesthetic depends on many factors including patient position during injection, posture after injection, dose and volume of drug used and specific gravity of the local anaesthetic solution in relation to CSF (baricity). The duration of action depends on the agent used. Bupivacaine, for example, acts for 120–180 min while lidocaine (lignocaine) acts for 60–90 min. Adding adjuvants like opioids or clonidine can prolong postoperative analgesia.

Intrathecal blocks can be performed with the patient in the sitting or lying (lateral decubitus) position. Strict asepsis has to be maintained throughout the procedure. The patient's back is cleaned with iodine or chlorhexidine solution. The line joining the highest points of the iliac crest passes through the spine of the 4th lumbar vertebra (L4) or the L4–L5 interspace. This line is taken as a guide to count intervertebral spaces upwards. Generally intrathecal injections are done below the L1 level. This is because the spinal cord ends at the L1 level in adults with the intrathecal space extending to S2. The skin over the chosen space is infiltrated in the midline with 2 ml of local anaesthetic, usually lido-caine (lignocaine). An appropriate spinal needle is introduced through this space and advanced until the dura and arachnoid mater are punctured. A give is usually felt on advancing the needle at this point. Needle position in the intrathecal space is confirmed by free flow of CSF through the needle. Local anaesthetic solution is then injected whilst holding the needle in position. A paramedian approach can be used in cases where the midline approach has failed. Both techniques require the skill and experience of an anaesthetist.

Complications of spinal blocks include hypotension, nausea, vomiting, urinary retention, failed blocks, headache and, very rarely, nerve damage. The incidence of headache is directly related to the size of the hole made in the dura. The use of small-diameter, pencil-point needles (typically 24-gauge or smaller) has significantly reduced the incidence of headache. Spinal anaes-thesia is excellent for shorter procedures (less than 2 h) below the umbilicus. Most Caesarean sections are done under spinal anaesthesia. The addition of opioids (e.g. diamorphine) provides longer-lasting analgesia. Spinal anaesthe-sia may not be suitable for prolonged surgery. Intrathecal microcatheters allow continuous local anaesthetic administration and, therefore, prolonged block-ade. This may be appropriate for some prolonged operations. Implantable intrathecal devices are useful in the management of chronic pain.

Epidural (extradural) blocks. The epidural space lies around the spinal cord between the dura mater and the vertebral canal. It extends from the foramen magnum to the sacrococcygeal membrane. This space contains spinal nerve roots, an epidural plexus of veins, spinal arteries, lymphatics and fat. The epidu-ral space is more voluminous than the intrathecal space and large amounts of local anaesthetic solution are required to achieve blocks of similar height when compared with spinal blocks. The advantage with epidural blocks is that cardio-vascular complications (e.g. hypotension) tend to be less dramatic.

Cervical, thoracic, lumbar or caudal epidural blocks can be done to obtain corresponding segmental blocks. The negative pressure seen in the epidural space is made use of in identifying the space using a loss of resistance tech-nique (Fig. 17.4). As with spinals, technical expertise is required and aseptic precautions need to be taken. Placement of epidural catheters allows prolonga-tion of analgesia either with intermittent boluses or continuous infusions of

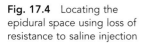
Fig. 17.4 Locating the epidural space using loss of resistance to saline injection

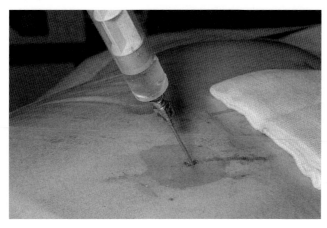

local-anaesthetic solutions. Epidurals are very effective and popular analgesic techniques for labour as well as postoperatively following major abdominal, thoracic or joint-replacement surgery. There is evidence that epidurals confer superior postoperative analgesia when compared to intravenous PCA.[19]

Patient-controlled epidural analgesia

Patient-controlled epidural analgesia (PCEA) is the epidural counterpart of intravenous patient-controlled analgesia (PCA). The technique is also occasionally used to test the response of chronic pain patients to neuraxial analgesia prior to considering implantable intrathecal drug-delivery systems. PCEA allows the patient to administer intermittent boluses of local anaesthetic solution (usually with an opioid) into the epidural space through a pump and catheter when needed. The bolus dose, lockout interval and background infusion can be programmed on the pump as with PCA. The advantage of PCEA over continuous infusions is the titration of agent to effect, thus minimising the dose of drug used (local anaesthetic and opioid).[20]

Implantable intrathecal drug-delivery systems[21]

Implantable intrathecal drug-delivery systems (IDDS) are small battery-powered pumps, which are implanted under the skin of the abdomen. They deliver small doses of morphine directly into the spinal fluid in the intrathecal space through a catheter that is tunnelled under the skin. The advantage of these devices is that pain relief can be achieved with much smaller doses than with oral and parenteral routes. IDDS improves clinical success in pain control, reduces pain, relieves common drug toxicities and improves survival in patients with refractory cancer pain.[21] IDDS are also used in failed back syndromes, phantom limb pain and complex regional pain syndromes.[22] Most pain physicians allow a trial period of 1–2 weeks with a temporary intrathecal catheter and portable pump to predict the potential success of an implanted device. Morphine is commonly used in these pumps, though bupivacaine and clonidine have also been tried. Baclofen is used in IDDS for treating painful spasms of multiple sclerosis and spinal cord injuries.[22] Pump refills will be needed when the drug runs out and can be done percutaneously.

Complications of implantable devices include infection, catheter dislodgement, disconnections, kinks and breakages and drug side effects like sedation, hypotension, nausea and vomiting.

Local anaesthetic infiltrations and field blocks

Subcutaneous infiltration with local anaesthetic is useful in herpes zoster, neuromas and other subcutaneous nodular or fibrotic pains.[23] Field blocks with local anaesthesia are less invasive, safe and provide good analgesia for various surgical procedures (e.g. inguinal hernia repair).[24] It is now customary to inject local anaesthetic solutions into the edges of the surgical wound at the end of surgery. This practice provides a significant reduction in postoperative pain and analgesic requirement.[24]

Trigger point injections

Myofascial pain syndrome is characterised by pain on movement of the affected muscles and reproduction of pain on palpation of well-localised trigger points within the muscle.[25] These are often located in the neck, back and shoulders. Small volumes of local anaesthetic (1–3 ml) are injected after palpation of these tender points. The mechanism of action of trigger point injections is not clearly known, but this technique can relieve pain and improve mobility.

Intravenous regional anaesthesia

Commonly known as Bier's block, this procedure provides anaesthesia for interventions of short duration (less than 1 h) in the forearm or foot. A vein is chosen as close as possible to the surgical site and a cannula inserted. A pneumatic tourniquet is placed around the arm or calf and inflated to 100 mmHg above the patient's systolic blood pressure. Local anaesthetic solution (20–40 ml) is injected slowly. Prilocaine 0.5% is the only local anaesthetic licensed for use in IVRA in the UK.

Complications are rare with this procedure if care is taken to make sure that the tourniquet is reliable and the cuff remains inflated for at least 20 min after injection of the local anaesthetic. Transient light headedness or tinnitus is sometimes noted. Bier's blocks using guanethidine is employed to diagnose sympathetically mediated pain. Their use in the treatment of sympathetic pain, however, lacks conclusive evidence.[26]

Ablative neuronal blockade

Cryoanalgesia

Cryoanalgesia is a technique of destruction of peripheral nerves by extreme cold for relief of pain. The physics behind cryoanalgesia is the Joule Thompson effect, which states that a drop in temperature is produced when a gas (nitrous oxide or carbon dioxide) under pressure is ejected through a nozzle.[27] Cryo-probe temperatures of as low as $-70°$ C are used to bring about degeneration of nerves. Since the nerve sheaths are not destroyed, the nerves eventually regenerate. The resultant conduction block provides analgesia lasting up to a few months. The nerves to be blocked are approached either percutaneously using a nerve stimulator or picked up under direct vision during surgery. Cryoanalgesia is simple to perform and economical.

Cryoanalgesia of branches of the trigeminal nerve is effective in providing pain relief for facial pain from head and neck cancers, trigeminal neuralgia and postherpetic neuralgia.[28] It also has a role in the treatment of neuropathic pain (e.g. pain from stump neuromas following amputations).

Percutaneous radiofrequency thermocoagulation

A radiofrequency current is employed with this technique to produce heat and destroy peripheral or central nerves.

The indications for RFTC are similar to cryoanalgesia. RFTC has been used for spinal facet joint denervations and thoracic and lumbar sympathectomies for conditions like hyperhidrosis, complex regional pain syndromes (CRPS), phantom limb pain and peripheral vascular disease.[29] RFTC involves placement of an insulated electrode shaft with an uninsulated tip into the nervous tissue. A generator source allows current to pass in and heat the surrounding tissues. The electrode itself does not get heated up. The RFTC machine is also capable of electrically stimulating the nerve and thereby helps in locating the nerve. Typically, temperatures of the order of 80–90°C are used for 60–90 s.[29] RFTC can be performed percutaneously on an outpatient basis with intravenous sedation and monitoring.

Complications are less frequent and procedures can be repeated if needed. RFTC destroys only the peripheral process of the axon and leaves the nerve architecture intact. Hence the nerve can regenerate with time. Neuropathic pain from nerve regeneration is a possibility that has raised concerns and paved the way for pulsed radiofrequency. This technique is currently under evaluation and involves application of pulses of radiofrequency current for a short duration (30 ms) with output adjusted to achieve temperatures not more than 42°C.[22]

Neurolytic blocks[29]

Neurolytic blocks use chemical agents to bring about destruction of nerve fibres or ganglia. Commonly used agents include phenol, ethyl alcohol and chlorocresol. They act by bringing about protein denaturation and extraction of membrane phospholipids. These agents are not selective and affect sensory, motor and autonomic nerve fibres. Nerve regeneration occurs as long as the cell body is intact. Nerve sprouting and neuroma formation are complications of these blocks. Pain, sometimes central, recurs in most patients in weeks to months. Motor block, autonomic dysfunction and unintentional destruction of adjacent tissues make these blocks unpopular for routine use. These blocks are reserved for patients who are unresponsive to noninvasive management and those who have terminal illnesses with limited life expectancy.

Peripheral nerve neurolysis has been employed successfully to treat pain from stump neuromas, intercostal neuralgias and entrapment syndrome. Neurolytic block via the interscalene or supraclavicular routes is useful in treating cancer pain involving the brachial plexus (e.g. Pancoast's tumour).[30] Trigeminal ganglion or peripheral branches of the trigeminal nerve can be ablated for treatment of trigeminal neuralgia or facial pain from inoperable cancers.[30] Intrathecal and epidural neurolytic blocks have been used for the treatment of pain and spasticity. With intrathecal neurolysis, there is a risk of permanent spinal cord damage with loss of motor, bowel, bladder and sexual functions.[29]

Neurolysis has been successfully used in the management of sympathetic pain of peripheral vascular disease, CRPS, Raynaud's disease and CREST syndrome. Sympathetic blockade can be achieved at the stellate ganglion, thoracic sympathetic or lumbar sympathetic levels. The coeliac plexus block prevents afferents and sympathetic fibres at the coeliac axis and is particularly effective in relieving pain from pancreatic and other upper abdominal cancers.

Fluoroscopy or computerised tomography (CT) guidance is often needed for successful administration of these blocks. Before embarking on neurolytic techniques, it is customary to do at least one diagnostic block with a local anaesthetic solution to confirm pain pathways and assess potential efficacy of neurolytic blockade.

Surgical techniques

In general, surgical techniques are used as a last resort as they are often irreversible and some of the results are very poor. They are reserved for patients who have not responded to noninvasive modes of treatment. Patients' consent and fitness for surgery are important. Very ill, debilitated patients may be unsuitable for surgical interventions. As with other neuroablative techniques, a diagnostic block should be performed to identify the involved pathways of pain and assess the value of surgical ablation. Some of the surgical interventions are briefly discussed below.

Neurectomies

Peripheral and cranial nerves have been severed surgically to treat cancer pain. Painful neuromas, loss of motor function and denervation hypersensitivity (development of severe pain and allodynia in the nerve territory) are some of the problems encountered with this technique.

Rhizotomies

These involve surgical division of the dorsal roots of spinal nerves. They are useful for painful malignancies, which are restricted to a particular dermatome.

Complications include infection, bleeding, spinal-cord infarction and CSF fistulae. Rhizotomies of trigeminal and glossopharyngeal nerves have been described for facial and oral cancers.[31]

Dorsal root entry zone lesions

These involve surgical lesioning of the dorsal horn of the spinal cord where neurones carrying nociceptive and thermal sensations enter. They are used mainly in the treatment of some types of neuropathic pain. These procedures are very invasive and evidence of benefit is lacking.

Cordotomy

This involves lesioning the anterolateral quadrant of the spinal cord that contain ascending tracts carrying pain and temperature signals to the brain.[32]

Cordotomies are indicated for unilateral cancer pain. Bilateral cordotomies can be performed for bilateral lesions. The procedure is usually performed percutaneously under fluoroscopic guidance with radiofrequency probes. Complications of this procedure include bladder and bowel dysfunction, sexual dysfunction, ataxia, paresis and sleep apnoea.

Microvasculature decompression

This is by far the most successful surgical procedure for trigeminal neuralgia.[32] It is reserved for patients who do not respond to medical management. It involves relieving compression of the trigeminal nerve by a branch of artery or vein at its point of entry in the pons. Complications of this procedure include hearing loss, CSF leak and transient cranial nerve palsies.

Stimulation analgesia

Transcutaneous electrical nerve stimulation

Small pulses of low-voltage electric current are used to stimulate the area of pain or ascending nerve tracts by placing electrodes on the skin. This usually results in the development of a pleasant paraesthesia in the field of stimulation. The mechanism of action of TENS remains unclear and is partly explained by the gate theory of pain.

The machine's stimulation frequency can be increased or decreased according to the patient's needs. The duration of each pulse of electricity can be adjusted along with its frequency. This can be used continuously or periodically several times a day. The equipment is easy to use and has few side effects. Caution must be exercised in patients with implanted cardiac pacemakers. TENS is widely used as an adjunct in analgesia during labour. It is used in many chronic pain states including myofascial syndromes, mechanical back and neck pain, joint pains and stump pains (Fig. 17.5). See also Chapter 10.

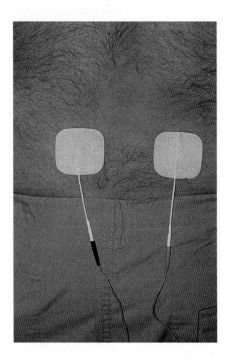

Fig. 17.5 Transcutaneous electrical nerve stimulation (TENS) electrodes applied for stimulation of the lower back in mechanical back pain.

Acupuncture

This method of pain relief has been used in China for over 2000 years. It involves insertion of needles into anatomically defined points called meridians. These points can be stimulated electrically or by digital pressure (acupressure). Acupuncture can be carried out in the area of pain or in entirely unrelated parts of the body that are thought to cause relaxation when stimulated. See also Chapter 10.

Spinal-cord stimulation[22]

This is also called dorsal-column stimulation. It involves insertion of electrodes into the epidural space and placement on the dura mater. When stimulated the patient feels paraesthesia in the area of their pain. An implanted impulse generator is used to stimulate the electrodes. The mechanism of action is unclear. It is thought to mobilise gamma-aminobutyric acid (GABA) and adenosine, restore GABA levels and inhibit afferent activity in the spinothalamic tracts. Though spinal-cord stimulation (SCS) has been tried for many conditions, clear indications are currently:

- intractable angina
- CRPS that has not responded to other treatments
- failed back surgery syndrome
- neuropathic pain
- nonreconstructable peripheral vascular disease.

A trial period with an external generator is often employed to assess the effectiveness of SCS undertaken before proceeding to an implanted generator.

Deep brain stimulation

This is a highly specialised neurosurgical technique that involves stereotactic implantation of electrodes into the periaqueductal/periventricular grey area or thalamic nuclei. They are usually kept as a last resort for intractable cancer pain and rarely used for nonmalignant pain. Intracranial haemorrhage and infection are potential complications of this procedure.

Physiotherapy

Pain often leads to reduction in activity and immobility and thereby muscle and joint stiffness, wasting and weakness of muscles, osteoporosis, physical impairment and disability. Encouragement of activity as early as possible and promotion of normal everyday living is the modern approach to pain as opposed to complete bed rest.

The physiotherapist plays a major role in achieving this objective. Massage, passive and active stretching of muscles, manipulation, mobilisation and exercise training are employed to enhance the range of joint movement and strengthen muscles. This is often supplemented with exercise programmes, and pacing and graded progression of activity to support the face-to-face work with the physiotherapist.

The use of analgesics and local anaesthetic injections can reduce pain and aid physiotherapy, which in turn improves physical function.

Psychological interventions

Pain is a sensory and emotional experience. There is subjective variation in individuals' responses to pain and pain management. Psychological and social factors play a major role in pain perception. Unresolved grief, stress and previous sexual abuse can adversely affect an individuals' ability to cope with pain. The majority of patients with pain, especially of a chronic nature have high levels of anxiety and distress. Management of pain will be successful only if these psychological components are addressed. Psychological interventions are not limited to chronic pain alone. There is evidence that cognitive behavioural methods can reduce pain and distress in acute pain.[18] Psychological preparation before surgery, for instance, can reduce postoperative analgesic requirements. For a more detailed discussion of psychology refer to Chapter 15.

Stress reduction and relaxation techniques[33]

A gentle, caring and supportive approach by physicians and nurses goes a long way in reducing some of the affective components of pain. Relaxation methods can be helpful in alleviating stress associated with pain. Some of the common relaxation techniques include calm or diaphragmatic breathing, muscle tension and release exercises, pleasant mental imagery (self-hypnosis) and meditation.

Cognitive behavioural therapy

This is a term applied to treatments that aim to reduce factors that maintain the patients' maladaptive behaviours, beliefs and thought patterns. Cognitive behavioural therapy (CBT) increases patients' coping and problem-solving skills, improves their health habits and helps them get along with their normal lives.[33] CBT programmes are conducted in an outpatient setting and usually consist of weekly sessions run over varying periods of time. There is considerable evidence that CBT is effective in reducing the distress associated with chronic pain.[34]

Marital/family psychotherapy

A dysfunctional family may be part of the reason for a patient's emotional problem. Sometimes, patients' illnesses and distresses can impact on their partners and children. Group- or family-based psychological interventions may be appropriate in such cases.[33]

Pain-management programmes

Multidisciplinary pain-management programmes have been developed in an effort to enhance patients' physical performance and help them with coping strategies. Most of these programmes use CBT to change patients' attitudes, beliefs and behaviour in relation to pain. These programmes include progressive muscle relaxation therapy, goal setting and pacing, group cognitive therapy, education about the physiology and the pharmacology of pain, and progressive supervised physiotherapy exercises.[2]

Summary

Pain is multidimensional. It has sensory, affective, cognitive, behavioural and social components. While analgesia is the primary aim in the treatment of acute pain, management of chronic pain involves a multidisciplinary approach that includes pharmacological, physical and psychological interventions.

Invasive methods of pain relief in general and surgical methods in particular have limitations with regard to benefit and have well-recognised complications. They should only be selected as part of a management strategy that will usually involve noninvasive interventions as well.

KEY POINTS

- Pain management is multimodal and may include analgesics, neuronal blockade, physiotherapy and psychological interventions
- PCA is extremely popular in the management of postoperative pain where its safety and efficacy are well established
- Peripheral nerve blocks are more commonly used in the management of acute pain especially in the perioperative setting
- In chronic pain a series of local nerve blocks are thought to break the cycle of pain, aid mobilisation and physiotherapy, thereby assisting in overall functional improvement[18]
- A thorough knowledge of anatomy is required to perform regional blocks
- Clinical dexterity is important when positioning regional block needles
- Surgical techniques are often used as a last resort as they are often irreversible and some of the results are very poor

References

1. Carr DB, Goudas LC Acute pain. *Lancet* 1999; **353**(9169): 2051–2058.
2. Nurmikko TJ, Nash TP, Wiles JR. Recent advances: control of chronic pain. *BMJ* 1998; **317**(7170): 1438–1441.
3. Dubner R, Ruda MA. Activity-dependent neuronal plasticity following tissue injury and inflammation. *Trends Neurosci* 1992; **15**(3): 96–103.
4. Wu CL et al. Correlation of postoperative pain to quality of recovery in the immediate postoperative period. *Reg Anesth Pain Med* 2005; **30**(6): 516–522.
5. Ashburn MA, Staats PS. Management of chronic pain. *Lancet* 1999; **353**(9167): 1865–1869.
6. Desborough JP. The stress response to trauma and surgery. *Br J Anaesth* 2000; **85**(1): 109–117.
7. Liu S, Carpenter RL, Neal JM. Epidural anesthesia and analgesia. Their role in postoperative outcome. *Anesthesiol* 1995; **82**(6): 1474–1506.
8. Anand KJ, Hickey PR. Pain and its effects in the human neonate and fetus. *N Engl J Med* 1987; **317**(21): 1321–1329.
9. Brodner G, Aken HV, Hertle L et al. Multimodal perioperative management – combining thoracic epidural analgesia, forced mobilization, oral nutrition – reduces hormonal and metabolic stress and improves convalescence after major urologic surgery. *Anesth Analg* 2001; **92**(6): 1594–1600.
10. World Health Organization. *National cancer control programmes: Policies and managerial guidelines*. Geneva: World Health Organization; 2002.
11. Amesbury B. Pain control in advanced cancer. In: Dolin SJ, Padfield NL (eds) *Pain medicine manual*, 2nd edn. Edinburgh: Butterworth-Heinemann; 2004: 257–266.
12. Macintyre PE. Safety and efficacy of patient-controlled analgesia. *Br J Anaesth* 2001; **87**(1): 36–46.
13. Ballantyne JC, Carr DB, Chalmers TC et al. Postoperative patient-controlled analgesia: meta-analyses of initial randomized control trials. *J Clin Anesth* 1993; **5**(3): 182–193.
14. McQuay HJ, Tramer M, Nye BA et al. A systematic review of antidepressants in neuropathic pain. *Pain* 1996; **68**: 217–227.
15. Onghena P, Van Houdenhove B. Antidepressant-induced analgesia in chronic non-malignant pain: a meta-analysis of 39 placebo-controlled studies. *Pain* 1992; **49**(2): 205–219.
16. Woolf CJ, Mannion RJ. Neuropathic pain: aetiology, symptoms, mechanisms, management. *Lancet* 1999; **353**(9168): 1959–1964.
17. Bonica JJ, Buckley FP. Regional analgesia with local anaesthetics. In: Bonica JJ (ed.) *The management of pain*, 2nd edn. Philadelphia: Lee and Febiger; 1990: 1883–1966.
18. McQuay HJ, Moore RA. *An evidence based resource for pain relief*. Oxford: Oxford University Press; 1998.
19. Wu CL, Cohen SR, Richman JM et al. Efficacy of postoperative patient-controlled and continuous infusion epidural analgesia versus intravenous patient-controlled analgesia with opioids: a meta-analysis. *Anesthesiol* 2005; **103**(5): 1079–88; quiz 1109–1110.
20. Cohen S, Amar D, Pantuck CB et al. Postcesarean delivery epidural patient-controlled analgesia. Fentanyl or sufentanil? *Anesthesiol* 1993; **78**(3): 486–491.
21. Smith TJ, Staats PS, Deer T et al. Randomized clinical trial of an implantable drug delivery system compared with comprehensive medical management for refractory cancer pain: impact on pain, drug-related toxicity, survival. *J Clin Oncol* 2002; **20**(19): 4040–4049.
22. Dolin SJ, Padfield NL. Invasive procedures: technical details. In: Dolin SJ, Padfield NL (eds) *Pain medicine manual*, 2nd edition. Edinburgh: Butterworth-Heinemann; 2004: 297–349.

23. Raj PP. Prognostic and therapeutic local anaesthetic blockade. In: Cousins MJ, Bridenbaugh PO (eds) *Neural blockade*, 2nd edition. Philidelphia: JB Lippincott; 1988: 899–933.

24. Dahl JB, Frederiksen HJ. Wound infiltration for operative and postoperative analgesia. *Curr Opinion Anesthesiol* 1995; **8**: 435–440.

25. Hogan QH, Abram SE. Neural blockade for diagnosis and prognosis. A review. *Anesthesiology* 1997; **86**(1): 216–241.

26. Jadad AR, Carroll D, Glynn C et al. Intravenous regional sympathetic blockade for pain relief in reflex sympathetic dystrophy: a systematic review and a randomized, double-blind crossover study. *J Pain Symptom Manage* 1995; **10**(1): 13–20.

27. Raj PP. Cryoanalgesia. In: Raj PP (ed.) *Practical management of pain*. Chicago: Yearbook Medical Publishers; 1986: 774–782.

28. Cousins MJ, Dwyer B, Gibb D. Chronic pain and neurolytic neural blockade. In: Cousins MJ, Bridenbaugh PO (eds) *Neural blockade*, 2nd edn Philidelphia: JB Lippincott; 1988: 1053–1084.

29. Shipton EA (ed.) *Interventional therapy*. In: *Pain – acute and chronic*, 2nd edition. London: Arnold; 1999: 232–247.

30. Budd K. Abortive nerve blocks and neurosurgical techniques. In: Nimmo WS, Smith G (eds) *Anaesthesia*. Oxford: Blackwell Scientific Publications; 1989: 1243–1264.

31. Loeser JD, Sweet WH, Tew JM. Neurosurgical operations involving peripheral nerves. In: Bonica JJ (ed.) *The management of pain*. Philidelphia: Lea and Febiger; 1990: 2044–2066.

32. Shipton EA. Surgical intervention. In: Shipton EA (ed.) *Pain – acute and chronic*, 2nd edn. London: Arnold; 1999: 270–281.

33. Skidmore JR. Psychological interventions for medical patients in pain. In: Dolin SJ, Padfield NL (eds) *Pain medicine manual*, 2nd edn Edinburgh: Butterworth-Heinemann; 2004: 281–287.

34. Eccleston C. Role of psychology in pain management. *Br J Anaesth* 2001; **87**(1): 144–152.

Keith Milligan

Management strategies

This chapter will look at clinical situations in various areas where pain management may be required and will highlight key learning points for each scenario.

Pain management in the community

The first point of contact for many patients in pain is the primary care team in the community and good pain management can often help avoid admission to secondary care.

Acute pain I

LEARNING POINT

Titrating intravenous opiates in this situation not only relieves pain but forms part of the early treatment of cardiac pain and should be given before hospital admission to try to reduce morbidity.

One of the commonest presentations is probably myocardial ischaemia and good pain management is essential to reduce the effects of increased catecholamine release, which can cause systemic hypertension, tachycardia, anxiety and breathlessness. Intravenous opiates form an integral part of the early management of acute cardiac pain and form part of the medical management of the condition.

Acute pain II

Many patients in the community have intermittent but regular acute, severe pain; for example, patients with persistent, infected leg ulcers that may require dressing changes two to three times a day. Between dressing changes there may be very little pain and it is, therefore, inappropriate to use large doses of long-acting opiates to manage 30-min episodes of acute pain. In this situation it is more appropriate to use *oramorph* (short-acting, quick-onset morphine) timed to have maximum effect at the anticipated time of the dressing change (administered 30 min before). If oral opiates are inadequate or limited by persistent side effects (e.g. nausea, vomiting and sedation) then consider the use of *entonox* (an inhaled analgesic consisting of oxygen and nitrous oxide as a 50:50 mixture) as an adjuvant to provide intense analgesia at the required time.

Chronic pain

Chronic pain is probably the commonest reason that patients consult with the general practitioner (GP) and the community team. As chronic pain by definition has been present for a long period of time (longer than 3 months) and is unlikely to suddenly get better it requires a different approach (mind-set) from the clinician. It is often difficult to gauge pain severity in the chronic pain patient, but pain scoring using a visual analogue scale (VAS) or verbal rating scale (VRS) may guide initial therapy. It is important to take a proper pain history as this can help differentiate between nociceptive and neuropathic pain and again may point the clinician towards different treatments.

Symptom control is important in chronic pain and should focus on appropriate drug management alongside functional restoration (e.g. sustained-release drugs as opposed to immediate release to provide background analgesia with or without co-analgesics). The clinician and patient must recognise that complete pain relief is an unrealistic goal and that the aim with any treatment is to get the *'best fit'* between pain relief and side effects. Many patients will comment that the therapy takes *'the edge off the pain'* but does not take it away.

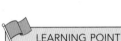

Some patients may benefit from a trial of opiate medication after appropriate screening. It is important that both the patient and doctor are aware of the risks and benefits. Other treatments could also include the use of transcutaneous electrical nerve stimulation (TENS). Longer term, the focus should be on pain management, which includes advice on appropriate exercise, pacing and reducing sickness behaviour. Onward referral to secondary care for expert advice on symptom management (which might include invasive therapies) and pain management (programmes including psychology and physiotherapy) should be considered where the patient fails to respond to simple measures.

Low back pain is the commonest form of chronic pain presentation and is usually triaged using a system of red and yellow flags to recognise the degree of medical seriousness of the condition and the level of psychosocial distress. If there is no requirement for further investigation (red flags) then functional restoration in conjunction with pain relief (yellow flags) and early return to work is the aim of treatment.

Simple neuropathic pain

LEARNING POINT

Sleep disturbance is a common feature of chronic pain in general and neuropathic pain in particular. If using tricyclic antidepressants they are best prescribed at night and titrated to 'best fit' for pain relief, sleep and side effects.

These pains are underdiagnosed and undertreated, apart from the obvious neuropathic pain syndromes (postherpetic neuralgia, trigeminal neuralgia and, to a lesser extent, diabetic neuropathy). Diagnosing neuropathic pain may be difficult, but is important, as the treatment can be completely different to nociceptive pain. The diagnosis is usually made on the history and symptoms such as burning, shooting pain, pins and needles, skin sensitivity, etc. There may be physical signs, such as allodynia, paraesthesia, altered temperature, sweating and colour indicative of a regional pain syndrome. Treatment options include a trial of tricyclic antidepressant medication in low dosage (amitriptyline 10–50 mg nocte) or an anticonvulsant (gabapentin 1200–1800 mg/day). Most clinicians start low and go slow when titrating. Neuropathic pain can also respond to opiate medication, but this is unlikely to be the first line of management.

Pain management in the Accident and Emergency Department

Patients often present in the Accident and Emergency Unit with acute pain following trauma. Pain should be assessed where possible using an appropriate tool, for example, 10 cm VAS, VRS or face, legs, activity, cry, consolability (FLACC)[1] scale in the case of younger children. This offers a baseline pain score and should indicate the appropriate analgesic intervention.

After minor trauma it is usually appropriate to administer oral analgesic including paracetamol and nonsteroidal anti-inflammatory drugs (NSAIDs) where not contraindicated.

If the more severely injured patient requires analgesia then opiates should be given intravenously and titrated against effect. It is difficult to justify the administration of intramuscular or subcutaneous analgesia in the trauma patient unless it is not possible to secure intravenous access. This is because the recently injured patient may be in shock and the intramuscular injection may not be released into the circulation for some hours, possibly after repeated injection due to persistent pain. These are the perfect conditions required to produce delayed respiratory depression and significant morbidity.

LEARNING POINT

The titration of intravenous opiates is the quickest and probably safest way of administering opiate medication.

The presentation of the patient will often dictate the type of intervention required. Special consideration of the use of opiates is required in the presence of a head injury as opiates can mask the signs of raised intracranial pressure.

Acute pain on the trauma ward

LEARNING POINT

Fractures are usually most painful before fixation and pain should be treated particularly if there is any delay before surgery.

Most inpatients on a trauma ward have suffered fractures, which may be single or multiple. As a rule of thumb – these will be very painful until immobilised by surgical fixation or put in a cast. Prior to fixation it is important to treat pain adequately. This is not so much of a challenge in the younger patient as they usually tolerate opiates by intravenous titration very well. However, the elderly patient with a fractured neck of femur is often frail and less tolerant of opiates and NSAIDs. A local nerve block in experienced (usually anaesthetic) hands can be administered in the form of a femoral 3-in-1 block, which allows movement of the patient prior to surgical fixation and reduces the amount of anaesthesia required during surgery.

Most fractures are managed with intravenous morphine either intermittently or with patient-controlled analgesia (PCA) after open reduction with internal fixation. Closed and manipulated fractures usually respond to simple intermittent oral analgesics.

Complex regional pain syndrome

Complex regional pain syndrome (CRPS) is a neuropathic pain syndrome that is frequently missed. There is often an injury or an event that causes immobilisation (type 1 CRPS). CRPS usually includes pain, allodynia (pain response to non-painful stimulus) or hyperalgesia (heightened response to a painful stimulus). There may be skin blood-flow changes and altered sweating in the affected area. Oedema is also a common feature of this condition.

Nerve injury may also include the above features and has been described as causalgia (type 2 CRPS) and the pain may extend beyond the area of the nerve distribution.

Pain and loss of function are the main features of this condition and it may progress through a hyperaemic phase into a more permanent dystrophic phase over weeks or months.

Treatment is difficult, but requires early recognition and a combination of measures to reduce pain, while intensive physiotherapy is utilised to try to restore function (reactivation and desensitisation). Pain-relieving measures include sympathetic nerve blocks (stellate ganglion and lumbar sympathetic nerve blocks) that may improve regional blood flow and reduce sudomotor disturbance. Drug treatments include use of tricyclic antidepressants and anticonvulsants titrated against pain relief, sleep and side effects. The drugs that are usually used include amitriptyline (10–75 mg at night) and gabapentin (1200–1800 mg/day in divided doses). If there is limited or no response then titration of conventional analgesics through the WHO analgesic ladder is recommended.[2]

As this syndrome is often characterised by increased autonomic activity, there is a place for the use of psychology and, in particular, cognitive behavioural therapy to try to suppress the adrenaline (epinephrine) response to pain or 'potential' pain. Fear of re-injury can be a potent barrier to recovery in certain patients.

> **LEARNING POINT**
>
> CRPS type 1 is often not recognised in the early phase and this can cause significant morbidity; early recognition and treatment is the key to successful resolution of symptoms.

Acute pain after day surgery

The anaesthetist will have considered the peri- and postoperative analgesic regimen required prior to surgery, using the concept of balanced analgesia, including one or more of the following combinations:

- Intravenous opiates
- NSAIDs
- Local anaesthetic blockade
- Adjuvant analgesic such as paracetamol.

In most cases the postoperative analgesic regimen will consist of simple oral analgesics, such as codeine paracetamol combinations (e.g. co-codamol 30/500) ± NSAIDs. These are suitable drugs to be used for take-home analgesia in day surgery.

The aim is to achieve the four 'A's prior to home discharge:

- Ambulant
- Alert
- Alimentation
- Analgesic.

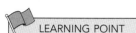

LEARNING POINT

Day surgery is becoming more prevalent and more complicated (hernias, varicose veins, cholecystectomy and spinal surgery) and can only be successful if the four 'A's are rigorously observed.

Patients must be eating and drinking and not be nauseous. They will be able to self-care, including basic hygiene and toileting. Patients need to be comfortable not just at rest, but also on movement. It is important that follow-on analgesia is prescribed and used especially if local anaesthetic blockade has allowed early discharge. Pain can increase rapidly as local anaesthetic wears off and analgesics should be readily available for the patient. Patient and carer both need to be advised in appropriate use of the analgesics prescribed.

Pain after major abdominal surgery

Poor pain management after abdominal surgery can have dire consequences for the patient and should never be ignored. The patient in pain after major surgery will not breathe well due to diaphragmatic splinting and will be relatively immobile. Lung atelectasis, pulmonary embolus, pneumonia, hypoxia, wound and anastomotic dehiscence, unscheduled further surgery and ITU admission may occur when pain is a major feature after big operations.

Nurse-controlled intramuscular injection

Nurse-controlled intramuscular injection is how pain has been traditionally managed over the years. The clinician prescribes the analgesia and the patient complains of pain to the nurse who administers the drug to the patient as prescribed. This is unreliable, as it requires appropriate prescribing by the clinician who may not see the patient at the time the drug is dispensed. It requires the nurse to recognise that the patient is in pain and to offer the right drug, in the right quantity, at the right interval and to monitor the response to treatment.

Nurse-controlled intravenous injection

Nurse-controlled intravenous injection has superseded the use of intramuscular injections in many establishments and is inherently safer, as the nurse is able to titrate the patient to comfort very quickly and observe for signs of overdose and manage them appropriately. This is usually protocol driven for safety and efficacy.

Patient-controlled analgesia

Patient-controlled analgesia (PCA) has become the standard technique in the management of postoperative pain. It requires the patient to be 'loaded' with analgesia at the start and then allows the patient to 'top-up' analgesia as required via a PCA machine. A typical adult regimen being 60 mg morphine diluted to 60 ml in 0.9% saline attached to a machine programmed to deliver 1 mg on demand with a 5 min lockout. The safety factor is that it is very difficult to keep pressing the demand button and the patient is likely to be sedated before delivering an overdose of morphine. There may be an added safety measure by limiting the amount of morphine that can be delivered in any 4-h period.

Patients need to be encouraged to self medicate so that they are comfortable not just at rest, but also on movement. The limiting factor with PCA has always been the nausea produced by the morphine and some patients may choose not to press the button because of this. It is important that the patient is monitored for this and appropriate antiemetics delivered before they get into the cycle of pain, hypoventilation, lung atelectasis, pneumonia and hypoxia.

Patient-controlled epidural analgesia

Patient-controlled epidural infusion analgesia (PCEA) has revolutionised major surgery over the last 10 years or so. The combination of low-dose opiate and local anaesthetic epidural infusion has become established practice in the UK. Most regimens also allow the patient a controlled bolus facility for top-up analgesia. With appropriate monitoring for side effects and complications (protocol driven) this has proved to be hugely beneficial in reducing morbidity and mortality.

Standard practice is for the anaesthetist to establish epidural analgesia just prior to surgery and use it alongside the anaesthetic, allowing much lower amounts of anaesthetic and also reducing the stress response to surgery. The level of insertion of the epidural is dictated by the level of surgery, but is usually high lumbar or low thoracic if an upper abdominal incision is used. A typical postoperative regimen might be an infusion of 0.1% bupivacaine with 2 μg per ml fentanyl at a rate of 8 ml/h with a bolus of 6 ml and a 20-min lockout before a further bolus can be delivered.

The most feared complication of delayed respiratory depression is very rare using regimens with fentanyl or diamorphine as the opiate and higher if epidural morphine is used. The most frequent complication is hypotension as a result of hypovolaemia and is simply managed with a fluid bolus before drastic measures, such as stopping the epidural infusion. Other concerns include a dense block, which could be due to epidural haematoma (patients on low-molecular-weight heparin) and this dictates when the catheter is removed. Under these circumstances more experienced assistance is urgently required from the acute pain team (often the duty anaesthetist).

Because the quality of the analgesia is so good, it is best to leave the epidural running until the patient can be transferred to an oral regimen. It is important to give oral medication at the time of discontinuing the infusion and not wait for pain to start. Some patients will complain of sore throat (anaesthetic complication) and shoulder-tip pain (pneumoperitoneum), which respond to supplementary paracetamol and NSAIDs (rectal or intravenous). It is important that oral opiates are not administered concurrently with the epidural infusion as this can increase the risk of respiratory depression.

Chronic pain after surgery

Hernia

Pain after inguinal hernia repair is a well-recognised complication of surgery and often has the features of neuropathic pain. The patient will often be told that they have a trapped nerve, but this implies that surgery can relieve the symptoms. The usual presentation is hypoaesthesia, with a burning sensation and very occasionally lancinating pain. Local anaesthetic and steroid combinations for scar pain may be successful in reducing symptoms, but generally this develops into a chronic pain problem that may require ongoing treatment with drugs for neuropathic pain. Further surgery is often unhelpful as the nerve injury is usually related to scar tissue and this will reform after re-exploration.

Post-vasectomy pain

This is a common complication of male sterilisation with pain ranging from mild to severe and is often debilitating. Simple analgesics are frequently insufficient, a range of other treatments are considered including trial of TENS, diagnostic lumbar sympathectomies and drug treatments in the form of tricyclic antidepressants and anticonvulsants.

Failed back-surgery syndrome

This typically presents early after operations on the lumbar spine and has two main features, which are chronic low back pain (often described as mechanical) and neuropathic leg pain. Treatment is dictated by the severity of the pain and disability, but usually involves efforts at pain control and rehabilitation. The back pain may be managed by transcutaneous electrical nerve stimulation (TENS) and conventional analgesic regimens progressing upwards through the analgesic ladder. Pain blocks, such as steroid epidurals, lumbar sympathectomies, nerve root blocks and facet blocks may be employed as a diagnostic and short-term therapeutic measure to try to encourage rehabilitation.

With increasing chronicity treatment focuses more on pain-management techniques, such as pain-management programmes, which require input from clinical psychology, occupational therapy and physiotherapy.

Post coronary artery bypass surgery

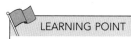

LEARNING POINT

Chronic pain after apparently successful surgical treatments can be a major cause of concern for the patient and can be extraordinarily difficult to manage, particularly as this did not form part of the patient's expectations prior to surgery.

Despite apparently successful surgery there are a small number of patients who continue to complain of chest pain after cardiac surgery. The pain is rarely 'angina' and can be due to a variety of causes including scar pain (characterised by an 'active'-looking keloid-type scar), sternal pain (often pain from the sternal wires) and neuropathic pain from the harvesting of the left internal mammary artery. Treatment usually focuses on differentiating between these and may involve repeated injection of the scar with steroid to desensitise the area. Local anaesthetic blockade of the sternum under X-ray control may indicate a problem with a sternal wire, which may need removing. The neuropathic pain is likely to be chronic and is managed with the use of tricyclic antidepressants and anticonvulsants.

Pain in Crohn's disease

These patients are often admitted to hospital with a flare up of the condition and may have cramping abdominal pain that requires analgesia. If the patient is nil by mouth in order to rest the bowel or in preparation for surgery, then the sensible option is to use intravenous analgesia to load the patient and then use a PCA for continuing analgesia. However, the acute flare up may last for several days or even weeks and the route of analgesia may need to be changed. If the switch is to oral analgesia the patient should be monitored to ensure that absorption is adequate. A Crohn's patient may be passing motions on an hourly basis and drugs like oral morphine, which have relatively poor bioavailability, may be ineffective. Slow-release preparations (e.g. MST slow-release morphine sulphate) may pass through the gastrointestinal tract very quickly (in under 12 hours) and thus not provide the expected analgesia. Consideration should be given in these circumstances to the use of topical analgesia (e.g. transdermal fentanyl or transdermal buprenorphine).

Pain management in patients with renal failure

Patients with chronic and end-stage renal failure will present at various times with pain problems the same as other patients. These will encompass the spectrum of nociceptive and neuropathic pain either as acute or chronic pain. The clinician has to be aware of the difficulties associated with the prescribing of various drugs due to the possible accumulation of drugs with active or toxic metabolites.

The use of NSAIDs should be avoided in patients with chronic renal failure so as not to worsen renal function. Also some drugs rely solely on renal function for drug elimination (e.g. morphine, which is metabolised to the water-soluble active metabolites morphine 6 and morphine 3 glucuronide). Significant opiate overdose is possible in these patients if treated with morphine. If in doubt, opiates that do not rely on renal excretion should be considered (e.g. transdermal fentanyl, transdermal buprenorphine and oxycodone). Gabapentin should be prescribed in a renal dose of 100–300 mg/day and the patient observed for possible side effects as it is excreted solely by the kidney.

Ischaemic limb pain

Commonly occurs due to arterial insufficiency and patients present with increasing ischaemic pain and progressively worsening skin blood flow leading to ulceration and gangrene. The patient typically has to keep the affected limb hanging down to try to increase the blood flow and finds the pain is worse at night. The symptoms are a combination of nociceptive and neuropathic pain, which usually requires revascularisation to relieve the symptoms.

Prior to surgery the nature and character of the pain should be determined on the history and appropriate treatment commenced.

Long-acting opiates are usually required in combination with a tricyclic antidepressant if nocturnal symptoms are prominent. If the pain is predominantly neuropathic in character then gabapentin should be added to the regimen. The clinician has to tailor the drug dose to the patient population, who are predominantly smokers with associated cardiac, renal and respiratory disease, or diabetics with poorly controlled blood sugars. They may be intolerant of conventional doses of drugs, and side effects in the form of confusion and hallucinations are common.

After surgical treatment, revascularisation or amputation the analgesic requirements usually drop and this requires a corresponding reduction in analgesia. It is common practice to reduce oral opiates by 50% postoperatively and thereafter reduce the dose more slowly to minimise the chances of a withdrawal syndrome.

Pain after amputation

Following amputation of a limb or body part there will be acute postoperative pain. This may also be accompanied by a 'phantom' limb or body part, which may be painful (up to 75% of patients).

Stump pain (pain localised to or in the stump) generally occurs after a noxious stimulus (nociceptive) and can be particularly troublesome when prosthetic limbs are being fitted. Occasionally surgical revision of the stump to provide better muscle coverage is helpful. It can persist long after surgery and may have some of the features of CRPS with sensitivity to light touch, burning pain and thermal reactivity with altered sudomotor activity (neuropathic).

Phantom pain (pain in the limb or body part that has been removed) may include shooting, stabbing and cramping pains in addition to those described for the stump pain and there may be a sensation of the 'limb' being twisted into an abnormal position. Most amputees report that the phantom shrinks with time but some will remain painful long term.

Treatment of this condition is predominantly symptom related and may include prolonged use of opiates, antidepressants and anticonvulsants. There is also a place for the use of cognitive behavioural therapy in the management of pain particularly after traumatic amputation (usually a younger population).

Post mastectomy many women experience a phantom breast, which can have similar symptoms to those of limb amputees and may require similar treatments. Phantom pains have also been described following removal of other body parts (e.g. digits, testical, rectum).

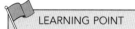

LEARNING POINT

Stump pain and phantom pain are different. Not all phantoms are painful.

Pain management for patients on opioids

Pain management in the drug abuser

Active drug abusers often appear in secondary care as a result of their addiction to controlled drugs; unfortunately they often present with groin infections leading to critical ischaemia in their lower limbs. They may also present with other common surgical emergencies and the results of trauma. They will often have pain, which may prove difficult to manage because they are used to 'industrial' quantities of opiates and also have reduced pain thresholds. In these situations careful consideration has to be given to the dose and route of drug administration, in many cases intravenous access may not be possible.

The clinician needs to be aware that some patients will have stopped illicit drugs and may be undertaking abstinence via naltrexone (blocks the effects of opiates) or disulfiram (produces toxic metabolites) or be on a maintenance programme with methadone (prevents withdrawal symptoms).

In the case of naltrexone the duration of action is of the order of 48–72 h and this needs to be discontinued prior to planned surgery if opiates are to be used for pain management. However, some patients have naltrexone implants and planned removal may not be an option. In the acute situation pain management is a particular problem as opiates will be ineffective and

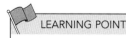

LEARNING POINT

Help and advice should always be sought from the acute pain team in these situations preferably before they get out of control. Addicts still feel pain.

alternatives, such as intravenous paracetamol and NSAIDs, need to be considered, possibly in conjunction with local anaesthetic nerve blocks or epidural analgesia with the addition of clonidine.

The patient who is on maintenance methadone will need to continue this peroperatively and will require top-up medication to deal with the acute pain being experienced. Even if epidural analgesia is employed the methadone should be continued to avoid the risk of a withdrawal syndrome.

Pain management in the patient on long-term opiates for chronic pain

These patients are easier than the drug abuser to manage, but will still experience acute pain after surgery. As with the patient on methadone maintenance, the normal dose of opiate should be continued and top-up medication delivered in addition to the maintenance. These patients are not opiate naïve and will usually require larger doses of opiate for acute-pain management (e.g. PCA bolus dose of morphine increased to 2 mg, normal dose 1 mg). Also consider adjuvant/co-analgesic drugs such as NSAIDs and paracetamol.

Complex neuropathic pain

Central pain

Pain due to damage to the central nervous system:

* The ventroposterolateral nucleus of the thalamus is connected to the spinothalamic tract and is an important part of the pain pathway. Damage to the thalamus after cerebral infarction can cause spontaneous peripheral pain on the opposite side of the body known as 'thalamic syndrome'. It is characterised by an unpleasant burning sensation.
* Spinal-cord damage due to MS, spinal-cord injury and tumour can all cause pain on the opposite side of the body to the lesion and again the pain is usually described as burning.

Treatments range from simple drug management with anticonvulsants, antidepressants and opiates, through to more complex treatments available in specialist centres. Drugs that have activity against the N-methyl-D-aspartate receptor (NMDA receptor), such as methadone or ketamine may be useful where other treatments have failed, but these drugs should only be used under the supervision of specialist centres. Nerve-stimulating and -blocking procedures have a limited place in the management of these conditions, but may be considered for discrete painful areas.

TENS has a limited place in the management of these conditions.

Peripheral neuropathic pain

Postherpetic neuralgia

Shingles occurs in the elderly and those that are immunocompromised. The previously dormant chickenpox virus (varicella zoster) attacks main nerve trunks causing demyelination and nerve damage. The incidence, duration and severity of postherpetic neuralgia increases with age and is often permanent. Patients will complain of burning, shooting pain with allodynia in the nerve distribution. The severity of the condition is much reduced with early antiviral treatment and many practitioners recommend the use of amitriptyline in low dosage (10–50 mg nocte) at the outset of symptoms before the rash has gone.

Refractory pain can be reduced with anticonvulsants such as gabapentin (1200–1800 mg day) or the use of opiates.

Topical treatment is available in the form of capsaicin cream, which depletes substance P at the C pain fibre ending. Unfortunately, a number of patients will be intolerant of this treatment because it causes burning pain on application and this can persist for 7–10 days. Other topical treatments that have been used include the use of topical local anaesthetic preparations, although their use may be limited by excess drug absorption.

Some patients respond to sympathetic nerve blocks (stellate ganglion block and lumbar sympathectomy), but the effect is often transitory lasting for, at most, 4–6 weeks and repeated nerve blocks are often impractical.

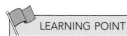

LEARNING POINT

Early treatment of the shingles pain will often reduce the severity of the postherpetic neuralgia.

Trigeminal neuralgia

The diagnosis is usually made clinically on the history, distribution of pain and the response to treatment. Further investigations are normally only carried out to plan surgical interventions and exclude an acoustic neuroma or other tumour.

The patient will complain of pain in the distribution of one branch of the trigeminal nerve and will describe an intense, shooting pain lasting 2–3 min, which may be triggered by eating, drinking, light touch or even a 'breath of air'. The patient will generally be pain free between attacks and may only experience one to two episodes a day, but may stop eating and drinking to avoid further episodes and may become suicidal.

Traditional treatment is with an increasing dose of carbamazepine titrated against pain relief and side effects, although refractory neuralgia may be treated with other anticonvulsants, including phenytoin and, more recently, gabapentin.

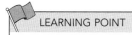

LEARNING POINT

The pain management of trigeminal neuralgia is considered by some to be a medical emergency, due to the intense nature of the pain and the psychological disturbance that often accompanies the onset of symptoms.

Referral to a pain specialist for invasive treatment can be considered in refractory cases and good results have been obtained with injection of glycerol into the foramen ovale at the base of the skull and selective radiofrequency lesioning of the Gasserian ganglion. Unfortunately, complications can occur, such as corneal anaesthesia and increased permanent pain in the form of 'anaesthesia dolorosa'. Alcohol injection is rarely used nowadays because of the latter complication.

Neurovascular decompression by a neurosurgeon carries the best hope of a cure and in expert hands the morbidity and mortality are low, even in elderly patients, and should be considered as an option if medical management fails.

Diabetic polyneuropathy

This involves diffuse nerve damage in multiple nerves, commonly a 'glove and stocking' distribution, reflecting the influence of the sympathetic nerves in the genesis of the pain. Patients will complain of burning pain that can be intolerable. Untreated pain may result in poor diabetic control and this often improves as pain recedes. This is a difficult condition to treat, with disease progression often leading to limb ischaemia and amputation.

Drug treatment includes the standard regimens of antidepressants, anticonvulsants, simple analgesics and opiates. More resistant pain requires referral to a specialist pain management centre for consideration of NMDA receptor antagonists (ketamine and methadone) or sympathetic nerve blocks.

AIDS, HIV and pain

Up to 60% of these patients will have pain either from the disease or that has been iatrogenically induced as a result of treatment. There may be a variety of symptoms including painful peripheral sensory neuropathy, pain due to extensive Kaposi's sarcoma, headache, pharyngeal and abdominal pain, arthralgias, myalgias, as well as painful dermatological conditions.

HIV-related peripheral neuropathy is often painful, affecting up to 30% of patients with AIDS. It is characterised by a sensation of burning, numbness or anaesthesia in the affected extremity. Several antiviral drugs, such as didanosine or zalcitabine, chemotherapy agents used to treat Kaposi's sarcoma (vincristine), as well as phenytoin and isoniazid, can also cause painful peripheral neuropathy.

Reiter's syndrome, reactive arthritis, and polymyositis are painful conditions reported in early HIV infection. Other painful rheumatologic manifestations of HIV infection include various forms of arthritis (painful articular syndrome, septic arthritis, psoriatic arthritis), vasculitis, Sjögren's syndrome, polymyositis, zidovudine (AZT) myopathy and dermatomyositis.

Conditions associated with chronic or intermittent pain include: intestinal infections with *Mycobacterium avium-intracellulare* and *Cryptosporidium*, which cause cramping and intermittent abdominal pain; hepatosplenomegaly resulting in abdominal distension and pain; oral and oesophageal candidiasis causing pain while the patient is eating and swallowing; and severe spasticity associated with encephalopathy, which causes painful muscle spasms.

HIV-related conditions that cause acute pain in children include: meningitis and sinusitis, which result in severe headaches, otitis media, shingles, cellulitis and abscesses, severe candida dermatitis and dental caries.

The principles of pain management in HIV/AIDS patients are the same as for cancer pain and the use of the WHO analgesic ladder is recommended.[2] The key to treatment is to take a careful pain history, because patients will complain of different types of pain in different locations at different times. Symptom management may require multimodal therapy to manage physical pain and psychological distress.

Social issues are also extremely relevant as this group of patients commonly includes intravenous drug abusers and children born with HIV.

Sickle cell disease and pain

Pain is the most frequent problem experienced by people with sickle cell disease. It profoundly affects their ability to function in work, school, play and social relationships. The frequency and severity of painful episodes are highly variable among patients. Some patients have pain every day where others may only experience occasional episodes. The majority of painful episodes have no clear precipitating cause, but may include dehydration, infection, stress and cold. Painful episodes may start in the first year of life and continue thereafter. These episodes last from hours to weeks followed by a return to baseline. Onset and resolution can be sudden or gradual. Patients experience a spectrum spanning acute and chronic pain; both the assessment and management must be suitable for both.

Simple analgesics and NSAIDs can be used for background analgesia, but care must be taken if there are any concerns about occult gastrointestinal bleeding and also nephropathy due to the disease.

A stepwise approach to pain management is recommended with the aim of relieving acute episodes within hours rather than days. This may require titration of intravenous analgesia as a hospital inpatient. If possible a home regimen should be adopted allowing the patient access to 'escape analgesia'. Unfortunately, owing to the frequency and severity of the episodes some patients are routinely undertreated and difficulties arise when the patient presents to the A&E department requesting drugs by name, route and dose to manage their pain!

The solution is to have a proper clinical assessment of the patient and to also address the psychological and physical issues around the problem. The spectrum of acute and chronic pain in these patients provides a treatment challenge that requires a sensitive approach to a lifelong condition.

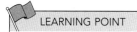

LEARNING POINT

Undertreatment of pain in these patients is common and is often the result of opiophobia on the part of the physician.

Pain in rheumatoid and other inflammatory conditions

Pain is a constant feature in these conditions and usually follows a relapsing course of acute or chronic pain. In general, the symptoms are usually well managed if the disease is in remission and simple analgesics (paracetamol $\pm$ codeine) and NSAIDs (if tolerated) are the mainstay of treatment.

Acute flare-ups often require a step up the analgesic ladder until disease management induces further remission. In severe cases and where there is loss of function the patient may opt for joint replacement as part of a pain-management strategy.

LEARNING POINT

Chronic pain with acute flare-ups often requires different types and strengths of analgesia.

Pain and the elderly

Pain, stiffness and lack of mobility, is a constant feature with most of the diseases affecting the elderly patient and is a particular feature of osteoarthritis. They may have pain in different parts of the body.

Treatment follows the same pathway as the WHO analgesic ladder, but is often limited by the side effects of the drugs used. In particular NSAIDs have to be used with caution due to the significant gastric and renal side effects, which can cause morbidity and even mortality due to gastrointestinal haemorrhage. The opiates including codeine all cause constipation, which usually requires active management alongside the pain management. Tricyclic antidepressants work well alongside the conventional analgesics and are generally well tolerated in this age group, acting as a co-analgesic.

Stimulation analgesia (TENS) offers significant advantages for this age group as there are no drug side effects, but its use is often limited by practical considerations.

As a group there is often a better response to interventions, such as steroid epidurals for back pain, than the younger patient and might be considered alongside conventional analgesia to try to maintain mobility.

The aim of treatment in this age group is to get the best fit between pain relief, function and side effects. It is important to recognise that this group of patients may have particular concerns about drug addiction with opiates and may be concerned that 'morphine' is an end of life drug. However, if the clinician 'starts low and goes slow' there is a good chance that the patient will tolerate opiates and other medications with adequate titration.

LEARNING POINT

Pain in the elderly is manageable if treated carefully and side effects are not ignored.

KEY POINTS

- Drugs should be titrated against benefit and side effect
- The WHO ladder is useful when considering painful nonmalignant conditions
- Regular assessment is required to optimise analgesic regimens
- Opioids have an important role and are safe if titrated and monitored properly
- Drug metabolism must be understood if side effects are to be minimised (e.g. renal excretion in renal insufficiency)
- Nonpharmacological interventions are important and should not be overlooked
- The psychological components of pain management must always be considered alongside other interventions

References

1. Voepel-Lewis T, Moore A, Edwards J et al. The reliability and validity of the face, legs, activity, cry, consolability observational tool as a measure of pain in children with cognitive impairment. *Anesth Analg* 2002; **95**(5): 1224–1229.
2. World Health Organization. *National cancer control programmes: policies and managerial guidelines*. Geneva: World Health Organization; 2002.

Further reading

Dolin SJ, Padfield NL (eds) *Pain medicine manual*, 2nd edn. Edinburgh: Butterworth-Heinemann; 2004.

Tait AR. *Bandolier's little book of pain*. Oxford: Oxford University Press; 2003.

Andrew Skinner

Pain, ethics and research

Introduction

Pain is well known to be a subjective phenomenon. Many doctors believe that some psychological illnesses will find their expression with pain as the major symptom. Many take a dichotomous view of pain, being worthy of attention where there is a clear-cut physical cause, yet in the absence of such a cause less worthy and the suffering consequent upon it less real. Most specialist pain physicians believe that entirely psychological pain is rare. What seems common is where there is a clear cause for pain (even if it is merely the aches and pains attending normal ageing), which is much more intrusive and harder to bear in the face of psychological co-morbidity and is itself often worsened by chronic ill health. Patients whose reported pain and suffering is disproportionate to their objective disease are often characterised as 'mad' or 'malingering'. Definitive psychiatric illness is rare in these patients and psychiatric referral almost invariably unhelpful. Whilst it is impossible to be certain ('How often have you failed to detect a deliberate lie, doctor?') conscious falsification of symptoms is also thought to be rare.

Unfortunately, the normal medical ('curative') paradigm, namely diagnosis leading to treatment and thus amelioration of symptoms, fails a significant number of patients. Despite the plain and obvious truth of this assertion, many doctors find purely symptomatic ('palliative') treatments if not an anathema, at least very much second best and, therefore, symptomatic treatments are poorly regarded, both in education and medical practice. Patients who are failed by the conventional medical paradigm are frustrating for doctors and these too are often described in deprecatory terms. Doctors will tend to take the view that the illness is, somehow, the patient's 'fault' and undertreat (or simply not treat) symptoms because of this. Whilst some of these patients will be difficult or impossible to treat, many will be improved by simple, conventional analgesics and the discomfiture of doctors is no reason not even to attempt treatment.

Why is pain undertreated?

- Clinicians fail to identify pain relief as a priority. Perhaps the curative paradigm is being slavishly followed to the exclusion of direct palliation of symptoms, perhaps some patients or their pains are seen as more worthy of treatment.
- Inadequate knowledge and skills amongst clinicians. Both ignorance of available treatments and an unreasonable fear that harm will arise from those treatments, lead to treatment failure.
- Fear of criticism or sanctions following apparently liberal prescribing. There are very specific fears surrounding those at the end of their lives (see below), but doctors worry that they might be seen as fuelling illicit drug use by supplying potent pain killers in the community. Unfortunately, the regulatory framework for the strong opioids is mainly intended to prevent illicit use rather than facilitate therapeutic use.
- Failure of hospitals, primary care organisations and licensing bodies to make pain relief a high priority.

Pain is often thought an inescapable accompaniment of illness, especially of injuries or surgery. Whilst the goal of high-quality pain relief for everyone is probably unachievable,[1] there is little doubt that considerable scope for improvement exists if treatment of pain is made a high priority.

Treating pain alone rarely improves long-term outcome (though there are obvious exceptions). It is important that treating the pain is essentially harm free, especially if the cause is relatively short lived, for example the pain after surgery.

Fear of harm is a potent cause of undertreatment of acute pain. Whilst some treatments do carry risk, this is often overestimated by junior colleagues, to whom the treatment of pain is usually delegated.

Long-term use of strong opioids

For the first 75 years of the 20th century opioids were rarely used in the UK, other than for a few days after acute injury or surgery. The reason that liberal use in the Victorian era gave way to effective prohibition is unclear, but until the mid 1970s the chronic use of opioids was virtually unknown in the UK. The main reason was probably an unreasonable fear of iatrogenic addiction.

The rise of palliative care and the hospice movement, championed by such pioneers as Dame Cicely Saunders, gave doctors both permission and confidence to use chronic oral opioids titrated to effect in patients with disseminated cancer. The principles established by Saunders and her co-workers were regular dosing at appropriate intervals with a sufficiently potent drug, at an adequate dose and use of the oral route. Synthesised into the WHO 'analgesic ladder'[2] these principles provide good pain relief, without recourse to specialist advice, for at least 75% of patients dying from disseminated malignancy.

The move in the 1980s to much more appropriate treatment in those approaching the end of their lives raised little in the way of serious ethical doubts. Physical dependence is not a significant problem, since stopping the drugs or dose reduction will rarely be required. Fears of obscure side effects in the very long term are also groundless for the same reasons. Tolerance seems unusual in treatment lasting for months or even a few years. The most common errors in treating pain from cancer are reluctance to start strong opioids, reluctance to escalate the dose or failure to manage side effects and constant swapping of opioids, which distracts from finding the correct dose of any one of them.

Unfortunately for patients with chronic pain and a long life expectancy, the decision to use strong opioids is less easy and, until recently, rarely recommended. The 'normal' opioid side effects (nausea, vomiting, itching, constipation and somnolence) limit treatment in many patients. Longer-term treatment may lead to less-well-known side effects, including weight gain or loss, hormonal effects such as reduced adrenal function, reduced sexual function and infertility. The immunological effects of using long-term opioids are well described; however, the clinical importance is not clear. Since many chronically painful conditions are very long lasting these side effects may become problematic with chronic treatment. What is plain is that psychological or physical dependence is rarely troublesome and illegal use and diversion of medically prescribed opioids is unusual. Whilst tolerance over the course of months or a few years is known to be rare, there are no follow-up data for very long-term use (perhaps several decades) for the treatment of chronic pain. At the time of writing we are in a transitional phase in the UK with the long-term use of strong opioids becoming less uncommon. In 2004 guidance (Recommendations for the appropriate use of opioids for persistent non-cancer pain: a consensus statement prepared on behalf of the Pain Society, the Royal College of Anaesthetists, the Royal College of General Practitioners and the Royal College of Psychiatrists) was published and is available on the web site of the British Pain Society.[3] It is comprehensive and well referenced. Whilst this guidance is wise, it is also clear that experience is too limited to unreservedly commend widespread prescription of strong opioids in those with long life expectancy. The author currently takes a pragmatic view, being relatively liberal in older non-cancer patients, but more conservative in the young.

Opioids, like other treatments aimed primarily at reducing nociceptive input, are relatively or absolutely ineffective in many chronic pain patients, since their pain and suffering (which is often obvious and severe) is usually at least partly driven by psychological factors rather than intense nociceptive input. Patients like this are often commenced on opioids with little improvement yet subsequent difficulty in stopping treatment. A few patients like this make the doctors who treat them much more cautious with these drugs.

Despite this rather gloomy view of chronic opioids in those with long life expectancy, there is no doubt that a subgroup of patients with primarily nociceptive pain and no adverse factors will do very well with long-term opioids, reducing pain, improving activities of daily living and overall quality of life. Patients who seem to be in this group can be offered a trial of opioids after frank discussion of their potential drawbacks. The general advice in this group of patients is to use long-acting drugs, to have the dose clearly under the control of a single prescriber and to avoid 'breakthrough' medication unless there are strong reasons to the contrary. This contrasts sharply with good practice in cancer pain.

Pain relief at the very end of life

For obvious reasons there are no controlled data as to whether or not appropriate therapeutic doses of opioid analgesics shorten patients' lives. However, most doctors who care for the dying take the view that appropriately administered opioids do not significantly curtail life. Opioids are often blamed for clouded consciousness towards the end of life, but increasing drowsiness is usually attributable to the disease itself and not a result of treatment. Patients whose pain is well controlled usually die without escalation of opioid doses, often on doses that have been well tolerated for many weeks. Thus the expert view, that opioids are relatively free from serious harm, seems correct. There is no doubt that the commonest error in prescribing opioids for patients approaching the end of their life is underdosing.

It is clear, however, that opioid analgesics are capable of killing. The mass murderer Harold Shipman, a GP in Greater Manchester, did just this to at least 200 of his patients. Doctors before and since have been accused and acquitted of such crimes, and there is little doubt that doctors in primary care especially have become much more cautious about the liberal use of opioids at the end of a patient's life. This has been exacerbated by a prosecution in County Durham in 2005 (trial of Dr Howard Martin) using the British National Formulary (BNF) suggested doses as a benchmark of appropriate practice. Whilst these doses are appropriate for many patients, especially the relatively opioid naïve, some patients will need doses considerably larger than normal. Several grams a day of morphine are unusual, but sometimes necessary, and fear of criticism or worse will undoubtedly make colleagues who are not pain specialists reluctant to explore higher doses even if clearly needed. The extent to which this will prevent effective pain relief or merely place demands upon specialist referral is unclear. We must all hope that good practice will make high-profile prosecutions rare, and colleagues in non-specialist practice feel able to continue to prescribe higher doses of opioids when indicated.

The law in England and Wales is actually very clear. It was effectively settled in the failed prosecution of John Bodkin Adams (in 1957), a GP in southern England. Bodkin Adams attended several elderly patients who died under his care after relatively liberal use of opioids; he being a beneficiary in several of their wills confused the situation. Bodkin Adams asserted that the doses he had used were solely to relieve suffering and any shortening of life an unwanted and unintended side effect. In accepting this defence the trial jury effectively settled English law, making this 'dual effect' an effective defence to unlawful killing, although as observed above, experts believe opioid doses needed to relieve pain rarely, if ever, shorten life. This defence was again successfully used in the prosecution in County Durham in 2005.

One area where 'dual effect' might still be an appropriate justification is the occasional use of sedation in addition to analgesia at the end of life. Very rarely pain and other symptoms, especially if complicated by agitation and anxiety, are very difficult to manage. Specialists in palliative medicine and, less often, pain specialists will from time to time advise sedation as the only practical means of relieving suffering. Chronic sedation (as distinct from analgesia) probably does shorten life, and is only ever appropriate in the final days of life. Colleagues who are not specialists in terminal care or symptom management should invariably take advice before chronically sedating patients, and should include nursing colleagues and the patient's family in making the decision. Some colleagues view sedation as, in effect, direct killing of patients, since few will survive many days after sedation has been started. This is not, of course, true for short-term use of sedatives to answer a specific clinical need such as an unpleasant procedure.

Research into pain treatments

Research into the treatment of pain is a difficult problem. Placebo therapy in the face of known pain will rarely be acceptable to a research ethics committee (REC) or, indeed, potential subjects. Unfortunately, since pain is subjective and unmeasurable randomisation between an experimental and a control group, where both subject and observer are blinded to which group each subject is in is essential. Pain research where this is not the case is almost worthless. Treatments, which appear effective in 'open label' trials, are often subsequently shown to be less so in properly blinded trials. Regulatory hurdles are formidable for the pain researcher. Controlled trials are now not only subject to ethical and institutional scrutiny, but most reputable journals require them to have been registered with a central register of trials (at a national or international level). This is to prevent publication and commercial bias and to make the results available to future investigators. On a depressing note, it is now almost impossible for a lone worker in an ordinary healthcare setting to conduct meaningful pain research. Successful research is almost always multicentre and sponsored by some large institution. Pharmaceutical companies sponsor a significant proportion of pain research, this is sometimes poorly disguised marketing and there is always concern about the independence of the investigators.

Acute pain

In acute pain an experimental intervention can be compared with a control intervention using some form of 'rescue' analgesia, such as 'as-required' oral analgesics or the number of patient-controlled analgesia (PCA) demands made. Analgesic consumption can be used as a surrogate for pain. Pain 'scores' are often used, either a rating scale (none, slight, significant, severe) or a visual analogue scale. Unfortunately, whilst these seem consistent for a patient describing how his/her pain changes, they are less reliable when used for comparisons between patients. Acute pain is rarely stable enough to allow a crossover design of trial where comparisons can be made between scores in the same patient.

A standard painful stimulus is a useful part of a pain trial. Experimental painful stimuli are described, but the relevance to clinical practice is not clear. Surgical removal of impacted third molar teeth has for many years been a standard experimental model for acute pain, and is almost invariably in young fit adults who are not taking other medicaments. Unfortunately, this procedure is being suggested less frequently than in the past, so this source of data is increasingly closed.

Chronic pain

Chronic pain research tends to score pain as one of its outcome measures. Crossover trials make scoring more useful and these are possible with the patient acting as their own control. However, side effects can make this design more difficult to 'blind' effectively. Measures of disability are also used in chronic pain research. There are numerous rating scales, which measure disability, if a validated scale exists for the area of research proposed, then this my be a useful strategy. One of the goals of chronic pain treatment is reduction of disability, so such an approach is clearly valid.

Pain in children

'Children' covers a huge range of patients, from the neonate, through the pre-vocal infant and toddler, the gradual maturation of the school years and finally the notoriously difficult years of adolescence. Whilst it is manifestly true that the brain develops hugely after birth the old assertion that neonates and infants have a blunted perception of pain is no longer thought sustainable. Pre-vocal children cannot describe pain. At least a dozen rating scales for acute pain in pre-vocal children exist, but none has gained universal acceptance, presumably since none is superior to the others.[4,5] A five modality rating scale using crying, facial expression, trunk and leg posture and motor activity has been described and this seems as useful as any.

Acute pain in children

Acute pain after surgery is well known and is probably the area in which we can and should be doing best. Treatment can be started under anaesthesia, by specialist anaesthetists and continued by specialist ward staff. A combination of paracetamol, non-steroidal anti-inflammatory drugs (NSAIDs) and opioids, is common. Rectal administration of the first two is usual, the latter by intravenous injection using a cannula placed under general anaesthesia.

Older children will use patient-controlled analgesia (PCA), those who cannot can have a similar device controlled by nursing staff. Some units use fixed-rate infusions of opioids, but these are attended by significant risk of overdose and need high-quality, frequent observations of the child if they are to be safe.

Local infiltration of the surgical wound is easy to practice (bupivacaine or levobupivacaine is the almost universal choice), but often poorly researched. Some nerve blocks are easy and safe in the hands of the generalist (Table 19.1), others appropriate only in specialist centres (Table 19.2). The only nerve block that has achieved widespread acceptance outside surgery is femoral nerve block for fractured femur. This is often combined with procedural analgesia to facilitate initial management in the accident department.

Nitrous oxide 50% with oxygen ('entonox') is widely used for procedural pain, as are systemic opioids. Ketamine is popular in paediatric practice,[6] but

TABLE 19.1 Some blocks for use in children by the non-specialist	
Block	Indication
Penile	Circumcision
Ilioinguinal	Herniotomy
Dental blocks	Dental extractions
Sub conjunctival bupivacaine	Strabismus surgery
Caudal epidural	Trunk surgery below the umbilicus
Axillary block	Hand and forearm surgery
Fascia illica block	Thigh and femoral surgery
Femoral nerve block	Femoral fracture

TABLE 19.2 **Some blocks for use in children, but only by specialists in paediatric practice**

Block	Indication
Intercostal block	Trunk surgery – especially unilateral
Paravertebral block	Trunk surgery – especially unilateral
Intra-pleural block	Trunk surgery – especially unilateral thoracic surgery
Lumbar epidural	Trunk surgery – especially abdominal surgery
Thoracic epidural	Trunk surgery – especially thoracic surgery

none of these should substitute for an appropriately administered general anaesthetic if that is what is really needed for a procedure; for example, in the repeated procedures for paediatric cancers, or for more unpleasant or protracted procedures. Enthusiasts will occasionally fall back on procedural analgesia where an anaesthetic is more appropriate.

Chronic pain in children

Children are prey to most of the causes of chronic pain that afflict adults. Clear-cut conditions are treated in similar ways to the same conditions in adults.

Like adults they also present with painful conditions that seem out of proportion to the physical problem or simply inexplicable in simple medical terms. It is clear that one determinant of chronic pain in children is their family's experience of chronic pain and chronic ill health. Children, especially as they become older, can use their health in a complex way to manage their interactions with their family, carers, teachers, friends and others. Chronic pain and disability in children is ill understood. Although chronic pain services for children exist in several tertiary centres in the UK and in other countries they are run on the basis of clinical judgement and experience rather than an extensive evidence base. Most will include a physician with an interest in children's pain, a children's psychologist and a specialist physiotherapist. The paradigm employed is generally one of rehabilitation and psychological support.

Pain in the elderly

In many ways the older patient is no different from other adults with pain. Chronic pain is somewhat more common in later life and surgery needed more often. The elderly are undoubtedly more sensitive to the effects of strong opioids, both because of increased CNS sensitivity and of lower volumes of distribution and slower clearance of the drugs. The extent of these changes varies between patients so, although initial doses need to be more conservative in the older patient, perhaps half that in the younger adult, adjustment in the light of the observed effects will be needed. This appears true irrespective of the route of administration. It also seems true of other drugs, such an anticonvulsants and antidepressants used for chronic pain.

Although it is often said that the elderly experience less pain, there is little science behind this. Pain thresholds in the elderly are not significantly higher than in younger adults. The elderly may bear pain more stoically, perhaps because of cultural factors, but this is not a justification for under-treatment.

Cognitive impairment in the older patient can make reporting and treatment of pain more difficult. A patient who is normally coherent can become confused following a change of location (to hospital) or during an acute illness. As in the preverbal child one is often forced to rely on behavioural assessment rather than direct report.

Elderly patients are more at risk from the gastric and renal side effects of NSAIDs. Ironically NSAIDs are often thought of as safe and opioids dangerous. As observed above it may be appropriate to use long-term opioids in the older patient when one might be reluctant in the younger patient.

References

1. Dolin SJ. Pain clinic. In: Dolin SJ, Padfield NL (eds). *Pain medicine manual*, 2nd edn. Edinburgh: Butterworth-Heinemann; 2004: 1–6.
2. World Health Organization. *National cancer control programmes: policies and managerial guidelines*. Geneva: World Health Organization; 2002.
3. The Pain Society. *Recommendations for the appropriate use of opioids for persistent non-cancer pain. A consensus statement prepared on behalf of the Pain Society, the Royal College of Anaesthetists, the Royal College of General Practitioners and the Royal College of Psychiatrists*. London: The Pain Society; 2004.
4. Suraseranivongse S, Kaosaard R, Intakong P et al. A comparison of postoperative pain scales in neonates. *Br J Anaesth* 2006; **97**(4): 540–544.
5. Suraseranivongse S, Santawat U, Kraiprasit K et al. Cross-validation of a composite pain scale for preschool children within 24 hours of surgery. *Br J Anaesth* 2001; **87**(3): 400–405.
6. Green SM, Krauss B. Ketamine is a safe, effective, and appropriate technique for emergency department paediatric procedural sedation. *Emerg Med J* 2004; **21**(3): 271–272.

Index

Note: Page numbers in *italics* refer to illustrations. Page numbers in **bold** refer to tables.

A

A-fibres, 9–10, **10**
  nociceptive activation, 54
  termination point in dorsal horn, 66, **66**
  thinly myelinated, 49
  WDR neurones, 73
  see also Aβ fibres; Aδ fibres
Abdomen
  pain prevalence in, 204
  surgery, 267–8
Aβ fibres, 9, **10**
  effect of nerve injury, 76
  primary afferent depolarisation
    (PAD), 75–6
  termination point in dorsal horn, 66, **66**
  WDR neurones, 73
Ablative neuronal blockade, 255–6
Absorption, drug, 38–42, 42–3
  factors affecting, 43
  local anaesthetics, 122–3
Accident and emergency
    department, 265–6
Acetaminophen *see* Paracetamol
Acetate, 13
Acetyl coenzyme-A, 13
Acetylcholine, 10–1, 13–4, 151
Acetylcholinesterase, 13
Acetylsalicylic acid *see* Aspirin
Acid sensitive ion channels (ASICs), *52*,
    53
Action potentials (APs), 6–9, *8*, 50–1, 66
  depolarisation, 8
  ionic fluxes during, 8–9
  propagation of, 9
  repolarisation, 9
Activated binding sites, 30, *31*
Active transport, 42
Acupuncture, 87–9, 173, **175**, 258
  complications, 88
  efficacy, 89
  mode of action, 87
  point location, 87
  Tao of Pooh, 174
  traditional Chinese vs. Western medical
    traditions, 87
  treatment sessions, 88–9

Acute pain
  in children, 282–3
  in the community, 263–4
  development to chronic pain, 188–90,
    189
  in general, 4
  NSAIDs and, 107
  research, 281
  on the trauma ward, 265–6
  vs. chronic pain, 187–8, 243
Aδ fibres, 21
  fast pain, 18
  termination point in dorsal horn, 66,
    66
  WDR neurones, 73
ADAPT, 100–1
Addiction, opioid, 247
Adenoma prevention with celecoxib
    study, 98
Adenomatous polyps
  adenomatous polyp prevention on
    vioxx trial, 98
  prevention of spontaneous
    adenomatous polyps trial, 99
Adenosine receptors, 35
Adenosine triphosphate (ATP), *52*
Adenosine triphosphate (ATP)-gated
    ion channel, 51, 53
Adenyl cyclase, 35, 71
Adenylate cyclase, 133
Adjuvant drugs, 143–58, 248, **248**
ADME acronym, 38
Adrenaline, 14
Aerosol drugs, 41
Afferent neurones, 58, 66, **66**
Age and pain, 204
  see also Elderly patients
Agonist ligands
  binding, 29, 30, *31*
  definition of, 28–9
  dose–response curve, 29–31, *30*
  inverse, 34
  vs. antagonist ligands, 34
AIDS, 274
Alkalinisation, local anaesthetics, 122–3
'All or none' law, 9

Allergic reactions
  to local anaesthetics, 121
  to TENS, 85, 86
  to topical treatments, 41
Allodynia
  complex regional pain syndrome, 266
  neuropathic pain, 58
  primary afferent depolarisation
      (PAD), 75
  WDR neurones, 73
α-adrenergic agonists, 150
α-adrenoceptors, 14
$α_2$-adrenoceptors, 77
$α_2$-agonists, **248**
Alzheimer's disease anti-inflammatory
      prevention trial, 100–1
Amethocaine, 177, **178**
Ametop®, 177, **178**
Amino acids, 15–6, 119
Amino-amides, 121
Amino-esters, 121
Amitriptyline, 145, **145**
  complex regional pain syndrome, 266
  migraine, **153**
  postherpetic neuralgia, 273
AMPA receptors, *11*, 36, 72
  central sensitisation, 74
  glutamate, 15, 55
Amputation, 271
  pain prevalence, **203**
Amygdala, 25
Anaesthesia, intradermal, 184
  see also Local anaesthetics
Anaesthesia dolorosa, 273
Analgesia, 4
  common analgesics, **4**
  conventional, 244, **247**
  miscellaneous drugs, 143–58
  opioid, 70, 137
  placebo, 70
  side effects, **247**
  stimulation, 257–59
  topical, 180–3
  unconventional analgesics, 247–48
  see also specific analgesic
Analgesic ladder, 244, *246*, 266, 278
Anatomical changes in nerve injury, 76
Angel dust, 148
Anger, 195, 234–5, 235
  cost of, 206
Ankle block, **250**
Antagonist ligands, 31–3
  definition of, 28–9
  vs. agonist ligands, 34
Anterior cingulate cortex (ACC), 69
Anticonvulsant drugs, 146–8, **148**
  migraine, **153**, 154

mode of action, 147
neuropathic pain, 248, 265
side effects, 147–8, **148**
trigeminal neuralgia, 273
Antidepressant agents, 144–6, **145**
  mode of action, 146
  neuropathic pain, 247–8
  and pain management, 144–5
  side effects, **145**, 146
  tricyclic, 145, **145**, **153**, 154, 265
Antihistamines for migraine, **153**
Antihypertensive medication, interaction
      with NSAIDs, 105
Anxiety, 195, 234, 235
  cost of, 206
  effect on pain experience, 70
Anxiolytics, **248**
APC study, 98
Approve trial, 98
Aqueous diffusion, 42
Arachidonic acid (AA), 53–4, 57, 92
Arterial insufficiency, 81
Arthritis
  celecoxib long-term arthritis safety
      study, 97
  corticosteroids, 152
  medal programme, 101
  NSAIDs and, 107
  therapeutic COX–189 arthritis research
      and gastrointestinal event
      trial, 97–8
Ascending pathways, 24–5
Aspirin, 107–9
  contraindications, 108
  gastrointestinal effects of, 106
  indications, 108
  mechanism of action, 107
  overdose, 108–9
Assessment of pain, 213–29
  barrier influencing, 214
  in children, 228
  in the elderly, 229
  history, 215–8
  investigations, 220
  measurement of pain *see* Measurement
      of pain
  objectives of, 214–5
  physical examination, 218–20
  process of, 215
  in special situations, 227–9
Asthma, effect of NSAIDs on, 103
Atropine, 14
Autogenic training, 238
Autonomic nervous system, effect of
      nerve injury on, 76–7
Axillary plexus block, 249–51, *250*
Axon telodendria, 6, *7*

Axons, 6, *7*
  function, 9–10
  types, 9–10, **10**
Axoplasmic transport, 11
Axotomy, 76–8
Azopropazone, 104

B

β-fibres, 9–10, **10**
Back beliefs questionnaire, 235
Back pain
  cost to society, 206–7
  genetics and, 205
  low, 188–90, **189**, 264
  radicular, corticosteroids, 152
  studies, 207–8, **208**
Baclofen, 150, **150**, 248, 254
Behavioural techniques, 237
Behaviours, pain promoting, 195–6
Beliefs, 235
Belonephobia, 177
Benzocaine, **122**
Benzodiazepines, 16
β-adrenoceptors, 14, 35, 77
β-blockers, **153**, 154
β-carbolines, 34
β-endorphin, 133
Bier's block, 125, 255
Bioavailability, 38, 270
Biofeedback, 239
Biogenic amines, 14–5
Bisphosphonates, **248**
Bladder nociceptors, 49, *49*
Blood–brain barrier, 42, 135–6
Bodkin Adams, John, 280
Body fluid compartments, 43–4
Bone, effect of NSAIDs on, 104
Botulinum toxin, 151
Botulism, 151
Brachial plexus block (axillary
      approach), 249–51, **250**, *251*
Bradykinin, 53, 55–6, 61
  inflammatory soup, *52*
  in neuropathic pain, 59–60
Brain, 25–6, 259
Brain-derived neurotrophic factor
      (BDNF), 54–5
Breathing, diaphragmatic, 238
Brief pain inventory (BPI), 225, *227*
Buccal drug administration, 39–41, *40*
Bupivacaine, 119, 120–1, **122**
  implantable intrathecal drug-delivery
      systems (IDDS), 254
  maximal safe dose of, **249**
  metabolism, 121

patient-controlled epidural analgesia
      (PCEA), 268
spinal (intrathecal) blocks, 252
toxicity, 122
Buprenorphine matrix-patch, 179, **181**

C

C-fibres, 9–10, **10**, 21
  effect of nerve injury, 76
  local anaesthetics, 121
  nociceptive activation, 54
  primary afferent depolarisation
      (PAD), 75
  slow pain pathway, 18
  termination point in dorsal horn, 66,
      66
  unmyelinated, 49
  WDR neurones, 73
Caffeine, 155
Calcitonin gene-related peptide
      (CGRP), 51, 60
Calcium, 72, 75
Calcium channels
  norepinephrine, 71
  voltage-gated, 59
Calcium ions
  central sensitisation, 74
  norepinephrine, 71
  role of, 9
Cancer pain, corticosteroids, 152
Cannabinoids, 57, 155–7
Capsaicin, 53
  postherpetic neuralgia, 273
  topical, 180–2, **184**
Carbamazepine, **148**, 273
Cardiovascular system
  and aspirin, 108
  effect of Coxibs on, 98–101
  effect of NSAIDs on, 100–1, 103, 106
  local anaesthetic toxicity, 121–2, 123
  neuraxial blocks, 251
Care planning, 209–10
Carrageenan, 54
Catapres TTS®, 180
Catastrophisation, 194, 236
Catecholamines, 14, 243
Categorical scales, 221
Cause of illness beliefs, 193
Celecoxib
  adenoma prevention with celecoxib
      study, 98
  cardiovascular risks of, 99
  celecoxib long-term arthritis safety
      study, 97
  in clinical practice, **114**

Central mechanisms, 65–78
Central nervous system (CNS)
    effect of opioids on, 137–8
    local anaesthetic toxicity, 121–2, 123
    opioids effect on, 133
Central neuraxial blocks, 251–4, **252**
Central pain, 272
Central sensitisation, 19, 73–8
Cerebral cortex, 25–6, *26*
Cerebrospinal fluid (CSF), 123–4
    see also Spinal (intrathecal) blocks
Cerebrovascular accident, 98
Character of pain, 216
Chemical stimuli, 49
Chemokines, 57–8
Chemosensitive fibres, 54
Chickenpox, 272–3
Children and pain, 204, 282–3
    assessment, 228
    nerve blocks, **282**, **283**
Chinese medicine, 87–9, 173
Chloride ions (Cl⁻), 12
Chlorocresol, 256
Chlorprocaine, **122**
Cholestyramine, 112
Choline, 13
Cholinergic neurones, 13
Chronic airway disease, effect of NSAIDs
    on, 103
Chronic pain, 3, 4, 198–9
    in children, 283
        prevalence, 204
    in the community, 264
    development from acute pain, 188–90,
        189
    emotional components of, 191–8, *192*
    immune cells and, 77
    long-term use of opioids, 278–9
    prevention of, 208–9
    psychological impact of, 230–41
    research, 281–2
    sensory components of, **190**, 190–1
    understanding the mechanisms
        of, 190–8
    vs. acute pain, 187–8, **188**, 243
Citruline, 75
CLASS study, 97
Classical conditioning, 196
Clinician-influenced assessment
    barriers, 214
Clinics, care planning in, 209–10
Clonidine, 150, **150**
    implantable intrathecal drug-delivery
        systems (IDDS), 254
    transdermal patch, 180, **181–2**
Clostridium botulinum, 151
Co-analgesics, 4, **4**

Coagulation, effect of NSAIDs on, 104
Cocaine, 118–9
    duration of action, **122**
    maximal safe dose of, **249**
Codeine
    metabolism, 136
    structure, 132
Cognitive-behavioural approach to
    pain, 192, *192*
Cognitive errors, 236
Cognitive restructuring, 236
Cognitive therapy, 236, 259–60
Cold haemoglobinuria, 81
Cold packs, **171**
Cold therapy, 81, 170, **171**
Cold-water immersion, **171**
Colorectal polyps, 98
Community pain management, 263–5
Competitive antagonism, *32*, 32–3
Complex neuropathic pain, 272–5
Complex regional pain syndrome, 266
Concentration–effect relationship, 30
Conductive heat therapy, 82
Confusion, opioid–induced, 137–8
Congenital insensitivity to pain with
    anhidrosis, 51
Conjugation, 44–5
Consequences of illness beliefs, 193
Constipation, opioid-induced, 138
Control
    of illness beliefs, 193–4
    loss of, 195
    of stress, 197
Coping, 197–8, 238–9
Cordotomy, 259
Coronary artery bypass grafting
    postoperative pain, 269
    valdecoxib/parecoxib in coronary
        artery bypass grafting trial, 99
Corticosteroids, 151–2, **248**
Cost of pain, 205–7
    to employers, 206
    to the individual, 205–6, *206*
    to society, 206–7
    treatment cost, 210
COX-2 inhibitors *see* Coxibs
COX inhibitors, 60
Coxibs, 96–101
    cardiovascular safety concerns of,
        98–9
    celecoxib long-term arthritis safety
        study, 97
    in clinical practice, **114–5**
    development of, 94
    in osteoarthritic patients, 106
    preliminary cardiovascular
        conclusions, 99–100

therapeutic COX-189 arthritis research and gastrointestinal event trial, 97–8

vioxx GI outcomes research study, 97, 98

see also NSAIDs

Cranial nerve neurectomies, 257

Crohn's disease, 269–70

Cross-sectional studies, 207

Cryoanalgesia, 255

Cryoglobulinaemia, paroxysmal, 81

Cryotherapy, 170, **171**

Culture and pain, 204–5

Cunate, 25

Cure/control of illness beliefs, 193–4

Cyclic adenosine monophosphate (cAMP), 35, 54, 55, 133, 140

Cyclic endoperoxides, 92

Cyclo-oxygenase (COX), 53–4, 92, 93–6

assays, 95–6

COX-1, 94–6, *95*

COX-2, 94–6, *95*

COX-3, 94

inhibitors, 60

selectivity, **95**, 95–6

see also Coxibs; NSAIDs

Cytochrome P450, 78, 110, *111*

Cytokines, 57–8, 60

D

Day surgery, 266–7

Deep brain stimulation, 259

Deep cervical plexus block, **250**

Deep heating treatments, 170, **171**

Definitions of pain, 1–2, **2**, 190, 213

δ-9-tetrahydrocannabinol, 155, 156

Aδ receptors, 134

Dendrites, 6, *7*, 60

Depolarisation, 8

Depot steroids, 152

Depression, 195, 206, 234, 235

Descending facilitation (DF), 68–9, 70

Descending inhibition (DI), 68–9, 70

Descending modulation, 68–71, **71**

mechanisms of, 70–1

role of, 70

supraspinal sites of origin, 69–70

Descending pathways, 25, *26*

Description of pain, 215

Desipramine, 145, **145**

Dexamethasone, 152

Dextro-bupivacaine, 119

Diabetic polyneuropathy, 273–4

Diacylglycerol (DAG), 35, 56

Diamorphine

patient-controlled epidural analgesia (PCEA), 268

structure, 131

Diaphragmatic breathing, 238

Dibucaine, 119, **122**

Diclofenac, 95, 97

cardiovascular safety advice, 106

in clinical practice, **112**

medal programme, 101

Digital nerve blocks, **250**

Dihydroxyeicosatetraenoic acids, 57

Direct coupling in DRG, 60

Disability, cost of, 206

Distal tubule, 45–6

Distribution of drugs, 42–4

Disuse syndrome, 235

Docking, 29, *30*

Dopamine, 14

Dorsal column pathway, 25

Dorsal-column stimulation, 258

Dorsal horn, *21*, 21–2, *23*, 25, 65–8, **66**

Dorsal reticular nucleus, 69

Dorsal root, *21*

entry zone lesions, 257

ganglion, 21, *21*, *22*, 65

cells, 51, 76

direct coupling, 60

Dose cycle, 31

Dose–response curve, 29–31, *30*

Doxepin, 145, **145**

Drawings, pain, 223–4

Drug abusers, 271–2

Drug(s), 4, **4**

absorption, 38–42, 42–3

biotransformation, 44–5

clearance, 45–6

CNS targets, 34–7

distribution, 42–4

dose cycle, 31

elimination/excretion, 45–6

interactions

NSAIDs, 105

paracetamol, 112

metabolism, 44–5

physico-chemical properties of, 42–3

routes of administration, 38–42, *40*

selectivity, 37

tolerance, 38

see also Pharmacodynamics; Pharmacology; *specific class; specific drug*

Dual effect of opioids, 280

Duration of pain, 189

Dynorphin, 133

Dynorphins, 132–3

E

EDGE, 101
EDGE II, 101
Eicosanoids, 92
Elderly patients, 283–4
    pain assessment, 229
    pain management strategies, 275–6
Electrical burns from TENS, 86
Electrical therapy, 172
Electroacupuncture, 88, 173
EMLA® (Eutectic Mixture of Local
        Anaesthetic), 177, **178**
Emotional components
    of chronic pain, 191–8, *192*
    in general, 4
Emphatic conduction, 58–9
End of life pain relief, 279–80
Endocannabinoid receptors, 35
Endocrine effects of central neuraxial
        blocks, 252
Endocrine response to pain, 243
Endogenous opioids, 132–3
Endorphins, 132–3, 226
Enkephalins, 17, 132–3
Enteral drug administration, 38–9
Entonox, 264, 282
Enzymes, 34
Ephatic coupling, 60
Epidemiology of pain, 201–11
Epidural blocks, 251, *253*, 253–4
    see also Patient-controlled epidural
        analgesia (PCEA)
Epidural injection, 124, 152
Epinephrine, 14
Erectile impotence, 146
Ergotamine, **153**, 155
Ethics, 277–84
Ethnicity and pain, 77–8
Ethyl alcohol, 256
Etidocaine, 122, **122**
Etodolac, 106
Etoricoxib, 101, **114**
Euphoria, opioid-induced, 137–8
European Organization for Research and
        Treatment of Cancer (EORTC)
        quality-of-life questionnaire, 225
Eutectic Mixture of Local Anaesthetic
        (EMLA®), 177, **178**
Exacerbating factors of pain, 217
Examination, physical, 160, *164*, 218–20
Excitatory chemical synapses, 11–2, 15
Excitatory interneurones, 68
Excitatory post synaptic potential
        (EPSP), 12, 66, 68, 72
Excitotoxicity, 15–6
Extracellular fluid, 42

Extracellular signal-related kinase
        (ERK), *52*, 56

F

Faces pain scale, 223–4, *223*
Facial nerve block, **250**
Facilitated diffusion, 42
Failed back-surgery syndrome, 269
Falsification of symptoms, 277
Family psychotherapy, 260
Fast pain pathways, 18
Fear, 195, 235–6
    effect on pain experience, 70
    fear avoidance beliefs
        questionnaire, 235
Feelings about pain, 194–5
    see also specific feeling
Females, pain prevalence, 203
Femoral nerve block, **250**
Fentanyl, **181**
    patient-controlled epidural analgesia
        (PCEA), 268
    transdermal, 178–9, **181**
Fibromyalgia prevalence, **203**, 204
Field blocks, 124, 254
First-pass metabolism, 39
Fluidotherapy, **171**
Focal pain, 216
Foetal anticonvulsant syndrome, 147–8
Fractures, 265–6
Frequency of pain, 202–3, **203**
Frustration, 195, 206
Functional status of pain, 218
Fusiform cells, 67

G

G-protein, 14
G-protein coupled receptors (GPCRs), 35,
        52, 54
    opioids, 133
    peripheral glutamate, 55
GABA_A receptor, 36, *37*, 150
Gabapentin, 59, **148**
    complex regional pain syndrome, 266
    migraine, **153**
    postherpetic neuralgia, 273
    trigeminal neuralgia, 273
Gaddum equation, 33
Galanin, 60
Gamma-aminobutyric acid (GABA),
        16, 36
    inhibitory interneurones, 68
    spinal-cord stimulation, 258
    see also GABA_A receptor
Gasserian ganglion block, **250**

Gastrointestinal system
  coxibs and, 96
  effect of aspirin on, 106
  effect of NSAIDs on, 102
  effect of opioids on, 138–9
  protection from NSAIDs, 106
Gate control theory, 23, 23–4, 80
Gender and pain, 77–8, 203
Genetics and pain, 77–8, 205
Glial cells, 77, 146
Glomerular filtration, 45
Glossopharyngeal nerve block, **250**
Glucuronide, 136
Glutamate, 15–6, 18, 36
  nociception and peripheral
    sensitisation, *52*
  nociceptor input effects, 72–3
  peripheral, 55
Glutamate/GABA$_B$ metabotropic
  receptors, 35
Glutathione, 111
Glycerol injection, 273
Glycine, 16, 68
Glycinergic neurones, 16
Golgi apparatus, 11
Gracile nuclei, 25
Grey matter, *21*, 21–2, *22*
Guanosine diphosphate (GDP), 35
Guanosine triphosphate (GTP), 35
Guanylyl cyclase, 37

H

Haemoglobinuria, cold, 81
Half-maximum effective dose, 122
Half-maximum lethal dose, 122
Head and neck nerve block, **250**
Headache syndromes
  anticonvulsants, 147
  prevalence, 204
  see also Migraine
Health-related quality of life
  measures, 224
Healthcare system influenced assessment
  barriers, 214
Heat-sensitive ion channels, 53
Heat stimuli, 49
Heat therapy, 82–3, 169–70, **171**
Hemp plant, 155
Hereditary sensory and autonomic
  neuropathy (HSAN) IV, 51, 77
Hernia, 268–9
History, patient, 160, *163*, 215–8
HIV, 274
Homeopathy, 89
Hospital anxiety and depression scale
  (HAD), 225, 233

Hot packs, **171**
Hydrolysis, 44
5-Hydroxytryptamine (5-HT),
  15, 35
5-Hydroxytryptamine receptor type 3
  (5-HT3), 109
Hyperalgesia, 51, 53–4
  complex regional pain syndrome,
    266
  cyclic adenosine monophosphate
    (cAMP), 55
  leukotriene B4, 57
  nerve growth factor, 57
  neuropathic pain, 58
  neurotrophins, 54–5
  referred, 67
Hypothalamus, 24, 69

I

Ibuprofen, 97–8
  cardiovascular safety advice, 106
  in clinical practice, **112**
Ice massage, **171**
Ice therapy, 81, **171**
Identity of illness beliefs, 192–3
Idiopathic pain, 191
Illness beliefs, 192–4
Imagery, 238–9
Imipramine, 145, **145**
Immobilisation and support, 83
Immune cells, *56*, 56–8, 61
  and chronic pain, 77
  in neuropathic pain, 60
Immunosuppression, opioid-
  induced, 138
Implantable intrathecal drug-delivery
  systems (IDDS), 254
Impotence, erectile, 146
In vitro assays, 96
Inactivated binding sites, 30, *31*
Incidence, 202
Indirect coupling, 60
Indometacin, **112–3**
Infiltrations, local anaesthetic, 254
Inflammation, 51
  neurogenic, 54
  in neuropathic pain, 59–60
Inflammatory conditions, 275
Inflammatory peripheral
  sensitisation, 51–8
  immune cells and cytokines, *56*,
    56–8
  inflammation, 51
  ion channels involved, 51–3
  mechanisms involving secondary
    messengers, 55–6

Inflammatory peripheral sensitisation
    (*Continued*)
    mediators, 53–5
Inflammatory soup, 51, *52*, 58, 61
Infra-red lamps, **171**
Inguinal hernia, 268–9
Inguinal nerve block, **250**
Inhaled drug administration, *40*, 41,
    246
Inhibitory chemical synapses, 12, *13*
Inhibitory interneurones, 68
Inhibitory post synaptic potential
    (IPSP), 12, 68
Injury, response to, 18–9
Inositol triphosphate (IP3), 35, 72
Inspection, 219
Insular cortex, 69
Insurmountable antagonism, 32, *32*
Intensity coding, 49, *49*
Intensity of pain, 216
Intercostal nerve blocks, **250**
Interferential therapy, 172
Interleukin-1 (IL-1), 78
Interleukin-1β (IL-1β), 57
Intermittent pain, 264
International Association for the Study of
    Pain (IASP), 1
Interneurones, 18, 22, 67–8, 150
Interventions, 242–60
    acute vs. chronic pain, 243
    pharmacological *see* Pharmacological
        interventions
    physical *see* Physical interventions
    psychological, 259–60
    systemic response to pain, 243–4
    therapeutic, 244–60, *245*
    treatment of pain, 243–4
Intervertebral disc prolapse, 152
Intra-articular drug administration, **246**
Intracellular fluid, 42
Intracellular receptors, 36–7
Intradermal anaesthesia, 184
Intramuscular drug administration, *40*,
    42, 244, **246**
    nurse-controlled, 267
    in trauma patients, 265–6
Intranasal drug administration, 41
Intrathecal injection, 123–4
Intravenous drug administration, 42,
    246, **246**
    local anaesthetics, 125–7
    nurse-controlled, 267
    in trauma patients, 265–6
Inverse agonist, 34
Investigations, 220
Ion channels, 51
    alterations in expression, 59

heat sensitive, 53
involved in nociception and peripheral
    sensitisation, 51–3, *52*
see also specific ion channel
Ion pore, 119, *120*
Ion-trapped drugs, 44
Ionotropic glutamate receptors, 15
Ionotropic receptors, 16
Ischaemia, tissue, 17–18
Ischaemic limb pain, 270–1
Itch, opioid-induced, 139

J

Joint pain prevalence, 204
Joule Thompson effect, 255
Juvenile rheumatoid arthritis, 108

K

Kainate receptors, 36
κ receptors, 134, 137
Kawasaki's disease, 108
Ketamine, 15, 148–9, **150**, 282–3
Ketoprofen, 106
Ketorolac
    cardiovascular safety advice, 106
    in clinical practice, **113**
Kidney(s)
    drug excretion, 45–6
    effect of NSAIDs on, 103
    failure, 270
Kwashiorkor, 43

L

L-Arginine, 75
L-Dopa, 14
Lactic acid, 18
Lamina, spinal cord *see* Rexed lamina,
    21–3, *22*, 67
Laser therapy, 172
Leu-enkephalin, 133
Leukaemia inhibitory factor (LIF), 60
Leukotriene B4 (LTB4), 57
Leukotrienes, 92, 103
Levobupivacaine, 119, **122**, **249**
Lidocaine, 119, 120–1, **122**
    EMLA, 177, **178**
    intradermal anaesthesia, 184
    maximal safe dose of, **249**
    metabolism, 121
    spinal (intrathecal) blocks, 252
    systemic administration, 126
    toxicity, 122
    transdermal patch, 179–80, **181**
Lidoderm patches, 179–80

Ligand-gated ion channels (LGICs), 36, *37*
Ligands *see* Agonist ligands; Antagonist ligands
Lignocaine *see* Lidocaine
Limb pain, ischaemic, 270–1
5-lipoxygenase (5-LOX), 57
Lissauer's tract, *22*, 66
Liver
  dysfunction with anticonvulsants, 147
  effect of NSAIDs on, 104
Local anaesthetics, 118–28
  chemistry, 120, **120**
  chronic pain management, 125–7
  classification, **122**
  clinical effect, 120–1
  history of, 118–9
  infiltrations, 254
  long-term blocks, 125
  maximal safe doses of, 249, **249**
  mechanism of action, 119, *120*
  metabolism, 121
  pharmacodynamics, 119–21
  pharmacokinetics, 121
  pharmacology, 119–23
  regional blocks, 123–5
  role in pain management, 123–8
  systemic absorption, 122–3
  systemic administration, 125–7
  systemic toxicity, 121–3
  topical creams, 177, **178**
Local interneurones, 66
Location of pain, 216
Lock and key principle, 29, *30*
Long-term local-anaesthetic blocks, 125
Long-term potentiation (LTP), 15, 75, 148–9
Longitudinal studies, 207–8, **208**
Loss due to pain, 232–3
Low back pain, 188–90, **189**, 264
Lower extremity nerve blocks, **250**
Lumiracoxib, 97–8, **114**

M

Magnesium ion, 74, *74*
Males, pain prevalence, 203
Management of pain
  in the community, 263–5
  interventions *see* Interventions
  pain management programmes, 239, 260
  strategies, 263–76
Manual therapy, 173–5
Marital psychotherapy, 260
Masked depression hypothesis, 144
Massage, 173–4, **176**

Mast cells, 57
McGill pain questionnaire, 224, *225*
Measurement of pain, 220–7
  multidimensional tools, 224–5
  other methods, 225–6
  unidimensional tools, 221–4
Mechanical stimuli, 49
Medal programme, 101
Medial prefrontal cortex, 69
Medial preoptic nucleus, 69
Medulla, 24, 25
Mefenamic acid, **113**
Meloxicam, 95
  cardiovascular safety advice, 106
  in clinical practice, **113**
Membrane barriers, drug movement through, 42
Membrane potentials, 6–9
  action potentials *see* Action potentials (APs)
  resting, 6, 8
Membrane stabilisers, **248**
Mepivacaine, **122**
Met-enkephalin, 133
Metabolic changes due to pain, 243
Metabolic effects of central neuraxial blocks, 252
Metabotropic glutamate receptors, 15, 73
Metabotropic receptors, 16
Methaemoglobinaemia, 123
Methylmorphine, 132
Methysergide, 154
Metoclopramide, 112, 184
Mexiletine, 126, 127–8
Microvasculature decompression, 257
Microwave diathermy (MWD), **171**
Migraine
  acute episodes, **153**, 154–5
  anticonvulsants, 147
  drug management of, 152–5, **153**
  prophylaxis, **153**, 154
Minitran®, 180
Misoprostol, 106
Mitochondria, 11
Mitogen activated protein kinase (MAPK), 56
Mode of onset of pain, 216
Models of pain, 231–2
Modulatory control, descending *see* Descending modulation
Monoamine oxidase (MAO), 14
Monoamine oxidase inhibitors (MAOI), 14, 144, 145
Monoaminergic neurotransmitters, 71
Mood, 189, 234–4
Morphine, 17

Morphine (*Continued*)
　implantable intrathecal drug-delivery
　　systems (IDDS), 254
　metabolism, 45, 136, *136*
　patient-controlled analgesia
　　(PCA), 267–68
　structure, 131, *131*
Motor examination, 219
Motor neurones, 6–17, *7*
　membrane potentials, 6–9
　nerve fibre types and function, 9–13
　neurotransmitters, 13–7
　propagation of action potentials, 9
Moxibustion, 88–9
μ receptors, 134, 137
Multidimensional pain measurement
　tools, 224–5
Muscarinic receptors, 14
Muscle relaxants, 149–50
Muscle relaxation, 82
Muscle spasm, 17–8, 149–50
Musculoskeletal conditions
　NSAIDs and, 106
　prevalence, 204
Musculoskeletal pain, 149–50, 152
Musculoskeletal physiotherapy, 174–5, **176**
Myelinated axons, 6
Myocardial infarction, 98
Myocardial ischaemia, 265
Myofascial pain syndrome, 254–5

N

N-acetyl-p-amino-benzoquinoneimine
　(NAPQ1), 110, 111, *111*
Nabilone, 155, 156
Nabumetone, 106
Naloxone, 139
Naltrexone, 139, 271–2
Naproxen, 97–8
　cardiovascular safety advice, 99, 106
　in clinical practice, **113**
Naratriptan, **153**, 155
Narcotic, definition of, 130
Nausea, opioid-induced, 138
$Na_v1.8$, *52*, 59
Needle phobia, 177
Nephron, 45
Nerve blocks
　in children, **282**, 282–3, **283**
　peripheral, 124–5, 248–51, **250**
　see also specific nerve
Nerve fibres *see* Axons
Nerve growth factor (NGF), 51, 54–5,
　146
　effect of nerve injury, 76
　neutrophil chemotaxis, 57

Nerve impulses, 118
Nerve injury, 58, 76–8
　anatomical changes, 76
　autonomic nervous system, 76–7
　genetics and pain, 77–8
　immune cells and chronic pain, 77
　nerve growth factor, 76
Neurectomies, 257
Neuro-psychiatric conditions, effect of
　NSAIDs, 105
Neuroanatomy, 20–7, 160, *162*
Neuroaxial blockade, 123–4
Neurogenic inflammation, 54
Neurokinin 1 (NK1), 72
Neurolytic blocks, 256
Neuromas, 18–9
Neuromatas, 18–9
Neuromuscular junction, *10*, 10–1
Neurones, 16–7
　see also specific neurone
Neuropathic pain, 191
　abnormal electrophysiology and, 58–9
　anticonvulsants, 147
　character of, 216
　complex, 272–5
　definition of, 2
　incidence, 3, **3**
　inflammatory processes in, 59–60
　ion channel expression alterations, 59
　local anaesthetics, 126
　management in the community, 265
　peripheral mechanisms of, 58–61
　sympathetic-sensory coupling, 60
　sympathetic sprouting, 60
Neuropeptide Y, 60
Neuropeptides, 54, 60
Neuropharmacology, 28–47
Neurophysiology, 6–19
Neurotransmitters, 13–7, 54
　see also specific neurotransmitter
Neurotrophins, 54–5, 146
Neutrophils, *56*, 56–7
Nicotinic receptors, 13
Nimesulide, 95, 106
Nitric oxide, 37, 75
Nitroglycerin patch, 180, **182**
Nitroplast®, 180
NMDA receptor antagonists, **248**
NMDA receptors, *11*, 36, 72
　central sensitisation, 73–4, *74*
　glutamate, 15
　ketamine, 148–9
　peripheral glutamate, 55
Nociceptive pain, 190–1
Nociceptive pathway, opioids, 133
Nociceptive-specific cells, 67
Nociceptive transduction, 61

Nociceptor specific neurones, 49, *49*
Nociceptors, 20, 61
  effects of input, 72–3
  peripheral, 21
  see also Primary afferent nociceptors
Node of Ranvier, 6, *7*
Non-monoaminergic
    neurotransmitters, 71
Non-nociceptive pain, 191
Non-pharmacological interventions, 80–
    90
Non-steroidal anti-inflammatory drugs
    (NSAIDs), 54, 91–109
  adverse effects of, 101–5, **102**
    bone, 104
    cardiovascular, 103–4
    coagulation, 104
    drug interactions, 105
    gastrointestinal, 102
    hepatic, 104
    pregnancy, 105
    rear, 105
    renal, 103
    respiratory, 103
    skin, 104
  cardiovascular safety and, 100–1
  clinical use of, 105–7, **112–5**
  in the elderly, 284
  pharmacokinetics of, 101
  side effects, **247**
  topical, 180, 182–3, **184**
  see also specific NSAID
Nonablative neuronal blockade, 248–55
Noradrenaline *see* Norepinephrine
Norepinephrine, 14, 71, *71*, 77, 243
Nortriptyline, 145, *145*, **153**
Nuclear receptors, 36–7
Nucleus tractus solitarius (NTS), 69
Numbness, **168**, 168–9
Numerical rating scales, 221–2, *222*
Nurse-controlled intramuscular
    injection, 267
Nurse-controlled intravenous
    injection, 267

O

O-toluidine, 123
Observational learning, 196
Odds ratio, 208, **208**
'OFF' cells, 70
Oligodendrocytes, 76–7
'ON' cells, 70
Operant learning, 196
Opiate, definition of, 130
Opioid peptides, 17
Opioid receptors, 25, 35, 133–4

Opioids, 70, 130–42
  absorption, 134–5
  addiction, 141, 247
  antagonists, 139
  common controversies, 139–42
  definitions, 130
  dependence, 140–1
  distribution, 135–6
  dual effect, 280
  effects on the CNS, 137–8
  in the elderly, 284
  end of life pain relief, 279–80
  endogenous, 132–3
  excretion, 136
  history, 130–1
  intravenous, 263–4
  long-term use of, 278–9
  mechanism of action, 133
  metabolism, 136, *136*
  pain management for patients
      on, 271–2
  peripheral effects, 138–9
  pharmacodynamics, 131–4
  pharmacokinetics, 134–6
  pharmacological actions, 137–9
  side effects, **247**
  structure, *131*, 131–2
  torrents, 139–40
  transdermal, 179
  withdrawal, 140
Oral drug administration, 38–9, **246**
  in trauma patients, 265–6
Oramorph, 264
Organ-bath, 31
Osteoarthritis, 106
Over-activity/under-activity cycle, 196,
    197
Oxidation, 44

P

Pain drawings, 223–4
Pain journey, 231
Pain-management programmes, 239, 260
Pain rating index (PRI), 224
Pain thresholds, 191
Palpation, 219
Papillary constriction, opioid-
    induced, 138
Parabrachial nucleus, 69
Paracetamol, 91, 109–15
  administration
    intravenous, 110
    oral, 109
    rectal, 109–10
  drug interactions, 112
  mechanism of action, 109

Paracetamol (*Continued*)
  metabolism, 110, *111*
  overdose, 111
  and pregnancy, 112
  side effects, 110
Paraffin baths, **171**
Paravertebral block, 124
Parecoxib
  in clinical practice, **114–5**
  contraindications, 107
  parecoxib/valdecoxib in coronary
    artery bypass grafting trial, 99
  skin effect of NSAIDs, 104
Parenteral drug administration, 38, 39–42
Paroxysmal cryoglobulinaemia, 81
Passive diffusion, 42
Patches, topical, 178–80, **181**
Patient-controlled analgesia (PCA), 247,
    267–68
Patient-controlled epidural analgesia
    (PCEA), 254, 268
Patient history *see* History, patient
Patient-influenced assessment
    barriers, 214
Perception of pain, 1, 213–4
Percussion, 219
Percutaneous radiofrequency
    thermocoagulation, 255–6
Periaqueductal grey matter (PAG), 24, 25,
    69
Period prevalence, 202
Peripheral glutamate, 55
Peripheral interventions, 159–84, *161*
  effect of, *176*
  pharmacological, *167*, 168–9
  physical, *166*, **168**, 168–75, **171**, **175**
Peripheral mechanisms, 48–61
Peripheral nerve
  blocks, 124–5, 248–51, **250**
  injury, 58–9
  neurectomies, 257
  neurolysis, 256
Peripheral nervous system, effect of
    opioids on, 138–9
Peripheral neuroanatomy, 21
Peripheral neuropathic pain, 272–5
Peripheral sensitisation, 61
  see also Inflammatory peripheral
  sensitisation
Personality influence on pain, 198
pH of drugs, 43
Phalens' sign, 220
Phantom limb pain/sensation, 271
  prevalence, **203**
Pharmacodynamics, 28–68
Pharmacokinetic antagonism, 34
Pharmacokinetics, 38–46

Pharmacological antagonism, 31–4
Pharmacological interventions, *167*,
    168–9, 175–84, 244–48, *245*
  see also Drug(s); *specific intervention*
Pharmacology, 28–47
Phase 1 drug metabolism, 44
Phase 2 drug metabolism, 44–5
Phencyclidine, 15, 148
Phenol, 256
Phenytoin, 105, 146, **148**, 273
Phospholipase, 92
Phospholipase C, 35, 71, 72
Phospholipid, 92
Phosphorylation, *52*, 56
Physical examination, 160, *164*, 218–20
Physical interventions, *166*, **168**, 168–75,
    171, **175**, 248–59
  see also specific intervention
Physiological antagonism, 34
Physiotherapy, 174–5, **176**, 259
Picture scales, 223, *223*
Pinocytosis, 43
Piroxicam
  cardiovascular safety advice, 106
  in clinical practice, **113**
Pizotifen, **153**, 154
pKa of drugs, 43, 120
Placebo effect, 70, 80, 281
Plasma protein binding, 43
Plasticity, 48, 61
Platelet aggregation, 104
Plexus blocks, 124
Point prevalence, 202
Polyethylene glycol, 152
Polymodal nociceptive cells, 67
Polypeptides, 35–6
Pons, 24, 25
Positron emission tomography (PET), 70
Post-synaptic cell, 10, 15, *16*
Post-vasectomy pain, 269
Postcentral gyrus, 69
Postherpetic neuralgia, 272–3
Postoperative pain, **203**, 227–8, 266–69
  abdominal surgery, 267–68
  acute, 266–7
  chronic, 268–9
Postsynaptic membrane ion
    channels, 12
Potassium and NSAIDs, 105
Potassium ions (K$^+$), 8
  excitatory chemical synapses, 12
  inhibitory chemical synapses, 12
  norepinephrine, 71
Potentiation, 89
  long-term, 15, 75, 148–9
Prefrontal cortex, 25
Pregabalin, **148**

Pregnancy
    anticonvulsants during, 147–8
    NSAIDs during, 105
    paracetamol in, 112
Preprodynorphin, 132–3
Preproenkephalin, 132–3
Preproopiomelanocortin, 132–3
Present pain intensity scale (PPIS), 224
PRESP trial, 99
Presynaptic cell, 10
Prevalence of pain, 202–3, **203**
Prevention of pain, 208–9
Prevention of spontaneous adenomatous
    polyps trial, 99
Prilocaine, **122**
    EMLA, 177, **178**
    maximal safe dose of, **249**
    metabolism, 121
    toxicity, 123
Primary afferent
    depolarisation (PAD), 73, 75–6
    fibres (PAF), 74
    neurones, 66, **66**
    nociceptors, 61
        biochemical differentiation, 50–1
        physiology of, 48–50
Primary complaints, 216
Primary nociceptive afferents, 22
Primary prevention of pain, 208
Primary sensitisation, 61
    see also Inflammatory peripheral
    sensitisation
Probenecid, 112
Progressive muscle relaxation, 238
Projecting neurones, 66
Propacetamol, 110
Propranolol, **153**, 154
Propriospinal neurones, 66
Prostaglandin E_2 (PGE$_2$), 52, 53–4
Prostaglandin-mediated pain, 93
Prostaglandins, 53–4, 92–3
    aspirin, 107
    bone effect of NSAIDs, 104
    in neuropathic pain, 60
    renal effect of NSAIDs, 103
    synthesis, 92, 93
Prostanoids, 92
Protein binding, 43
Protein C, 35
Protein kinase A, 35, 51, 52, 55
    central sensitisation, 74
    opioids, 133
Protein kinase C, 51, 52, 55–6
    central sensitisation, 74
Proton pump inhibitors, 106
Provocative tests, 220
Proximal tubule, 46

Psychodynamic therapy, 238
Psychogenic pain, 191
Psychological assessment, 218
Psychological impact of chronic
        pain, 230–41
    factors influencing wellbeing, 233–7
    interventions, 236–39
    seeing the psychologist, 231–3
Psychological interventions, 259–60
    see also specific intervention
Psychologists, seeing, 231–3
Psychometric tests, 233–4
Psychotherapy, 260
Pulmonary route of administration, 40,
        41, **246**
Purinergic receptors, 53
Pyramidal cells, 67

Q

Quality of life, 232–3
Qui, 173

R

Radiant heat, 82
Radiation, pain, 216
Radicular pain, 124, 152
Radiofrequency thermocoagulation,
        percutaneous, 255–6
Range of motion, 219
Ranitidine, 106
Raynaud's disease, 81
Re-uptake sites, 34
Receptor tyrosine kinases (RTKs), 35–6
Receptors
    drug, 28–9
    pain, 17–8
    plasticity, 38
    subtypes, 37
    see also specific receptor
Recovery, effects on, 188–90
Rectal drug administration, 39, **246**
Reduction, 44
Referred pain, 67, 216
Reflexes, 220
Regional blocks, 123–5
    neuroaxial blockade, 123–4
    peripheral nerve blocks, 124–5
Relaxation, 237, 259
Relieving factors of pain, 217
Renal route of drug excretion, 45–6
Repolarisation, 9
Research, 277–84
Respiratory system
    effect of NSAIDs on, 103
    effect of opioids on, 137

Respiratory system (*Continued*)
  neuraxial blocks, 251–2
Respondent learning, 196
Resting membrane potential (RMP), 6, 8
Rexed lamina, spinal cord, 21–3, *22*, 66, **66**, 67
Reye's syndrome, 108
Rheumatoid conditions, 275
Rhizotomies, 257
Rhodopsin/beta-adrenergic receptor-like receptors, 35
RICE protocol, 81
Ring block, 124
Rofecoxib, 97, 98
  cardiovascular risks of, 99
Ropivacaine, **122**
  maximal safe dose of, **249**
Rostroventral medulla, 70
Routes of administration, 38–42, *40*, 246
  see also specific route
Rubefacients, 180, **184**

S

Salicylate, topical, 182, **184**
Salicylic acid, 107
  see also Aspirin
Saturday night palsy, 10
  see Sunday morning palsy
Schild analysis, 32–3, *33*
Schild plot, 33, *33*
Schwann cells, *7*
Sciatic nerve block, **250**
Second-order neurones, 24, 66, 67
Secondary complaints, 216
Secondary messengers, 55–6, 61
Secondary prevention of pain, 209
Secretin receptor-like receptors, 35
Sedation, 137–8, 280
Selective COX-2 inhibitors *see* Coxibs
Selective nerve root block, 124
Selective serotonin reuptake inhibitors (SSRIs), 145
Self-efficacy, 194
Sensation of pain, **168**, 168–9
Sensory components of chronic pain, **190**, 190–1
Sensory examination, 220
Serotonin, 14–5, 146
Serotonin/noradrenaline reuptake inhibitors (SNRIs), 145, **145**
Serotonin syndrome, 146
Severity of pain, 216
Sexual dysfunction, 146
Shingles, 272–3
Short wave diathermy (SWD), **171**

Sickle cell disease, 81, 274–5
σ receptors, 134
Silent nociceptors, 50, 61
Site of pain, 216
Skeletal muscle relaxants, 149–50
Skin
  effect of NSAIDs on, 104
  rashes with anticonvulsants, 147
Sleep, 233, 265
Slow pain pathways, 18
Social learning, 196
Social withdrawal, 189
Socioeconomic class and pain, 204
Sodium channels
  Nav, 1.8, *52*, 59
  nerve damage, 59
  nociception and peripheral sensitisation, 51–3, *52*
  voltage-gated, 51–3, *52*, 59, 118, 119, *120*
Sodium ions (Na$^+$), 8
  central sensitisation, 74
  excitatory chemical synapses, 12
  nerve impulses, 118
Sodium valproate, 147, **148**
Solubility, drugs, 43
Somatic pain, 17–9, 48–9, 217
  definition of, 2
  sensory components of chronic, 191
Somatic peripheral neuroanatomy, 160, *162*
Spasm, muscle, 149–50
Spasticity, 149–50, 151
Spinal-cord, *21*, 21–2, *22*
  cordotomy, 257
  Rexed lamina of, 21–3, 66, **66**, 67
  stimulation, 258
Spinal (intrathecal) blocks, 251, 252–3
Spinal nerve rhizotomies, 257
Spinal pain, 149–50
Spinomesencephalic pathway, 24, *26*
Spinoreticular pathway, 24, *26*
Spinothalamic pathway, 24, *26*, 67
Splanchnic perfusion, 252
Stevens-Johnson syndrome, 147
Still's disease, 108
Stimulation analgesia, 257–59
Stimulation therapy, 172–3
Stress, 196–8, 259
  cost of, 206
  response, 243
Strychnine, 16
Studies, pain, 207–8
Stump pain, 271
  prevalence, **203**
Subcutaneous drug administration, *40*, 41, 244, **246**

in trauma patients, 265–6
Sublingual drug administration, 39–41, 40
Substance P, 17, 51
    central sensitisation, 74
    in neuropathic pain, 60
    nociceptor input effects, 72
Sumatriptan, **153**, 155
Sunday morning palsy, 10
    see Saturday night palsy
Superficial cervical plexus block, **250**
Superficial heat treatments, 170, **171**
Superior colliculus, 24
Support and immobilisation, 83
Suppositories, 39
Suprascapular nerve block, **250**
Surgery, pain after see Postoperative pain
Surgical techniques, 256–7
Sympathectomy, 60
Sympathetic nervous system, hypothalamic activation of, 243
Sympathetic-sensory coupling, 60
Sympathetic sprouting, 60
Sympathetically maintained pain (SMP), 76
Synapses, *10*, 10–2
    excitatory chemical, 11–2
    inhibitory chemical, 12, *13*
Systemic administration of local anaesthetics, 125–7
Systemic response to pain, 243–4

T

Tachykinin receptors, 35
Taoism, 173, **174**
TARGET trial, 97–8
Telodendria, axon, 6, 7
Temporal features of pain, 217
Tendon jerk, 12, *13*
Tendon reflexes, 220
TENS see Transcutaneous electrical nerve stimulation (TENS)
Terminal buttons, 6, 7
Tertiary prevention of pain, 209
Tetracaine, **122**, 177, **178**
    maximal safe dose of, **249**
Tetrodotoxin (TTX), 51–3
Thalamus, 24
Therapeutic COX-189 arthritis research and gastrointestinal event trial, 97–8
Therapeutic heat, 169–70
Therapeutic ratio, 37
Therapeutic window, 122
Thermoreceptive-specific cells, 67
Thermotherapy, 169–70

Thiopental, 44
Third day instillation, 125
Thoughts, 192–4
Thromboxane, 95
Thromboxane A_2, 104
Time-line of illness beliefs, 193
Tinel's sign, 219
Tissue ischaemia, 17–8
Tizanidine, 150
Tocainamide, 126
Tolerance to opioids, 139–40
Topical analgesics, 180–3, **246**
Topical drug administration, 41, 177, **178**
Topical patches, 178–80, **181**
Topiramate, **153**
Tramadol, 184
Transcellular fluid, 42
Transcription factors, 36–7
Transcutaneous drug administration, 41
Transcutaneous electrical nerve stimulation (TENS), 83–6, 173, **175**, 257, *258*
    chronic pain, 264
    complications, 86
    contraindications, 84
    gate control theory, 24
    indications, 84
    pads, 85
    use of, 85–6
    WDR neurones, 73
Transdermal drug administration, 178–80, **181**, **246**
Transdermal fentanyl, 178–9, **181**
Transduction, 49
Transient receptor potential channel 1 receptors (TRPV1), *52*, 53, 57
    nerve injury, 59, 76
Transmission, pain, 18–9
Transmitter receptors, 34–7
Transmucosal drug administration, **246**
Transocular drug administration, 41
Trauma, 265–6
Treatment of pain, 243–4
    see also Management of pain
Treatment planning, 160–8, *165*, 209–10
    see also Care planning
Tricyclic antidepressants, 145, **145**
    migraine, **153**, 154
    neuropathic pain, 265
Trigeminal ganglion, 256
Trigeminal neuralgia, 257, 273
Trigger point injections, 254–5
Triptans, **153**, 155
Trunk nerve blocks, **250**
Tryptophan, 14
Tubular re-absorption, 45–6
Tubular secretion, 46

Tumour necrosis factor α (TNFα), 56, 57
Tyrosine, 14
Tyrosine hydroxylase, 14
Tyrosine kinase, 35–6
Tyrosine kinase A (trkA), 51, *52*

U

Ultrasound, 170, **171**
Unconventional analgesics, 247–48
Undertreatment, 278–80
Unidimensional pain measurement
        tools, 221–4
Upper extremity nerve blocks, **250**
Urinary system
    effect of opioids on, 138–9
    neuraxial blocks, 252

V

Valdecoxib
    risks of, 100
    skin effect of NSAIDs, 104
    valdecoxib/parecoxib in coronary
        artery bypass grafting trial, 99
Vanilloid receptors *see* Transient receptor
        potential channel 1 receptors
        (TRPV1)
Vapocoolant sprays, **171**
Varicella zoster, 272–3
Vasectomy, pain after, 269
Vasoconstrictors, 122
Vasodilatation, 54
Vasodilation, 82
Venlafaxine, 145, **145**
Ventral column, *22*
Ventral horn of grey matter, *21*
Ventral root, *21*
Verbal rating scales, 221
VIGOR study, 97, 98
Vioxx
    adenomatous polyp prevention on
        vioxx trial, 98

vioxx GI outcomes research study, 97
Visceral pain, *49*, 49–50, 217
    definition of, 2
    sensory components of chronic, 191
Visual analogue scales, *222*, 222–3
Visual disturbance, 105
Visualisation, 238–9
Voltage-gated ion channels, 34, 50–1
    calcium, 59
    sodium, 51–3, *52*, 59, 118, 119, *120*
Voltage-gated Na$^+$ currents
        (VGSCs), 51–3, *52*
Volume of distribution (Vd), 44
Vomiting, opioid-induced, 138

W

Warfarin
    interaction with NSAIDs, 105
    interaction with paracetamol, 112
Wax/paraffin baths, **171**
Wellbeing, factors influencing, 233–7
White matter, *22*
Wide dynamic range (WDR)
        neurones, 67, 69, 73
    central sensitisation, 73–4, *74*
'Wind-up', 19, 73
Withdrawal syndromes, 38
Work absenteeism, 206
Wound irrigation, 183–4
Wrist block, **250**

Y

Yang, 173
Yellow flags, 188
Yin, 173

Z

Zolmitriptan, **153**, 155